Design and Quality Considerations for Developing Mobile Apps for Medication Management:

Emerging Research and Opportunities

Kevin Yap
La Trobe University, Australia

Eskinder Eshetu Ali
Addis Ababa University, Ethiopia

Lita Chew
National University of Singapore, Singapore

A volume in the Advances in Medical Technologies and Clinical Practice (AMTCP) Book Series

IGI Global
PUBLISHER of TIMELY KNOWLEDGE

Published in the United States of America by
IGI Global
Medical Information Science Reference (an imprint of IGI Global)
701 E. Chocolate Avenue
Hershey PA, USA 17033
Tel: 717-533-8845
Fax: 717-533-8661
E-mail: cust@igi-global.com
Web site: http://www.igi-global.com

Library of Congress Cataloging-in-Publication Data

Names: Yap, Kevin, 1977- author. | Ali, Eskinder, 1984- author. | Chew, Lita, 1967- author.
Title: Design and quality considerations for developing mobile apps for medication management : emerging research and opportunities / by Kevin Yap, Eskinder Ali, and Lita Chew.
Description: Hershey, PA : Medical Information Science Reference, [2020] | Includes bibliographical references and index. | Summary: "This book explores the concepts of pharmaceutical care and medication adherence and the role of m-health technologies in improving medication management"-- Provided by publisher.
Identifiers: LCCN 2019060012 (print) | LCCN 2019060013 (ebook) | ISBN 9781799838326 (hardcover) | ISBN 9781799838333 (ebook)
Subjects: MESH: Telemedicine | Mobile Applications | Medication Adherence | Medication Errors--prevention & control | Health Behavior
Classification: LCC R858 (print) | LCC R858 (ebook) | NLM W 83.1 | DDC 610.285--dc23
LC record available at https://lccn.loc.gov/2019060012
LC ebook record available at https://lccn.loc.gov/2019060013

This book is published in the IGI Global book series Advances in Medical Technologies and Clinical Practice (AMTCP) (ISSN: 2327-9354; eISSN: 2327-9370)

British Cataloguing in Publication Data
A Cataloguing in Publication record for this book is available from the British Library.

All work contributed to this book is new, previously-unpublished material.
The views expressed in this book are those of the authors, but not necessarily of the publisher.

For electronic access to this publication, please contact: eresources@igi-global.com.

Advances in Medical Technologies and Clinical Practice (AMTCP) Book Series

ISSN:2327-9354
EISSN:2327-9370

Editor-in-Chief: Srikanta Patnaik, SOA University, India & Priti Das, S.C.B. Medical College, India

MISSION

Medical technological innovation continues to provide avenues of research for faster and safer diagnosis and treatments for patients. Practitioners must stay up to date with these latest advancements to provide the best care for nursing and clinical practices.

The **Advances in Medical Technologies and Clinical Practice (AMTCP) Book Series** brings together the most recent research on the latest technology used in areas of nursing informatics, clinical technology, biomedicine, diagnostic technologies, and more. Researchers, students, and practitioners in this field will benefit from this fundamental coverage on the use of technology in clinical practices.

COVERAGE

- Neural Engineering
- Telemedicine
- Diagnostic Technologies
- Clinical Nutrition
- Patient-Centered Care
- Nursing Informatics
- Biometrics
- Clinical High-Performance Computing
- Biomechanics
- E-Health

IGI Global is currently accepting manuscripts for publication within this series. To submit a proposal for a volume in this series, please contact our Acquisition Editors at Acquisitions@igi-global.com or visit: http://www.igi-global.com/publish/.

The Advances in Medical Technologies and Clinical Practice (AMTCP) Book Series (ISSN 2327-9354) is published by IGI Global, 701 E. Chocolate Avenue, Hershey, PA 17033-1240, USA, www.igi-global.com. This series is composed of titles available for purchase individually; each title is edited to be contextually exclusive from any other title within the series. For pricing and ordering information please visit http://www.igi-global.com/book-series/advances-medical-technologies-clinical-practice/73682. Postmaster: Send all address changes to above address.

Titles in this Series

For a list of additional titles in this series, please visit:
http://www.igi-global.com/book-series/advances-medical-technologies-clinical-practice/73682

Mobile Devices and Smart Gadgets in Medical Sciences
Sajid Umair (The University of Agriculture, Peshawar, Pakistan)
Medical Information Science Reference • © 2020 • 363pp • H/C (ISBN: 9781799825210) • US $245.00

Applications of Deep Learning and Big IoT on Personalized Healthcare Services
Ritika Wason (Bharati Vidyapeeth's Institute of Computer Applications and Management (BVICAM), India) Dinesh Goyal (Poornima Institute of Engineering and Technology, India) Vishal Jain (Bharati Vidyapeeth's Institute of Computer Applications and Management (BVICAM), India) S. Balamurugan (QUANTS IS and Consultancy Services, India) and Anupam Baliyan (Bharati Vidyapeeth's Institute of Computer Applications and Management (BVICAM), India)
Medical Information Science Reference • © 2020 • 248pp • H/C (ISBN: 9781799821014) • US $275.00

Communicating Rare Diseases and Disorders in the Digital Age
Liliana Vale Costa (University of Aveiro, Portugal) and Sónia Oliveira (University of Aveiro, Portugal)
Medical Information Science Reference • © 2020 • 412pp • H/C (ISBN: 9781799820888) • US $295.00

Artificial Intelligence Paradigms in Smart Health Informatics Systems
Abdel-Badeeh M. Salem (Ain Shams University, Egypt) and Senthil Kumar A V (Hindusthan College of Arts and Science, India)
Medical Information Science Reference • © 2020 • 300pp • H/C (ISBN: 9781799811015) • US $265.00

Incorporating the Internet of Things in Healthcare Applications and Wearable Devices
P. B. Pankajavalli (Bharathiar University, India) and G. S. Karthick (Bharathiar University, India)
Medical Information Science Reference • © 2020 • 288pp • H/C (ISBN: 9781799810902) • US $285.00

For an entire list of titles in this series, please visit:
http://www.igi-global.com/book-series/advances-medical-technologies-clinical-practice/73682

IGI Global
PUBLISHER of TIMELY KNOWLEDGE

701 East Chocolate Avenue, Hershey, PA 17033, USA
Tel: 717-533-8845 x100 • Fax: 717-533-8661
E-Mail: cust@igi-global.com • www.igi-global.com

Table of Contents

Foreword

Since introducing the term 'Digital Health' to Wikipedia in 2012, the lead author of this book (Dr Kevin Yap) has been exploring the opportunities for technology to improve health outcomes in several research areas, including medication and medication management.

As pharmacists, the authors know that the implications of poor medication management can be devastating. Patients who fail to adhere to their medications are in danger of having adverse health events that have the potential to impact on their quality of life. It is often the more vulnerable patients that are less likely to take medications as prescribed, leading to this group having an increased risk of hospitalisations and poorer clinical outcomes.

With a large proportion of chronic patients failing to adhere to their treatment regimes, it is important to explore new options to help patients manage medications. Innovative methods that can be used to increase patient compliance and the effectiveness of pharmaceutical interventions can help improve clinical outcomes and reduce the cost of care.

This book provides a great overview of how to develop digital applications, and specifically how the growth and maturity of digital health technologies can provide mobile health applications that support individuals taking routine medications. The advent of smartphones, and their prevalence in the population, has enabled the development of personalised mobile technology-based pharmaceutical interventions easily located with the patient. These apps can be designed to improve medication management across a variety of patient groups.

The intention of the book is to guide the development of effective digital applications and the book explores design principles and factors which make some apps more successful than others. It also explores the factors involved in disrupting medication management and the strategies that can be adopted to improve adherence within the population.

In this book, the authors explore the challenges of designing mobile technology to improve pharmaceutical care and medication adherence. The authors have a background in pharmacy, pharmacoepidemiology and digital technology, and understand the challenges associated with designing mobile technology and the need to change patient behavior.

I know this book will be valuable to health professionals, medical researchers and developers who are interested in improving medication management through mobile applications.

James Boyd
La Trobe University, Australia

Preface

In the last decade, the emergence of various technologies, such as the internet, World Wide Web, mobile and hand-held devices (e.g. tablets and iPads), smartphones and mobile social media, has affected the way in which health-related information is distributed and accessed by both patients and healthcare professionals. The increasing popularity of the internet and World Wide Web as an online repertoire of health-related, disease-related and drug-related information has also increased exponentially. A new model of healthcare has emerged in which the focus is now on long term conditions, preventive and continuing care; integrating healthcare with people's lives in the homes and communities; enabling a team-based and shared-record system; and empowering patients to act as a partner in their own care.

Inevitably, the digital revolution has also led to an evolution of patients in the digital age. A new generation of individuals are emerging due to their digital connectedness to technologies, internet and the World Wide Web. Known as the "Generation Cs", this group is constantly plugged into technology, and they communicate more quickly and effectively via text messaging, social networks and emails through their smartphones and handheld gadgets. Originally defined as the group of 25 to 41-year-olds belonging to the Generation Ys (The Nielsen Company (US) LLC, 2012), a new school of thought has now classified the "Gen Cs" as not being bound by any demographic age group, but by the their "psychographics" of similar values, interests, attitudes and behavior (Energy Resourcing, n.d.; Pickett, 2019). Therefore, the Gen Cs can encompass the Generations X and Y, or even the Millennials (Energy Resourcing, n.d.; Pickett, 2019). They thrive on instant communication technologies (e.g. instant messaging and chats) and have constant access to the Web. It is not uncommon to see this group of people "googling" for health information and constantly being on their smartphones. On the other hand, the growing elderly population, often referred to as the "Silver Tsunami", are also catching up in the digital world.

Many of them have turned to the internet (or mobile internet) to search for information regarding their drug therapies and the need for their medications, thus earning them the name "Silver Surfers" (Dailey, Kalis, & Sather, 2015; Manovel & Sather, 2017).

The use of mobile technologies has become one of the most promising healthcare innovations that is directed at improving healthcare quality and outcomes – giving rise to the area of mHealth (mobile health). Mobile apps, short message services (SMS), automated sensing, media capabilities and video conferencing are some of the functionalities of mobile devices with healthcare applications. Healthcare professionals can use their mobile devices to look up drug and treatment resources, learn about new treatments and clinical research, help them educate and diagnose patients, as well as choose appropriate treatment paths for patients. The Quantified Self movement has also provided another dimension to mHealth by incorporating the use of sensors, wearables and the Internet-of-Things to acquire and track health-related data, so that patients can be empowered to make the necessary changes in their lifestyles or behavior to maintain their health. It is no doubt that mobile technologies have significant contributions in day-to-day life. Reports show that there were about 325,000 mHealth apps listed in the major app stores in 2017 (Research2Guidance, 2017). This number is expected to rise due to the continued increase in investments in health apps. Moreover, future advancements in mobile technologies are expected to provide more flexibility in the use of mobile devices for healthcare by way of functionalities embedded in the devices or connectivity to external devices. With the ubiquity of mobile technologies and their flexibility to incorporate multiple personalisable strategies, there is a considerable potential for the development and implementation of mHealth-based interventions.

In a world where mHealth apps for healthcare professionals and patients are rapidly increasing, it is important that the quality of such apps is not compromised in terms of efficacy, usability and safety. There is a disparity in the way clinicians and patients view mHealth apps. Many healthcare professionals tend to have serious doubts regarding the trustworthiness of mHealth apps and systems. In contrast, patients tend to trust the "star" ratings and user reviews of mHealth apps in the app stores – this is despite the disclaimers provided by some app developers that the apps should not replace a healthcare professionals advice and clinical judgement. Therefore, in recent years, many professional organizations have taken a stand on trying to improve the quality of mHealth apps. For example, the US Food and Drug Administration (FDA) has published regulations to guide developers design their apps and clinicians to evaluate such apps (Shuren, Patel, & Gottlieb, 2018; US Food and Drug Administration, 2019). However, these regulations are general and do not guarantee efficacy or safety. Furthermore, the agency has largely concentrated on medical apps – defined as those that "are intended to treat, diagnose, cure, mitigate or prevent disease or other conditions". The American Medical Association (AMA) has also followed suit by creating an alliance, called Xcertia, with the American Heart Association and the Healthcare Information and Management Systems Society (HIMSS) to set guidelines on evaluating the quality, effectiveness and safety of mHealth apps (American Medical Association, 2016; Xcertia, 2019). Similarly, the American Psychological Association (APA) has introduced a 5-step evaluation process to help clinicians make more informed choices on recommending mHealth apps (American Psychiatric Association, 2020). However, there is a gap in terms of determining what makes a good quality mHealth app that targets pharmaceutical care and medication management, particularly medication adherence.

There is a need to develop digital health tools and mHealth applications that are usable and affordable by patients and healthcare professionals, as well as being practical and clinically relevant. For example, ease-of-use associated with mobile app interfaces can be more important to patients than the number and type of functionalities. Similarly, app developers, healthcare professionals and patients should also understand the advantages and limitations of mHealth apps. With the growing numbers of mHealth interventions, there is a need to evaluate the quality of existing apps based on quality assessment criteria that are grounded in published literature and health behavior research. These criteria can help identify the quality of mHealth apps from the perspectives of reliability, feature usefulness and feature convenience. From the designer's or developer's perspective, understanding how health behavior theories and patient-centered approaches can be applied to mHealth can potentially lead to the development of clinically-relevant digital health systems and mHealth apps.

Although much research has been done on evaluating the usefulness of mHealth interventions, at the point of publishing this book, there is no authoritative resource that guides developers to design and develop mHealth tools for pharmaceutical care, medication management and adherence, as well as for end-users to evaluate such tools. Books on medication adherence have generally focused on methods of enhancing adherence and patient communication strategies. For example, Bosworth talks about the causes of medication non-adherence and how healthcare professionals can determine if a patient is non-adherent (Bosworth, 2012). In addition, Shea introduces various patient interviewing techniques and strategies on how healthcare practitioners can better communicate with patients to increase their interest in taking their medications (Shea, 2018). Martin and colleagues also advocate a model for healthcare professionals to use as a guide to enhance their patients' medication adherence through health-related behavior changes (Martin, Haskard-Zolnierek, & DiMatteo, 2010). On the other hand, books on mHealth have generally focused on regulatory trends (Malvey & Slovensky, 2014), mHealth research (Moumtzoglou, 2016), and on upcoming technological trends (Cerrato & Halamka, 2019; Eren & Webster, 2017; R. Istepanian, Laxminarayan, & Pattichis, 2007; R. S. H. Istepanian & Woodward, 2017), such as wireless and mobile communication technologies, wearable sensors for monitoring and tracking health, telehealth and telemedicine applications, and even on the Internet-of-Things and blockchain technologies. The closest books that are related to quality of mHealth innovations and their relation to patient care are by Moumtzoglou (Moumtzoglou, 2019), and Donner and Mechael (Donner & Mechael, 2013). In Moumtzoglou's book, various applications of mHealth in a variety of healthcare settings (e.g. cancer, obesity, wound management, emergency medicine, etc) are described, with the aim of helping designers understand how mobile technologies can be applied to healthcare practices. In contrast, Donner and Mechael focus on how mHealth can motivate and influence health behavioral changes. Despite the tremendous potential of mHealth apps in addressing health-related problems, there is currently no book that has targeted the clinical gap of how mHealth technologies can improve pharmaceutical care, medication management and medication adherence in particular. The importance of medication management and adherence in patients with chronic diseases, such as cancer, cannot be denied. Thus, the opportunity for mHealth apps to be used for the pharmaceutical care of patients is indeed appealing.

The success of medication management and adherence apps depends on user acceptance and usage of the apps in their daily lives. It is essential for app developers to gain an in-depth understanding of the factors that can influence the acceptance of mHealth apps for pharmaceutical care. It has been suggested that end users' acceptance of a technology-based health intervention can be studied through evaluation of their behavioral intention to use the intervention. As such, this book aims to demonstrate to readers how mHealth technologies can be designed and developed for the purposes of improving pharmaceutical care, medication management and medication adherence. Targeting two common drug-related problems of drug interactions and medication non-adherence, this book will guide the reader through the process of identifying the healthcare problem; conducting research through engagement with stakeholders; co-designing, developing and testing the mHealth solutions; evaluating the solutions and generating evidence; and finally, implementing the solution in clinical practices. To this end, it is clear that various specialties have to be integrated with the medical, pharmaceutical and health sciences in order for such technologies to work in healthcare – such as health systems engineering, human factors engineering, human-computer-environment interactions, computer sciences and the psychological sciences. Furthermore, in order to ensure the potential effectiveness of mHealth-based pharmaceutical interventions, health behavior change frameworks and pharmaco-cybernetic approaches must be considered during the process of development. As such, this book is aimed at a wide variety of target audiences, including designers and developers of mHealth apps, healthcare professionals, clinical/medical informaticists, health service administrators, pharmacy managers, informatics pharmacists and patient care providers. At a broader level, this book will definitely be of interest to students, researchers, patients and anyone who wants to know about the considerations and approaches to designing, developing and evaluating mobile technology-based interventions for improving the quality of pharmaceutical care.

Thus, this book is organized into seven distinct chapters that introduces the reader to the concepts of pharmaceutical care, as well as the role of mHealth technologies in improving medication management. Chapter 1 introduces the concept of drug interactions and its impact on patients with cancer. It then leads into the concept of medication adherence, the prevalence of non-adherence and how it can impact the pharmaceutical care of patients with cancer. This chapter also provides an insight to the factors influencing medication adherence, issues behind non-adherence and the types of intervention strategies that have targeted non-adherence. In order for such intervention strategies to work, there is a need for collaboration between healthcare professionals and patients. In addition, the need to address the intervention strategies, not just at the patient level, but also from a macro-, meso-, and micro-level are discussed.

Chapter 2 provides a chronological overview of the trends in mHealth research in terms of the types of mobile devices used, their functionalities and the medical conditions that the interventions have been carried out. Based on several reviews, distinct trends include a shift from communicable diseases to non-communicable diseases, as well as from supporting healthcare services to other purposes, such as preventive care and health promotion. The advent of smart devices, such as smartphones, tablet PCs, iPhones and iPads have also seen a rise in mHealth research on short message services (SMS), internet-based interventions and mobile apps. Other smartphone functionalities like the camera/video, Bluetooth, near-field communication sensors, and image and motion sensors, among others, have also been harnessed for diagnosis and monitoring. Through several examples of mHealth apps, this chapter also illustrates the need for mHealth apps to have an evidence base in order to show a positive impact on disease and medication management.

Chapter 3 begins by providing an overview on how the roles of patients and healthcare professionals have evolved with the digital age. The domains of digital health and pharmaco-cybernetics/cyber-pharmacy are introduced together with several pharmaco-cybernetic frameworks that are relevant for designing digital health innovations. Concepts such as the digital health innovation process cycle, Pharmaco-cybernetic Maxims, user-centered (UCD), experience-centered (ECD) and activity-centered designs (ACD), and the Ecological Systems Theory applied to technological and mHealth systems are explained in more detail. In addition, the key considerations for designing Android and iOS apps, as well as in UCD, ECD and ACD approaches to technological product design are provided. Furthermore, the later part of the chapter discusses the role of health behavior theories in the development of mHealth apps. The Intervention Mapping (IM) approach and the Behavioral Intervention Technology (BIT) model are used to demonstrate how an mHealth intervention can be developed for medication adherence, and the methods and considerations for usability testing of the mHealth intervention are also described.

Chapter 4 aims to provide guidance to mHealth app developers, clinicians and patients on the types of quality parameters to consider in apps designed for pharmaceutical care and medication management. Based on two quality assessment tools developed by the authors for medication management and adherence apps, the general quality criteria for reliability, usability and privacy of mHealth apps are described. In addition, feature usefulness criteria for tele-monitoring apps, interaction checkers, dose calculators, medication information provision apps, medication record apps and medication adherence apps; as well as other criteria related to tele-support, tele-collaboration and personalization/contextualization are discussed. A list of top-ranking medication management apps evaluated using the quality assessment tools is also provided together with some security and privacy recommendations for mHealth app design.

Chapter 5 provides an overview of the models that facilitate the adoption of mHealth technologies – primarily focusing on the Technology Acceptance

Model (TAM) and the Unified Theory of Acceptance and Use of Technology (UTAUT) model – so as to provide readers with an insight to the determinants of patients' acceptance of technological systems. The origins and evolution of the models are discussed through various constructs, such as behavioral intention to use the technology, usage behavior, performance expectancy (perceived usefulness) and effort expectancy (perceived ease of use), among others. In addition, the application of these models to determine the factors that influence user acceptability and adoption of mHealth-based interventions among healthcare professionals is demonstrated through a case study of pharmacists in Singapore.

Chapter 6 demonstrates the application of the IM framework, BIT model and UCD principles through a case example of the design and development of an in-house medication adherence app prototype for oral anticancer medications, called MedFC. This prototype was designed to help oncology clinicians monitor their patients for *Med*ication adherence through near-field communication (N*FC*) technologies. The chapter describes how patients' medication adherence needs, mobile app usage patterns, perceptions of medication adherence strategies and experiences with the prototype helped inform the development of MedFC. Additionally, based on several studies conducted by the authors, this chapter guides the reader through the 6 steps in the IM framework to showcase how MedFC was designed, developed, implemented and evaluated in its target audience of patients with cancer and their caregivers.

Chapter 7 provides another case example of how OncoRx-MI, a drug interaction database for *Onco*logy drug prescriptions (*Rx*) accessible on the *M*obile *I*nternet, was designed and developed from a pharmaco-cybernetics approach. The uniqueness of this database is its ability to provide interaction information of conventional western drugs and complementary and alternative medicines for both anticancer drugs and combination chemotherapy regimen cocktails. Following the 5 activities in the digital health innovation process cycle, this chapter provides a step-by-step guide on how the healthcare problem was identified in oncology practice all the way through to designing, developing and implementing the database platform in clinical practice, and generating evidence of its relevance and credibility.

In summary, the pharmaco-cybernetic frameworks and behavioral models described in this book are meant to provide some guidance to app developers, healthcare professionals and patients regarding the design and quality considerations needed to develop good quality mHealth systems that will appeal to end-users. Of course, safety and efficacy are crucial aspects for choosing appropriate mHealth apps for medication management. However, these should not be the only metrics used for adopting mHealth apps. Dimensions of usability (e.g. app flexibility, usefulness, user satisfaction, attractiveness), reliability (e.g. operability, consistency and error rates), as well as user and field testing are just as important. From the identification of design requirements to the applications of the various pharmaco-cybernetic frameworks and approaches, we hope that readers will understand the critical issues surrounding the development and implementation of mHealth applications and systems that target pharmaceutical care and medication management.

Finally, this book has been inspired by the PhD work of two of the co-authors, Dr Kevin Yap and Dr Eskinder Eshetu Ali. Through our work, we felt that there was a need to translate the evidence base of our findings to something that is more applicable and understandable in the practice setting. We would like to acknowledge the La Trobe University Social Research Platform Grant for its support, without which this book would not have been possible. Additionally, we would like to thank Dr Michael Liem for his insightful help and contribution to the publication of this book. Lastly, we would like to thank our families for their tremendous support and the Lord for His enduring love, care and strength throughout this period.

"And now these three remain: faith, hope and love. But the greatest of these is love." — Holy Bible: King James Version

Kevin Yap
La Trobe University, Australia

Eskinder Eshetu Ali
Addis Ababa University, Ethiopia

Lita Chew
National University of Singapore, Singapore

REFERENCES

American Medical Association. (2016, 12 Dec). *Alliance forms to develop guidelines for evaluation of mHealth apps*. Retrieved 27 Mar, 2020, from https://www.ama-assn.org/press-center/press-releases/alliance-forms-develop-guidelines-evaluation-mhealth-apps

American Psychiatric Association. (2020). *App evaluation model*. Retrieved 27 Mar, 2020, from https://www.psychiatry.org/psychiatrists/practice/mental-health-apps/app-evaluation-model

Bosworth, H. B. (2012). *Enhancing Medication Adherence: The Public Health Dilemma*. London, UK: Springer Healthcare Ltd. doi:10.1007/978-1-908517-66-1

Cerrato, P., & Halamka, J. (2019). *The Transformative Power of Mobile Medicine: Leveraging Innovation, Seizing Opportunities and Overcoming Obstacles of mHealth*. Academic Press.

Dailey, J., Kalis, B., & Sather, T. (2015). The next eHealth wave for silver surfers: Health management. *Accenture Insight Driven Health*, 1-4. Retrieved from https://www.accenture.com/_acnmedia/accenture/conversion-assets/dotcom/documents/global/pdf/dualpub_15/accenture-health-management-silver-surfers-pov.pdf

Donner, J., & Mechael, P. (Eds.). (2013). mHealth in Practice: Mobile Technology for Health Promotion in the Developing World (1st ed.). London, UK: Bloomsbury Academic.

Energy Resourcing. (n.d.). *6 Things you need to know about Generation C*. Retrieved 27 Mar, 2020, from https://energyresourcing.com/blog/6-things-you-need-to-know-about-generation-c/

Eren, H., & Webster, J. G. (2017). *Telehealth and Mobile Health* (1st ed.). CRC Press.

Istepanian, R., Laxminarayan, S., & Pattichis, C. S. (Eds.). (2007). *M-Health: Emerging Mobile Health Systems*. Springer Science & Business Media.

Istepanian, R. S. H., & Woodward, B. (2017). *M-Health: Fundamentals and Applications*. John Wiley & Sons, Inc.

Malvey, D., & Slovensky, D. J. (2014). mHealth: Transforming Healthcare. Springer US.

Manovel, I., & Sather, T. (2017). Silver surf's up: Senior citizens are riding the digital health wave. *Accenture Insight Driven Health*, 1-9. Retrieved from https://www.accenture.com/t00010101t000000__w__/au-en/_acnmedia/pdf-47/accenture-health-silver-surfers-in-australia.pdf#zoom=50

Martin, L. R., Haskard-Zolnierek, K. B., & DiMatteo, M. R. (2010). *Health Behavior Change and Treatment Adherence: Evidence-Based Guidelines for Improving Healthcare*. Oxford University Press.

Moumtzoglou, A. (2016). *M-Health Innovations for Patient-Centered Care*. IGI Global. doi:10.4018/978-1-4666-9861-1

Moumtzoglou, A. (2019). *Mobile Health Applications for Quality Healthcare Delivery*. IGI Global. doi:10.4018/978-1-5225-8021-8

Pickett, P. (2019). *The characteristics of Generation C*. Retrieved 27 Mar, 2020, from https://www.thebalancecareers.com/who-is-generation-c-and-what-are-they-all-about-2071937

Research2Guidance. (2017). *mHealth economics 2017: Current status and future trends in mobile health*. Retrieved from https://research2guidance.com/product/mhealth-economics-2017-current-status-and-future-trends-in-mobile-health/

Shea, S. C. (2018). *The Medication Interest Model: How to Talk With Patients About Their Medications* (2nd ed.). Lippincott Williams & Wilkins.

Shuren, J., Patel, B., & Gottlieb, S. (2018). FDA Regulation of Mobile Medical Apps. *Journal of the American Medical Association*, *320*(4), 337–338. doi:10.1001/jama.2018.8832 PMID:29971339

The Nielsen Company (US) LLC. (2012). *Introducing Generation C Americans 18-34 are the most connected.* Retrieved 28 Jul, 2019, from https://www.nielsen.com/us/en/insights/article/2012/introducing-generation-c/

US Food and Drug Administration. (2019). *Device software functions including mobile medical applications.* Retrieved 27 Mar, 2020, from https://www.fda.gov/medical-devices/digital-health/device-software-functions-including-mobile-medical-applications

Xcertia. (2019). *Xcertia mHealth app guidelines*. Retrieved 27 Mar, 2020, from https://xcertia.org/the-guidelines/

Acknowledgment

The authors acknowledge that this project was completed with the assistance of the La Trobe University Social Research Platform Grant. The authors would also like to thank Dr Michael Liem from La Trobe University for his insightful help and contribution to the success of this book.

Chapter 1
Introduction to Pharmaceutical Care and Medication Adherence

ABSTRACT

Pharmaceutical care is a concept that involves identifying, solving and preventing drug-related problems, such as drug interactions, with regards to a patient's drug therapy. Cancer patients are at high risk of drug interactions due to the complex pharmacological profiles and narrow therapeutic indices of anticancer drugs. Furthermore, these patients tend to consume complementary and alternative medicines, thus predisposing them to a risk of herb-drug interactions. This can impact their adherence to anticancer therapies. Various factors are involved in medication non-adherence, such as the cost of medications and patients' beliefs about the value of their treatments. There is a need to understand the impact of non-adherence and optimize intervention strategies from a macro-, meso-, and micro-level. Chapter 1 introduces the concept of pharmaceutical care and the impact of oncology drug interactions and medication non-adherence in patients with cancer. The chapter will also provide an insight to the factors influencing medication adherence and the intervention strategies that have targeted non-adherence.

DOI: 10.4018/978-1-7998-3832-6.ch001

INTRODUCTION

The provision of pharmaceutical care is a concept that involves identifying, solving, and preventing potential or actual drug-related problems (DRPs) with regards to a patient's drug therapy (American Society of Hospital Pharmacists, 1993). In general, DRPs can be categorized into problems and causes, and are related to factors such as drug choices, drug doses, drug interactions, adverse drug events due to drug administration, medical errors of omission, and patient-related factors (Anderson; Pharmaceutical Care Network Europe). As a system of healthcare delivery to patients, pharmaceutical care requires the coordinated efforts of all healthcare professionals, including physicians, pharmacists, nurses, and other health practitioners. In the clinical setting, various healthcare professionals work in tandem to provide pharmaceutical care to patients. Certain therapeutic decisions, such as dose adjustments, are made on the basis of experience and trial-and-error methods, which is subjective and time-consuming. Healthcare professionals are responsible for patient treatment outcomes that result from their actions, but it is not always possible to achieve desirable therapeutic outcomes in patients as a result of DRPs.

One of the DRPs that is common in patients with cancer is drug interactions. Many of them receive multiple medications to treat their co-morbid conditions and toxicities that are associated with anticancer treatments and cancer-related syndromes. A drug interaction is defined as a change in the way a drug acts in the body when taken with certain other drugs, herbs, foods, or when taken with certain medical conditions (U.S. National Institutes of Health). It may cause the drug to be more or less effective or cause a unique response that does not occur when either agent is given alone. Approximately 20-30% of all adverse drug reactions (ADRs) are due to drug interactions (Beijnen & Schellens, 2004; Kuhlmann & Muck, 2001). The potential for an interaction is about 6% when 2 drugs are prescribed together and the risk increases markedly to 84% when the number of concomitant medications is increased to 6 (Karas, 1981; Kuhlmann & Muck, 2001). At least one potential drug-drug interaction (DDI) occurs in 27% of patients with cancer, of which 13% involves an anticancer drug (ACD), and 86% are classified as being of moderate or major severity (Riechelmann et al., 2007). The complex pharmacological profiles of ACDs, their narrow therapeutic indices and steep dose-toxicity curves, predispose patients with cancer to high incidences of DDI-related adverse events. In addition, patient-related factors, such as age-related renal and/or hepatic insufficiencies, malnutrition and malabsorption, and patients' pharmacogenetic characteristics, can also alter the metabolism and elimination of ACDs, thus causing elderly patients with cancer to become more susceptible to DDI effects (Delafuente, 2003; Riechelmann & Saad, 2006). Such effects are relevant clinically in up to 80% of the elderly (Beijnen & Schellens, 2004).

In general, DDIs can be classified into pharmacokinetic, pharmacodynamic and pharmaceutical interactions (Chan & Yap, 2010). Pharmacokinetic interactions involve alterations in the absorption, distribution, metabolism or elimination properties of a drug, which can be due to enzyme induction or inhibition, or protein displacement. On the other hand, pharmacodynamic interactions can be due to additive, antagonistic or synergistic effects of the individual drugs. The last type of DDIs – pharmaceutical interactions – occur when chemically incompatible drugs are co-administered, leading to precipitation and inactivation of the therapeutic effects of the drugs (Chan & Yap, 2010; Yap, Chui, & Chan, 2008). There are 3 scenarios in which DDIs can potentially affect a patient's cancer therapy: adding an interacting drug to the patient's existing chemotherapy treatment, administering chemotherapy treatment to the patient when he is concurrently on an interacting drug, and removing an interacting drug from the patient's chronic chemotherapy (Yap, et al., 2008). Clinicians need to be vigilant when treating cancer patients who are concurrently on both chemotherapy and non-ACDs.

Patients manifesting certain cancer types, such as brain tumours and metastases, tend to receive long-term antiepileptic drugs. These antiepileptic drugs are prone to interactions with ACDs, hence leading to higher risks of DDI events. Although antiepileptic drug monotherapy can be effective in ~60-70% of newly diagnosed patients (Patsalos, Froscher, Pisani, & van Rijn, 2002; Patsalos & Perucca, 2003; Emilio Perucca, 1997), up to 50% of patients who fail initial antiepileptic treatment can be managed by switching to an alternative antileptic drug (Patsalos, et al., 2002; Emilio Perucca, 1997). Epileptic patients who do not respond to monotherapy can be given a combination of antiepileptic drugs to optimize seizure control, but this comes at the expense of an increased risk of adverse effects (Patsalos, et al., 2002; Patsalos & Perucca, 2003; Emilio Perucca, 1997; E. Perucca, 2006).

On the other hand, prophylaxis with antiepileptics in patients with brain tumours without documented seizures has been a controversial issue. Based on a meta-analysis of 12 studies, the American Academy of Neurology has advised against the use of antiepileptic drug prophylaxis in such patients, since none of the studies found efficacy of prophylactic antiepileptics in preventing first seizures in patients with brain tumors (Glantz et al., 2000).

However, a large majority of neurosurgeons (82%), neurologists (53%), and medical (50%) and radiation (33%) oncologists have reported to prescribe AED prophylaxis (Glantz, et al., 2000), possibly either based on personal preference, training and experience; or to avoid malpractice claims brought by patients or family members of patients who might experience seizures (Elkayam, 2005).

Furthermore, cancer patients often experience psychological distress, which may predispose them to psychiatric illnesses or exacerbated pre-existing psychiatric conditions (Bailey et al., 2005). The prevalence rates of psychological distress in cancer patients are high, ranging from 30% to 43%, and can include conditions like anxiety and post-traumatic stress (25-48%), psychological disorders (major depressive disorder, 5-42%), schizophrenia (0.5-1.5%) and bipolar disorder (0.4-1.6%) (Akizuki et al., 2003; Miovic & Block, 2007; Zabora, BrintzenhofeSzoc, Curbow, Hooker, & Piantadosi, 2001). These patients are often prescribed with psychotropic drugs – medications that are capable of altering the mind, emotions and behavior (Stedman, 2005) – such as antidepressants, antipsychotics, sedatives and/or hypnotics (Clarke Institute of Psychiatry, 2007). Concurrent use of ACDs and psychotropic drugs can result in potential DDIs that are harmful in clinical practice. This is concerning because cancer patients are generally more likely to receive psychotropic agents than patients in general hospitals. For example, in a study examining psychotropic drug prescribing patterns of physicians in the US, over 80% of 200 hospitalised patients with cancer were prescribed with at least one psychotropic drug, among which 36% were prescribed with 3 or more psychotropics (Stiefel, Kornblith, & Holland, 1990). In a similar study in Spain, the proportion prescribed with psychotropic drugs increased from 82% in 2002 (198/241 patients) to 90% (293/325 patients) in 2009 (Farriols et al., 2012). Patients with newly diagnosed cancers on psychotropics had a 30% higher rate of physician visits, 18% higher rate of hospitalizations and a 30% higher rate of outpatient visits (Aroke, Vyas, Buchanan, & Kogut, 2019). The odds of cancer patients being prescribed psychotropic drugs were higher than the general population (adjusted odds ratio for benzodiazepines=1.70, antidepressants=1.38 and antipsychotics=1.70) (Ng, Boks, Smeets, Zainal, & de Wit, 2013).

In the course of cancer therapy, an increasing number of patients are also consuming complementary and alternative medicines (CAMs), including traditional Chinese medicines (TCMs) (Boon, Olatunde, & Zick, 2007; Bressler, 2005). CAM usage in the general United States (US) population has increased over the past 20 years, reaching 45% in 2012 (Bishop et al.,

2019). A similar trend is seen in the cancer population. There is ~36-80% of cancer patients in the US who use CAMs to relieve treatment-related symptoms (Subramani & Lakshmanaswamy, 2017). A particularly large proportion of Asian patients also use CAMs concurrently with their cancer therapies, ranging from 45% of Japanese (Hyodo et al., 2005), 12-62% of Taiwanese (Kuo et al., 2018; Yen, Lai, Muo, & Sun, 2017), 75-80% of Chinese in China (Sun, Mao, Vertosick, Seluzicki, & Yang, 2018), and 55-67% of Singaporeans (Chow et al., 2010; C. M. Lim, Ng, & Loh, 2010; J. Lim et al., 2006; Shih, Chiang, & Chan, 2009). These CAMs are usually taken without the physician's knowledge, and patients tend to be resistant to discussions of their CAM use with their physicians, possibly due to clinician indifference or opposition to CAM use, their clinician's emphasis on scientific evidence, or their anticipation of a negative response from the clinician (Institute of Medicine (US) Committee on the Use of Complementary and Alternative Medicine by the American Public, 2005; Tasaki, Maskarinec, Shumay, Tatsumura, & Kakai, 2002). Moreover, the effects of many CAMs are not well-documented due to the lack of well-designed safety and efficacy studies (Kinsel & Straus, 2003; Tabish, 2008). As a result, DRPs such as herb-drug interactions (HDIs) between ACDs and CAMs may occur, which can lead to a compromise in the safety and efficacy of the chemotherapy treatment.

DDIs with ACDs may potentially be harmful to patients due to the narrow therapeutic indices of ACDs and the interacting non-ACDs. While pharmacodynamic interactions form the basis of improving the clinical responses of cancer patients on combination chemotherapy cocktails, other undesirable clinical consequences may also occur in these patients (Scripture & Figg, 2006; Yap, et al., 2008). Furthermore, some CAM products may contain multiple pharmacologically-active constituents, which may further increase the risk of ACD-CAM interactions (Yap, See, & Chan, 2010). Although there are more than 2000 DDIs that have been identified, only a limited number are of interest from a clinical standpoint (Bjerrum, Andersen, Petersen, & Kragstrup, 2003). By knowing the magnitude of the DDIs, clinicians can avoid unwanted toxicities and inadequate drug exposures due to the interactions, so as to better manage their patients' drug therapies.

The manifestation of drug-related problems such as DDIs can impact the medication adherence patterns of patients. The World Health Organization (WHO) defines medication adherence as the "extent to which a person's behavior-taking medication, following a diet, and/or executing lifestyle changes, corresponds with agreed recommendations from a healthcare provider" (Sabaté & Sabaté, 2003). There are three phases of medication adherence: (i) the time the first dose is taken (initiation), (ii) the extent to which a patient's actual dosing corresponds to the prescribed dosing regimen (implementation), and (iii) the end of therapy (discontinuation) (Hugtenburg, Timmers, Elders, Vervloet, & van Dijk, 2013; Vrijens et al., 2012; Zullig & Bosworth, 2017). Patients may intentionally or unintentionally fail to adhere to their medication regimens at any of these phases (Gadkari & McHorney, 2012; Osterberg & Blaschke, 2005). When patients fail to fill their prescription for a new medication or do not begin taking medications after filling their prescription (i.e. at the initiation phase), it is called primary non-adherence (F. Seal, Cave, & Atkinson, 2017; Solomon & Majumdar, 2010). On the other hand, secondary non-adherence is when the patients' non-adherence behavior occurs between initiation and discontinuation (Solomon & Majumdar, 2010). Non-adherence can also be intentional or unintentional. While intentional non-adherence involves an active decision by the patient not to follow treatment recommendations; unintentional non-adherence refers to the patients' passive deviation from treatment recommendations due to forgetfulness or not knowing how to take their medications. Many studies on the prevalence of adherence do not differentiate between intentional and unintentional non-adherence (Hugtenburg, et al., 2013), thus in this book, we do not differentiate between the two types of non-adherence as well.

Medication non-adherence is a primary concern of health systems worldwide due to its adverse effects on clinical outcomes and healthcare costs (Brown & Bussell, 2011; Iuga & McGuire, 2014; National Council on Patient Information and Education, 2013). The WHO estimates that, on average, only about 50% of patients with chronic diseases are adherent to their medications (Brown & Bussell, 2011; World Health Organization, 2003; Zullig & Bosworth, 2017). Non-adherence has multifaceted impacts on the clinical and economic outcomes of healthcare (Benjamin, 2012; National Council on Patient Information and Education, 2013; Rosen, Fridman, Rosen, Shane, & Pevnick, 2017; van Boven et al., 2014; Viswanathan et al., 2012). The clinical impacts of non-adherence include reduced survival, avoidable hospitalizations and death (Currie et al., 2012; Eells et al., 2016; Neiheisel, Wheeler, & Roberts, 2014; Scheel et al., 2017), while the economic impacts are generally associated with the direct costs of managing morbidities and complications caused by non-adherence and the indirect costs of lost productivity (Cutler, Fernandez-Llimos, Frommer, Benrimoj, & Garcia-Cardenas, 2018; Iuga & McGuire, 2014). For example, the US healthcare system spends between 100 and 300 billion US Dollars (USD) annually for hospitalization and other health service-related costs due to medication non-adherence (Iuga & McGuire, 2014). Similarly, the annual costs to countries in the European Union are also estimated to be approximately 125 billion Euros (Khan & Socha-Dietrich, 2018).

Various theories have been proposed to understand and predict medication non-adherence behavior. However, most of these theories have showed low predictive accuracy (Rickles, 2010). Therefore, an integrated framework that accounts for the complexity of cognitive and dynamic behavior of adherence behavior has been proposed – called the Dynamic Exchange Model for Medication Adherence Levels and Comparison of Outcomes (DEMMALCO). This framework relates how patients attribute their medication use to treatment outcomes, as well as choose future actions based on their expectations and alternatives available (Rickles, 2010). The framework includes concepts on the attribution of control, self-efficacy and patient's beliefs about their treatment outcomes (Kjos, Vaughan, & Bhargava, 2019). The Locus of Control (LOC) is a concept that is based on the belief that a health outcome is dependent on one's behavior. A belief in greater self-influence means a higher internal LOC, while a belief in greater external influences (e.g. fate) means a higher external LOC (Kjos, et al., 2019; Wallston, Stein, & Smith, 1994). On the other hand, self-efficacy in medication adherence, which is defined as the knowledge and skills to use the medication properly, can be predicted using the Medication Understanding and Use Self-Efficacy Scale (MUSE) (Rosenbaum & Ben-Ari Smira, 1986). In the MUSE model, a lack of self-efficacy implies an increase of non-adherence behavior (Rickles, 2010).

Medication adherence is of crucial importance in cancer patients due to the increasing number of oral anticancer medications (OAMs) in recent years (Barillet, Prevost, Joly, & Clarisse, 2015; Greer et al., 2016; Huang, Chen, Lin, & Chang, 2016). The responsibility of self-managing complex dosing regimens and serious side-effects can be overwhelming for many patients and may lead to non-adherence (Banna et al., 2010; D'Amato, 2008; Davey, 2013; Geynisman & Wickersham, 2013; B. S. Seal, Anderson, & Shermock, 2016; Weingart et al., 2008). Non-adherence to OAMs significantly reduces patients' progression-free survival (Shafrin et al., 2017). An evaluation study of the relationship between adherence and disease-free survival (DFS) showed that breast patients who were non-adherent to their hormonal therapy had a significantly higher risk of a DFS event (invasive recurrence at any site) (Chirgwin et al., 2016). The healthcare costs of non-adherence to OAMs ranged between USD$48,598 and USD$162,699 per patient per year, and the cost variation was double that of all other disease groups (Cutler, et al., 2018; Latremouille-Viau et al., 2017). According to studies that have used indirect methods of adherence measurements (e.g. questionnaire-based scales), the levels of OAM adherence range from 23% to almost 100% (Huang, et al., 2016). Levels of adherence can vary depending on the type of OAM and the point of time in a long duration of therapy (Ayres, Baldoni Ade, Borges, & Pereira, 2014; Chlebowski, Kim, & Haque, 2014; Greer, et al., 2016). As an example, adherence levels of oral endocrine therapy can range between 60% and 90% in the first year of treatment, but decreases to as low as 50% in the fifth year of therapy (Greer, et al., 2016). In non-endocrine OAM therapy, patients' adherence rates can vary between 69% and 100% in the first year of therapy (Greer, et al., 2016; Newman-Casey, Dayno, & Robin, 2016). On the other hand, non-adherence rates are only up to 41% in patients taking targeted therapies (Geynisman & Wickersham, 2013). All these data put to question the common belief that patients with cancer will be adherent to their medications because of the gravity of their condition (Davey, 2013; Noens et al., 2009; Weingart, et al., 2008).

Various interventions strategies have been applied to improve medication adherence and clinical outcomes for chronic illness management. These strategies can be introduced at the macro-, meso- micro- or patient-level (Berben, Dobbels, Engberg, Hill, & De Geest, 2012; De Geest, Ruppar, Berben, Schonfeld, & Hill, 2014). Macro-level interventions deal with the improvement of health policies, changes in insurance coverage and medication reimbursement methods (Niteesh K. Choudhry et al., 2011; De Geest, et al., 2014; González López-Valcárcel et al., 2017; Lauffenburger & Choudhry, 2018). Meso-level interventions focus on modification of practice patterns, healthcare professionals' competencies and skill mix of the healthcare team at healthcare facilities (Berben, et al., 2012). Micro-level interventions involve providing continuing education to healthcare professionals in adherence-enhancing programs so as to maximize their competencies (Berben, et al., 2012; De Geest, et al., 2014).

Patient-level adherence-enhancing interventions can be classified as informational, behavioral, and psychological/affective (Berben et al., 2011; Kirsch et al., 2014; Kripalani, Yao, & Haynes, 2007). Informational interventions usually involve the provision of written or audio-visual materials and telephone or face-to-face education conducted by healthcare professionals (Axelsson & Lötvall, 2012; Newman-Casey, Weizer, Heisler, Lee, & Stein, 2013). On the other hand, behavioral interventions typically involve reminder systems using pillboxes, calendars or electronic reminders; simplification of dosage schedules; skill-building activities conducted by healthcare professionals; and other interventions that involve rewards and reinforcement (Costa et al., 2015; Kim et al., 2014; Kreyenbuhl, Record, & Palmer-Bacon, 2016). In contrast, psychological/affective interventions focus on the emotions and feelings of patients and utilize support groups or peer mentor programs that involve family members, colleagues and/or fellow patients (Gu et al., 2017; Haynes, Ackloo, Sahota, McDonald, & Yao, 2008; Nieuwlaat et al., 2014). Many adherence-enhancing interventions involve combinations of two or more of these strategies because of the multiplicity of patient-related factors associated with medication non-adherence (N. K. Choudhry et al., 2017; Marcum, Sevick, & Handler, 2013; Mathes, Antoine, Pieper, & Eikermann, 2014; Newman-Casey, et al., 2016; Nieuwlaat, et al., 2014). These strategies can also be combined across the macro-, meso- micro- and patient-levels of interventions (Bosworth, 2012; Conn, Ruppar, Chase, Enriquez, & Cooper, 2015; Peterson, Takiya, & Finley, 2003).

The factors influencing patients' medication adherence patterns can also be classified under the macro-, meso-, micro- and patient-levels (Foulon, Schoffski, & Wolter, 2011; Hershman, 2016; Ruddy, Mayer, & Partridge, 2009; Schneider, Hess, & Gosselin, 2011). At the macro-level, decisions such as those regarding the amount of co-payment influence patients' adherence behavior. These macro-level interventions help reduce the financial barriers to medicine access using relevant policy initiatives (Hershman, 2016). For example, studies have shown that an increase in co-payment amount can lead to a decrease in the level of adherence (Dusetzina, Winn, Abel, Huskamp, & Keating, 2014; Neugut et al., 2011). Meso-level factors, such as the skill mix of healthcare professionals in a healthcare facility can also influence patients' medication adherence – higher adherence levels were observed in cancer patients receiving prescriptions from medical oncologists than primary care or other physicians (Murphy, Bartholomew, Carpentier, Bluethmann, & Vernon, 2012; Neugut, et al., 2011; Partridge, Wang, Winer, & Avorn, 2003). The addition of an oncology pharmacist was also found to improve OAM adherence significantly (Walter et al., 2016). At the micro-level, interventions have focused on improving the communication between patients and their doctors about the financial and therapeutic aspects of their treatments (Bestvina et al., 2014; O'Rourke, 2016), thus resulting in a more satisfying and collaborative patient-physician communication and a high patient adherence (Bestvina, et al., 2014; Chlebowski, et al., 2014; Jacobs et al., 2017; O'Rourke, 2016). At the patient level, factors such as the complexity of regimens, experience of adverse effects, disease stage, patient's age and their beliefs about the value of their treatment have significant influence over their medication adherence (Chirgwin, et al., 2016; Demissie, Silliman, &

Lash, 2001; Fink, Gurwitz, Rakowski, Guadagnoli, & Silliman, 2004; Irwin & Johnson, 2015; Lash, Fox, Westrup, Fink, & Silliman, 2006; Z. Moon, Moss-Morris, Hunter, & Hughes, 2017; Neugut, et al., 2011; Timmers et al., 2014; Winterhalder et al., 2011; Yagasaki, Komatsu, & Takahashi, 2015). Although there are conflicting findings on the influence of socio-economic factors (e.g. education level, income), these factors still play a significant role in patients' adherence behavior (Bourmaud et al., 2015; Chirgwin, et al., 2016; Partridge, Avorn, Wang, & Winer, 2002; Puts et al., 2014).

Given the complexity of the factors influencing medication adherence, the design and implementation of effective interventions that address the underlying macro-, meso-, micro- and patient-level factors is important (Chirgwin, et al., 2016; Hershman, 2016). Throughout the years, various digital strategies have been conceived and used as aids by healthcare professionals for delivering optimum pharmaceutical care and health-related outcomes. For example, audio and video programs have been used in the public health education of chronic diseases, such as cancer (Lederer, 2007). Organizations, such as the American Cancer Society, have also released several cancer education films to the general public (Cantor, 2007). The usefulness of video tapes in improving the knowledge and awareness of prostate-cancer screening in African-American men has also been demonstrated in a randomized intervention trial (Taylor et al., 2006). However, adherence interventions from the literature have largely focused on patient-level factors (Greer, et al., 2016), such as face-to-face, print or telephone-based education (Hadji et al., 2013; Kav & Tokdemir, 2017; Kirsch, et al., 2014; J. H. Moon et al., 2012; Neven et al., 2014; Simons et al., 2011; Sommers, Miller, & Berry, 2012; Tschida et al., 2012), pharmacist- or nurse-facilitated and telephone-based monitoring of side-effects (Gebbia et al., 2013; Khandelwal, Duncan, Ahmed, Rubinstein, & Pegus, 2012), tailoring adherence strategies to patients' needs (Schneider, Adams, & Gosselin, 2014), pillboxes prefilled with patient's daily medications (Macintosh, Pond, Pond, Leung, & Siu, 2007), automated voice response systems for symptom management (Spoelstra et al., 2013), and short messaging service (SMS) for delivery of reminders and motivating messages (Spoelstra et al., 2016). While some studies have reported the effectiveness of these adherence strategies, most of the evidence is inconclusive (Greer, et al., 2016; Mathes, et al., 2014). According to a systematic review by Greer et al.(2016), interventions involving multi-disciplinary pharmaceutical care and treatment monitoring programs were found to be effective in improving adherence, but other interventions involving educational support, pharmacy-based programs, counseling, prefilled pill boxes and automated voice response systems did not have any significant impact in improving adherence. Often, adherence interventions that showed promises of effectiveness had employed multiple adherence-enhancing strategies and were expensive to implement in routine clinical practice (N. K. Choudhry, et al., 2017; Greer, et al., 2016; Leporini, De Sarro, & Russo, 2014; Mathes, et al., 2014; Nieuwlaat, et al., 2014).

The integration of information technology and internet technologies has changed the way in which healthcare is practised. The internet is rapidly gaining importance for both healthcare professionals and patients as a means to search for health-related and drug-related information. Patients are becoming more well-informed about health-related issues through information that they receive over the internet. The advancement of technology has also led to the development of many pharmaco-informatics applications that can help reduce DRPs. Studies on the effectiveness of support systems for clinical decisions, e-prescribing, and drug-order entry have shown benefits in reducing medication errors, and in the prevention and management of chronic diseases (Bates et al., 1999; Dexter et al., 2001; Overhage, Tierney, Zhou, & McDonald, 1997). For example, the error rate detected in outpatients with cancer was lowest at a site that had a complete electronic medical record system and a computerized order-entry system, with only one chemotherapy error detected in 500 visits (Walsh et al., 2009). Bar-coded inpatient drug orders can minimize the probability of medication and dispensing errors, and electronic medical records can decrease the risk of DRPs, such as errors of omission, which can result in failure to provide required medications to the patient (Anderson; Larrabee & Brown, 2003). E-prescribing systems can also remind clinicians about potential drug interactions or a patient's drug allergies (Bates & Komaroff, 2006).

However, the ubiquitous nature of the internet and the World Wide Web has also led to several issues that can affect the quality of pharmaceutical care for patients in the digital age (Yap, Chan, & Chui, 2009). The lack of emotion and interconnectedness in digital communication modes, such as emails, can obscure non-verbal cues between the patient and the practitioner, thus resulting in a digital dehumanization in the patient–practitioner relationship. Furthermore, virtual conflicts of recommendation can occur due to the patient misinterpreting general information that is not applicable or tailored towards his personal needs, or the patient obtaining erroneous information on the internet. This conflict of recommendation can cause a sense of confusion and uncertainty in the patient, resulting in him turning to other inappropriate forms of therapy or a delay of his treatment. Lastly, the easy dissemination of health-related and drug-related information has led to the emergence of online pharmacies which can provide drugs at a more attractive and cheaper price, thus resulting in the phenomenon of online self-prescribing. The main concern regarding these online pharmacies is the lack of appropriate professional qualifications or healthcare expertise, as well as the lack of quality and efficacy controls in the drugs supplied, thus resulting in substandard or fake medicines (Veronin & Nguyen, 2008). All these issues may lead to patients' non-adherence to their medications, which in turn can result in other DRPs, such as dosing problems or potential drug interactions; and consequently, lead to a cascade of events that might substantially compromise their safety. The advent of mobile health (mHealth) technologies can help facilitate the efficient implementation of strategies that target DRPs such as DDIs (Bredrup, 2012; Yap, Chui, & Chan, 2011; Yap, See, Kuo, Chui, & Chan, 2012) and medication adherence (Agboola et al., 2014; Ali, Leow, Chew, & Yap, 2018; Fishbein et al., 2017; Hsu et al., 2017). The rest of this book will discuss the roles of mHealth interventions in improving pharmaceutical care, particularly in relation to oncology drug interactions and medication adherence.

REFERENCES

Agboola, S., Flanagan, C., Searl, M., Elfiky, A., Kvedar, J., & Jethwani, K. (2014). Improving outcomes in cancer patients on oral anti-cancer medications using a novel mobile phone-based intervention: Study design of a randomized controlled trial. *JMIR Research Protocols*, *3*(4), e79. doi:10.2196/resprot.4041 PMID:25537463

Akizuki, N., Akechi, T., Nakanishi, T., Yoshikawa, E., Okamura, M., Nakano, T., ... Uchitomi, Y. (2003). Development of a brief screening interview for adjustment disorders and major depression in patients with cancer. *Cancer*, *97*(10), 2605–2613. doi:10.1002/cncr.11358 PMID:12733160

Ali, E. E., Leow, J. L., Chew, L., & Yap, K. Y. (2018). Patients' perception of app-based educational and behavioural interventions for enhancing oral anticancer medication adherence. *Journal of Cancer Education*, *33*(6), 1306–1313. doi:10.100713187-017-1248-x PMID:28707206

American Society of Hospital Pharmacists. (1993). ASHP statement on pharmaceutical care. *American Journal of Hospital Pharmacy*, *50*(8), 1720–1723. doi:10.1093/ajhp/50.8.1720 PMID:8427270

Anderson, G. K. (2004, Nov 12). *Preventive medicine and the electronic health record*. Retrieved 17 Feb, 2020, from https://www.medscape.com/viewarticle/492842

Aroke, H. A., Vyas, A. M., Buchanan, A. L., & Kogut, S. J. (2019). Prevalence of psychotropic polypharmacy and associated healthcare resource utilization during initial phase of care among adults with cancer in USA. *Drugs - Real World Outcomes*, *6*(2), 73–82. doi:10.100740801-019-0153-5 PMID:31020617

Axelsson, M., & Lötvall, J. (2012). Recent educational interventions for improvement of asthma medication adherence. *Asia Pacific Allergy*, *2*(1), 67–75. doi:10.5415/apallergy.2012.2.1.67 PMID:22348209

Ayres, L. R., Baldoni Ade, O., Borges, A. P., & Pereira, L. R. (2014). Adherence and discontinuation of oral hormonal therapy in patients with hormone receptor positive breast cancer. *International Journal of Clinical Pharmacy*, *36*(1), 45–54. doi:10.100711096-013-9833-5 PMID:23934310

Bailey, R. K., Geyen, D. J., Scott-Gurnell, K., Hipolito, M. M., Bailey, T. A., & Beal, J. M. (2005). Understanding and treating depression among cancer patients. *International Journal of Gynecological Cancer*, *15*(2), 203–208. doi:10.1136/ijgc-00009577-200503000-00003 PMID:15823100

Banna, G. L., Collova, E., Gebbia, V., Lipari, H., Giuffrida, P., Cavallaro, S., ... Ferrau, F. (2010). Anticancer oral therapy: Emerging related issues. *Cancer Treatment Reviews*, *36*(8), 595–605. doi:10.1016/j.ctrv.2010.04.005 PMID:20570443

Barillet, M., Prevost, V., Joly, F., & Clarisse, B. (2015). Oral antineoplastic agents: How do we care about adherence? *British Journal of Clinical Pharmacology*, *80*(6), 1289–1302. doi:10.1111/bcp.12734 PMID:26255807

Bates, D. W., & Komaroff, A. L. (2006). Digital age. Next: paperless medicine. *Newsweek, 148*(16), 63.

Bates, D. W., Teich, J. M., Lee, J., Seger, D., Kuperman, G. J., Ma'Luf, N., ... Leape, L. (1999). The impact of computerized physician order entry on medication error prevention. *Journal of the American Medical Informatics Association*, *6*(4), 313–321. doi:10.1136/jamia.1999.00660313 PMID:10428004

Beijnen, J. H., & Schellens, J. H. (2004). Drug interactions in oncology. *Lancet Oncology*, *5*(8), 489–496. doi:10.1016/S1470-2045(04)01528-1 PMID:15288238

Benjamin, R. M. (2012). Medication adherence: Helping patients take their medicines as directed. *Public Health Reports*, *127*(1), 2–3. doi:10.1177/003335491212700102 PMID:22298918

Berben, L., Bogert, L., Leventhal, M. E., Fridlund, B., Jaarsma, T., Norekval, T. M., ... De Geest, S. (2011). Which interventions are used by health care professionals to enhance medication adherence in cardiovascular patients? A survey of current clinical practice. *European Journal of Cardiovascular Nursing*, *10*(1), 14–21. doi:10.1016/j.ejcnurse.2010.10.004 PMID:21095160

Berben, L., Dobbels, F., Engberg, S., Hill, M. N., & De Geest, S. (2012). An ecological perspective on medication adherence. *Western Journal of Nursing Research*, *34*(5), 635–653. doi:10.1177/0193945911434518 PMID:22309989

Bestvina, C. M., Zullig, L. L., Rushing, C., Chino, F., Samsa, G. P., Altomare, I., ... Zafar, S. Y. (2014). Patient-oncologist cost communication, financial distress, and medication adherence. *Journal of Oncology Practice*, *10*(3), 162–167. doi:10.1200/JOP.2014.001406 PMID:24839274

Bishop, F. L., Lauche, R., Cramer, H., Pinto, J. W., Leung, B., Hall, H., ... Adams, J. (2019). Health behavior change and complementary medicine use: National Health Interview Survey 2012. *Medicina (Kaunas, Lithuania)*, *55*(10), E632. doi:10.3390/medicina55100632 PMID:31554323

Bjerrum, L., Andersen, M., Petersen, G., & Kragstrup, J. (2003). Exposure to potential drug interactions in primary health care. *Scandinavian Journal of Primary Health Care*, *21*(3), 153–158. doi:10.1080/02813430310001806 PMID:14531506

Boon, H. S., Olatunde, F., & Zick, S. M. (2007). Trends in complementary/alternative medicine use by breast cancer survivors: Comparing survey data from 1998 and 2005. *BMC Women's Health*, *7*(1), 4. doi:10.1186/1472-6874-7-4 PMID:17397542

Bosworth, H. B. (2012). *Enhancing Medication Adherence: The Public Health Dilemma*. London, UK: Springer Healthcare Ltd. doi:10.1007/978-1-908517-66-1

Bourmaud, A., Henin, E., Tinquaut, F., Regnier, V., Hamant, C., Colomban, O., ... Chauvin, F. (2015). Adherence to oral anticancer chemotherapy: What influences patients' over or non-adherence? Analysis of the OCTO study through quantitative-qualitative methods. *BMC Research Notes*, *8*(1), 291. doi:10.118613104-015-1231-8 PMID:26142140

Bredrup, T. (2012, Mar 9). *iPhone app manages dangerous interactions between chemotherapy and alternative medications*. Retrieved 18 Feb, 2020, from https://www.imedicalapps.com/2012/03/iphone-app-dangerous-chemothearpy-alternative-medications/#

Bressler, R. (2005). Herb-drug interactions: Interactions between kava and prescription medications. *Geriatrics*, *60*(9), 24–25.

Brown, M. T., & Bussell, J. K. (2011). Medication adherence: WHO cares? *Mayo Clinic Proceedings*, *86*(4), 304–314. doi:10.4065/mcp.2010.0575 PMID:21389250

Cantor, D. (2007). Uncertain enthusiasm: The American Cancer Society, public education, and the problems of the movie, 1921-1960. *Bulletin of the History of Medicine*, *81*(1), 39–69. doi:10.1353/bhm.2007.0002 PMID:17369662

Chan, A., & Yap, K. Y. (2010). Detection and management of oncology drug interactions: Can we do better? *Maturitas*, *65*(3), 181–182. doi:10.1016/j.maturitas.2009.12.001 PMID:20036470

Chirgwin, J. H., Giobbie-Hurder, A., Coates, A. S., Price, K. N., Ejlertsen, B., Debled, M., ... Thurlimann, B. (2016). Treatment adherence and Its impact on disease-free survival in the breast international group 1-98 trial of tamoxifen and letrozole, alone and in sequence. *Journal of Clinical Oncology*, *34*(21), 2452–2459. doi:10.1200/JCO.2015.63.8619 PMID:27217455

Chlebowski, R. T., Kim, J., & Haque, R. (2014). Adherence to endocrine therapy in breast cancer adjuvant and prevention settings. *Cancer Prevention Research*, *7*(4), 378–387. doi:10.1158/1940-6207.CAPR-13-0389 PMID:24441675

Choudhry, N. K., Avorn, J., Glynn, R. J., Antman, E. M., Schneeweiss, S., Toscano, M., ... Shrank, W. H. (2011). Full coverage for preventive medications after myocardial infarction. *The New England Journal of Medicine, 365*(22), 2088–2097. doi:10.1056/NEJMsa1107913 PMID:22080794

Choudhry, N. K., Krumme, A. A., Ercole, P. M., Girdish, C., Tong, A. Y., Khan, N. F., ... Franklin, J. M. (2017). Effect of reminder devices on medication adherence: The REMIND randomized clinical trial. *JAMA Internal Medicine, 177*(5), 624–631. doi:10.1001/jamainternmed.2016.9627 PMID:28241271

Chow, W. H., Chang, P., Lee, S. C., Wong, A., Shen, H. M., & Verkooijen, H. M. (2010). Complementary and alternative medicine among Singapore cancer patients. *Annals of the Academy of Medicine, Singapore, 39*(2), 129–135. PMID:20237735

Clarke Institute of Psychiatry. (2007). *Clinical Handbook of Psychotropic Drugs* (17th ed.). Toronto, Canada: Hogrefe and Huber Publishers.

Conn, V. S., Ruppar, T. M., Chase, J.-A. D., Enriquez, M., & Cooper, P. S. (2015). Interventions to improve medication adherence in hypertensive patients: Systematic review and meta-analysis. *Current Hypertension Reports, 17*(12), 94. doi:10.100711906-015-0606-5 PMID:26560139

Costa, E., Giardini, A., Savin, M., Menditto, E., Lehane, E., Laosa, O., ... Marengoni, A. (2015). Interventional tools to improve medication adherence: Review of literature. *Patient Preference and Adherence, 9*, 1303–1314. doi:10.2147/PPA.S87551 PMID:26396502

Currie, C. J., Peyrot, M., Morgan, C. L., Poole, C. D., Jenkins-Jones, S., Rubin, R. R., ... Evans, M. (2012). The impact of treatment noncompliance on mortality in people with type 2 diabetes. *Diabetes Care, 35*(6), 1279–1284. doi:10.2337/dc11-1277 PMID:22511257

Cutler, R. L., Fernandez-Llimos, F., Frommer, M., Benrimoj, C., & Garcia-Cardenas, V. (2018). Economic impact of medication nonadherence by disease groups: A systematic review. *BMJ Open, 8*(1), e016982. doi:10.1136/bmjopen-2017-016982 PMID:29358417

D'Amato, S. (2008). Improving patient adherence with oral chemotherapy. *Oncology Issues, 23*(4), 42–45. doi:10.1080/10463356.2008.11884291

Davey, M. P. (2013). Improving adherence to oral anticancer therapy. *Nursing, 43*(9), 31–36. doi:10.1097/01.NURSE.0000432915.51753.0c PMID:23963388

De Geest, S., Ruppar, T., Berben, L., Schonfeld, S., & Hill, M. N. (2014). Medication non-adherence as a critical factor in the management of presumed resistant hypertension: A narrative review. *EuroIntervention, 9*(9), 1102–1109. doi:10.4244/EIJV9I9A185 PMID:24457281

Delafuente, J. C. (2003). Understanding and preventing drug interactions in elderly patients. *Critical Reviews in Oncology/Hematology, 48*(2), 133–143. doi:10.1016/j.critrevonc.2003.04.004 PMID:14607376

Demissie, S., Silliman, R. A., & Lash, T. L. (2001). Adjuvant tamoxifen: Predictors of use, side effects, and discontinuation in older women. *Journal of Clinical Oncology, 19*(2), 322–328. doi:10.1200/JCO.2001.19.2.322 PMID:11208822

Dexter, P. R., Perkins, S., Overhage, J. M., Maharry, K., Kohler, R. B., & McDonald, C. J. (2001). A computerized reminder system to increase the use of preventive care for hospitalized patients. *The New England Journal of Medicine, 345*(13), 965–970. doi:10.1056/NEJMsa010181 PMID:11575289

Dusetzina, S. B., Winn, A. N., Abel, G. A., Huskamp, H. A., & Keating, N. L. (2014). Cost sharing and adherence to tyrosine kinase inhibitors for patients with chronic myeloid leukemia. *Journal of Clinical Oncology, 32*(4), 306–311. doi:10.1200/JCO.2013.52.9123 PMID:24366936

Eells, S. J., Nguyen, M., Jung, J., Macias-Gil, R., May, L., & Miller, L. G. (2016). Relationship between adherence to oral antibiotics and postdischarge clinical outcomes among patients hospitalized with Staphylococcus aureus skin infections. *Antimicrobial Agents and Chemotherapy, 60*(5), 2941–2948. doi:10.1128/AAC.02626-15 PMID:26926634

Elkayam, E. S. (2005). Seizure prophylaxis and liability. *Mayo Clinic Proceedings, 80*(2), 288. doi:10.4065/80.2.288 PMID:15704787

Farriols, C., Ferrandez, O., Planas, J., Ortiz, P., Mojal, S., & Ruiz, A. I. (2012). Changes in the prescription of psychotropic drugs in the palliative care of advanced cancer patients over a seven-year period. *Journal of Pain and Symptom Management, 43*(5), 945–952. doi:10.1016/j.jpainsymman.2011.05.010 PMID:22436835

Fink, A. K., Gurwitz, J., Rakowski, W., Guadagnoli, E., & Silliman, R. A. (2004). Patient beliefs and tamoxifen discontinuance in older women with estrogen receptor-positive breast cancer. *Journal of Clinical Oncology*, *22*(16), 3309–3315. doi:10.1200/JCO.2004.11.064 PMID:15310774

Fishbein, J. N., Nisotel, L. E., MacDonald, J. J., Amoyal Pensak, N., Jacobs, J. M., Flanagan, C., ... Greer, J. A. (2017). Mobile application to promote adherence to oral chemotherapy and symptom management: A protocol for design and development. *JMIR Research Protocols*, *6*(4), e62. doi:10.2196/resprot.6198 PMID:28428158

Foulon, V., Schoffski, P., & Wolter, P. (2011). Patient adherence to oral anticancer drugs: An emerging issue in modern oncology. *Acta Clinica Belgica*, *66*(2), 85–96. doi:10.2143/ACB.66.2.2062525 PMID:21630604

Gadkari, A. S., & McHorney, C. A. (2012). Unintentional non-adherence to chronic prescription medications: How unintentional is it really? *BMC Health Services Research*, *12*(1), 98. doi:10.1186/1472-6963-12-98 PMID:22510235

Gebbia, V., Bellavia, M., Banna, G. L., Russo, P., Ferrau, F., Tralongo, P., & Borsellino, N. (2013). Treatment monitoring program for implementation of adherence to second-line erlotinib for advanced non-small-cell lung cancer. *Clinical Lung Cancer*, *14*(4), 390–398. doi:10.1016/j.cllc.2012.11.007 PMID:23313173

Geynisman, D. M., & Wickersham, K. E. (2013). Adherence to targeted oral anticancer medications. *Discovery Medicine*, *15*(83), 231–241. PMID:23636140

Glantz, M. J., Cole, B. F., Forsyth, P. A., Recht, L. D., Wen, P. Y., Chamberlain, M. C., ... Cairncross, J. G. (2000). Practice parameter: Anticonvulsant prophylaxis in patients with newly diagnosed brain tumors. Report of the Quality Standards Subcommittee of the American Academy of Neurology. *Neurology*, *54*(10), 1886–1893. doi:10.1212/WNL.54.10.1886 PMID:10822423

González López-Valcárcel, B., Librero, J., García-Sempere, A., Peña, L. M., Bauer, S., Puig-Junoy, J., ... Sanfélix-Gimeno, G. (2017). Effect of cost sharing on adherence to evidence-based medications in patients with acute coronary syndrome. *Heart (British Cardiac Society)*, *103*(14), 1082–1088. doi:10.1136/heartjnl-2016-310610 PMID:28249992

Greer, J. A., Amoyal, N., Nisotel, L., Fishbein, J. N., MacDonald, J., Stagl, J., ... Pirl, W. F. (2016). A systematic review of adherence to oral antineoplastic therapies. *The Oncologist*, *21*(3), 354–376. doi:10.1634/theoncologist.2015-0405 PMID:26921292

Gu, L., Wu, S., Zhao, S., Zhou, H., Zhang, S., Gao, M., ... Tian, D. (2017). Association of social support and medication adherence in Chinese patients with type 2 diabetes mellitus. *International Journal of Environmental Research and Public Health*, *14*(12), 1522. doi:10.3390/ijerph14121522 PMID:29211039

Hadji, P., Blettner, M., Harbeck, N., Jackisch, C., Luck, H. J., Windemuth-Kieselbach, C., ... Kreienberg, R. (2013). The patient's anastrozole compliance to therapy (PACT) program: A randomized, in-practice study on the impact of a standardized information program on persistence and compliance to adjuvant endocrine therapy in postmenopausal women with early breast cancer. *Annals of Oncology*, *24*(6), 1505–1512. doi:10.1093/annonc/mds653 PMID:23378537

Haynes, R. B., Ackloo, E., Sahota, N., McDonald, H. P., & Yao, X. (2008). Interventions for enhancing medication adherence. *Cochrane Database of Systematic Reviews*, *2*, CD000011. doi:10.1002/14651858.CD000011.pub3 PMID:18425859

Hershman, D. L. (2016). Sticking to it: Improving outcomes by increasing adherence. *Journal of Clinical Oncology*, *34*(21), 2440–2442. doi:10.1200/JCO.2016.67.7336 PMID:27217447

Hsu, G. I.-H., Crawford, S. Y., Paolella, G., Cuellar, S., Wirth, S. M., Venepalli, N. K., ... Boyd, A. D. (2017). Design of customized mobile application for patient adherence to oral anticancer medications utilizing user-centered design. *The Journal of Biocommunication*, *41*(1), 5–14. doi:10.5210/jbc.v41i1.7499

Huang, W. C., Chen, C. Y., Lin, S. J., & Chang, C. S. (2016). Medication adherence to oral anticancer drugs: Systematic review. *Expert Review of Anticancer Therapy*, *16*(4), 423–432. doi:10.1586/14737140.2016.1159515 PMID:26935964

Hugtenburg, J. G., Timmers, L., Elders, P. J., Vervloet, M., & van Dijk, L. (2013). Definitions, variants, and causes of nonadherence with medication: A challenge for tailored interventions. *Patient Preference and Adherence*, *7*, 675–682. doi:10.2147/PPA.S29549 PMID:23874088

Hyodo, I., Amano, N., Eguchi, K., Narabayashi, M., Imanishi, J., Hirai, M., ... Takashima, S. (2005). Nationwide survey on complementary and alternative medicine in cancer patients in Japan. *Journal of Clinical Oncology*, *23*(12), 2645–2654. doi:10.1200/JCO.2005.04.126 PMID:15728227

Institute of Medicine (US) Committee on the Use of Complementary and Alternative Medicine by the American Public. (2005). *Complementary and Alternative Medicine in the United States*. Retrieved from https://www.ncbi.nlm.nih.gov/books/NBK83794/ doi:10.17226/11182

Irwin, M., & Johnson, L. A. (2015). Factors influencing oral adherence: Qualitative metasummary and triangulation with quantitative evidence. *Clinical Journal of Oncology Nursing*, *19*(3Suppl), 6–30. doi:10.1188/15.S1.CJON.6-30 PMID:26030389

Iuga, A. O., & McGuire, M. J. (2014). Adherence and health care costs. *Risk Management and Healthcare Policy*, *7*, 35–44. doi:10.2147/RMHP.S19801 PMID:24591853

Jacobs, J. M., Pensak, N. A., Sporn, N. J., MacDonald, J. J., Lennes, I. T., Safren, S. A., ... Greer, J. A. (2017). Treatment satisfaction and adherence to oral chemotherapy in patients with cancer. *Journal of Oncology Practice*, *13*(5), e474–e485. doi:10.1200/JOP.2016.019729 PMID:28398843

Karas, S. Jr. (1981). The potential for drug interactions. *Annals of Emergency Medicine*, *10*(12), 627–630. doi:10.1016/S0196-0644(81)80085-6 PMID:7305093

Kav, S., & Tokdemir, G. (2017). The effect of structured education to patients receiving oral agents for cancer treatment on medication adherence and self-efficacy. *Asia-Pacific Journal of Oncology Nursing*, *4*(4), 290. doi:10.4103/apjon.apjon_35_17 PMID:28966956

Khan, R., & Socha-Dietrich, K. (2018). Investing in medication adherence improves health outcomes and health system efficiency. *OECD Health Working Paper No. 105*. Retrieved from http://www.oecd.org/officialdocuments/publicdisplaydocumentpdf/?cote=DELSA/HEA/WD/HWP(2018)2&docLanguage=En

Khandelwal, N., Duncan, I., Ahmed, T., Rubinstein, E., & Pegus, C. (2012). Oral chemotherapy program improves adherence and reduces medication wastage and hospital admissions. *Journal of the National Comprehensive Cancer Network: JNCCN, 10*(5), 618–625. doi:10.6004/jnccn.2012.0063 PMID:22570292

Kim, K. B., Han, H.-R., Huh, B., Nguyen, T., Lee, H., & Kim, M. T. (2014). The effect of a community-based self-help multimodal behavioral intervention in Korean American seniors with high blood pressure. *American Journal of Hypertension, 27*(9), 1199–1208. doi:10.1093/ajh/hpu041 PMID:24671049

Kinsel, J. F., & Straus, S. E. (2003). Complementary and alternative therapeutics: Rigorous research is needed to support claims. *Annual Review of Pharmacology and Toxicology, 43*(1), 463–484. doi:10.1146/annurev.pharmtox.43.100901.135757 PMID:12540748

Kirsch, M., Berben, L., Johansson, E., Calza, S., Eeltink, C., Stringer, J., ... De Geest, S. (2014). Nurses' practice patterns in relation to adherence-enhancing interventions in stem cell transplant care: A survey from the Nurses Group of the European Group for Blood and Marrow Transplantation. *European Journal of Cancer Care, 23*(5), 607–615. doi:10.1111/ecc.12172 PMID:24393127

Kjos, A. L., Vaughan, A. G., & Bhargava, A. (2019). Impact of a mobile app on medication adherence and adherence-related beliefs in patients with type 2 diabetes. *Journal of the American Pharmacists Association, 59*(2S), S44-S51 e43. doi:10.1016/j.japh.2018.12.012

Kreyenbuhl, J., Record, E. J., & Palmer-Bacon, J. (2016). A review of behavioral tailoring strategies for improving medication adherence in serious mental illness. *Dialogues in Clinical Neuroscience, 18*(2), 191–201. PMID:27489459

Kripalani, S., Yao, X., & Haynes, R. B. (2007). Interventions to enhance medication adherence in chronic medical conditions: A systematic review. *Archives of Internal Medicine, 167*(6), 540–550. doi:10.1001/archinte.167.6.540 PMID:17389285

Kuhlmann, J., & Muck, W. (2001). Clinical-pharmacological strategies to assess drug interaction potential during drug development. *Drug Safety, 24*(10), 715–725. doi:10.2165/00002018-200124100-00001 PMID:11676300

Kuo, Y. T., Chang, T. T., Muo, C. H., Wu, M. Y., Sun, M. F., Yeh, C. C., & Yen, H. R. (2018). Use of complementary traditional Chinese medicines by adult cancer patients in Taiwan: A nationwide population-based study. *Integrative Cancer Therapies*, *17*(2), 531–541. doi:10.1177/1534735417716302 PMID:28665160

Larrabee, S., & Brown, M. M. (2003). Recognizing the institutional benefits of bar-code point-of-care technology. *Joint Commission Journal on Quality and Safety*, *29*(7), 345–353. doi:10.1016/S1549-3741(03)29042-0 PMID:12856556

Lash, T. L., Fox, M. P., Westrup, J. L., Fink, A. K., & Silliman, R. A. (2006). Adherence to tamoxifen over the five-year course. *Breast Cancer Research and Treatment*, *99*(2), 215–220. doi:10.100710549-006-9193-0 PMID:16541307

Latremouille-Viau, D., Guerin, A., Gagnon-Sanschagrin, P., Dea, K., Cohen, B. G., & Joseph, G. J. (2017). Health care resource utilization and costs in patients with chronic myeloid leukemia with better adherence to tyrosine kinase inhibitors and increased molecular monitoring frequency. *Journal of Managed Care & Specialty Pharmacy*, *23*(2), 214–224. doi:10.18553/jmcp.2017.23.2.214 PMID:28125373

Lauffenburger, J. C., & Choudhry, N. K. (2018). A call for a systems-thinking approach to medication adherence: Stop blaming the patient. *JAMA Internal Medicine*, *178*(7), 950–951. doi:10.1001/jamainternmed.2018.0790 PMID:29799994

Lederer, S. E. (2007). Dark victory: Cancer and popular Hollywood film. *Bulletin of the History of Medicine*, *81*(1), 94–115. doi:10.1353/bhm.2007.0005 PMID:17369664

Leporini, C., De Sarro, G., & Russo, E. (2014). Adherence to therapy and adverse drug reactions: Is there a link? *Expert Opinion on Drug Safety*, *13*(Suppl 1), S41–S55. doi:10.1517/14740338.2014.947260 PMID:25171158

Lim, C. M., Ng, A., & Loh, K. S. (2010). Use of complementary and alternative medicine in head and neck cancer patients. *The Journal of Laryngology and Otology*, *124*(5), 529–532. doi:10.1017/S0022215109992817 PMID:20163747

Lim, J., Wong, M., Chan, M. Y., Tan, A. M., Rajalingam, V., Lim, L. P., ... Tan, C. L. (2006). Use of complementary and alternative medicine in paediatric oncology patients in Singapore. *Annals of the Academy of Medicine, Singapore*, *35*(11), 753–758. PMID:17160187

Macintosh, P. W., Pond, G. R., Pond, B. J., Leung, V., & Siu, L. L. (2007). A comparison of patient adherence and preference of packaging method for oral anticancer agents using conventional pill bottles versus daily pill boxes. *European Journal of Cancer Care*, *16*(4), 380–386. doi:10.1111/j.1365-2354.2006.00758.x PMID:17587364

Marcum, Z. A., Sevick, M. A., & Handler, S. M. (2013). Medication nonadherence: A diagnosable and treatable medical condition. *Journal of the American Medical Association*, *309*(20), 2105–2106. doi:10.1001/jama.2013.4638 PMID:23695479

Mathes, T., Antoine, S. L., Pieper, D., & Eikermann, M. (2014). Adherence enhancing interventions for oral anticancer agents: A systematic review. *Cancer Treatment Reviews*, *40*(1), 102–108. doi:10.1016/j.ctrv.2013.07.004 PMID:23910455

Miovic, M., & Block, S. (2007). Psychiatric disorders in advanced cancer. *Cancer*, *110*(8), 1665–1676. doi:10.1002/cncr.22980 PMID:17847017

Moon, J. H., Sohn, S. K., Kim, S. N., Park, S. Y., Yoon, S. S., Kim, I. H., ... Kim, D. H. (2012). Patient counseling program to improve the compliance to imatinib in chronic myeloid leukemia patients. *Medical Oncology (Northwood, London, England)*, *29*(2), 1179–1185. doi:10.100712032-011-9926-8 PMID:21472487

Moon, Z., Moss-Morris, R., Hunter, M. S., & Hughes, L. D. (2017). Understanding tamoxifen adherence in women with breast cancer: A qualitative study. *British Journal of Health Psychology*, *22*(4), 978–997. doi:10.1111/bjhp.12266 PMID:28850763

Murphy, C. C., Bartholomew, L. K., Carpentier, M. Y., Bluethmann, S. M., & Vernon, S. W. (2012). Adherence to adjuvant hormonal therapy among breast cancer survivors in clinical practice: A systematic review. *Breast Cancer Research and Treatment*, *134*(2), 459–478. doi:10.100710549-012-2114-5 PMID:22689091

National Council on Patient Information and Education. (2013). *Accelerating progress in prescription medicine adherence: The adherence action agenda. A national action plan to address America's "Other Drug Problem"*. Retrieved 10 May, 2018, from https://goo.gl/iSsPB3

Neiheisel, M. B., Wheeler, K. J., & Roberts, M. E. (2014). Medication adherence part one: Understanding and assessing the problem. *Journal of the American Association of Nurse Practitioners*, *26*(1), 49–55. doi:10.1002/2327-6924.12099 PMID:24382862

Neugut, A. I., Subar, M., Wilde, E. T., Stratton, S., Brouse, C. H., Hillyer, G. C., ... Hershman, D. L. (2011). Association between prescription co-payment amount and compliance with adjuvant hormonal therapy in women with early-stage breast cancer. *Journal of Clinical Oncology*, *29*(18), 2534–2542. doi:10.1200/JCO.2010.33.3179 PMID:21606426

Neven, P., Markopoulos, C., Tanner, M., Marty, M., Kreienberg, R., Atkins, L., ... Deschamp, V. (2014). The impact of educational materials on compliance and persistence rates with adjuvant aromatase inhibitor treatment: First-year results from the compliance of aromatase inhibitors assessment in daily practice through educational approach (CARIATIDE) study. *The Breast*, *23*(4), 393–399. doi:10.1016/j.breast.2014.02.009 PMID:24675394

Newman-Casey, P. A., Dayno, M., & Robin, A. L. (2016). Systematic review of educational interventions to improve glaucoma medication adherence: An update in 2015. *Expert Review of Ophthalmology*, *11*(1), 5–20. doi:10.1586/17469899.2016.1134318 PMID:27134639

Newman-Casey, P. A., Weizer, J. S., Heisler, M., Lee, P. P., & Stein, J. D. (2013). Systematic review of educational interventions to improve glaucoma medication adherence. *Seminars in Ophthalmology*, *28*(3), 191–201. doi:10.3109/08820538.2013.771198 PMID:23697623

Ng, C. G., Boks, M. P., Smeets, H. M., Zainal, N. Z., & de Wit, N. J. (2013). Prescription patterns for psychotropic drugs in cancer patients; A large population study in the Netherlands. *Psycho-Oncology*, *22*(4), 762–767. doi:10.1002/pon.3056 PMID:22351591

Nieuwlaat, R., Wilczynski, N., Navarro, T., Hobson, N., Jeffery, R., Keepanasseril, A., ... Haynes, R. B. (2014). Interventions for enhancing medication adherence. *Cochrane Database of Systematic Reviews*, *11*, CD000011. doi:10.1002/14651858.CD000011.pub4 PMID:25412402

Noens, L., van Lierde, M. A., De Bock, R., Verhoef, G., Zachee, P., Berneman, Z., ... Abraham, I. (2009). Prevalence, determinants, and outcomes of nonadherence to imatinib therapy in patients with chronic myeloid leukemia: The (ADAGIO) study. *Blood*, *113*(22), 5401–5411. doi:10.1182/blood-2008-12-196543 PMID:19349618

O'Rourke, K. M. (2016). *'Nonadherence may be the norm': Why cancer patients don't take their medications.* Retrieved 28 May, 2018, from https://wb.md/2sgC9Bf

Osterberg, L., & Blaschke, T. (2005). Adherence to medication. *The New England Journal of Medicine*, *353*(5), 487–497. doi:10.1056/NEJMra050100 PMID:16079372

Overhage, J. M., Tierney, W. M., Zhou, X. H., & McDonald, C. J. (1997). A randomized trial of "corollary orders" to prevent errors of omission. *Journal of the American Medical Informatics Association*, *4*(5), 364–375. doi:10.1136/jamia.1997.0040364 PMID:9292842

Partridge, A. H., Avorn, J., Wang, P. S., & Winer, E. P. (2002). Adherence to therapy with oral antineoplastic agents. *Journal of the National Cancer Institute*, *94*(9), 652–661. doi:10.1093/jnci/94.9.652 PMID:11983753

Partridge, A. H., Wang, P. S., Winer, E. P., & Avorn, J. (2003). Nonadherence to adjuvant tamoxifen therapy in women with primary breast cancer. *Journal of Clinical Oncology*, *21*(4), 602–606. doi:10.1200/JCO.2003.07.071 PMID:12586795

Patsalos, P. N., Froscher, W., Pisani, F., & van Rijn, C. M. (2002). The importance of drug interactions in epilepsy therapy. *Epilepsia*, *43*(4), 365–385. doi:10.1046/j.1528-1157.2002.13001.x PMID:11952767

Patsalos, P. N., & Perucca, E. (2003). Clinically important drug interactions in epilepsy: General features and interactions between antiepileptic drugs. *Lancet Neurology*, *2*(6), 347–356. doi:10.1016/S1474-4422(03)00409-5 PMID:12849151

Perucca, E. (1997). Pharmacologic advantages of antiepileptic drug monotherapy. *Epilepsia*, *38*(s5), S6–S8. doi:10.1111/j.1528-1157.1997.tb04598.x

Perucca, E. (2006). Clinically relevant drug interactions with antiepileptic drugs. *British Journal of Clinical Pharmacology*, *61*(3), 246–255. doi:10.1111/j.1365-2125.2005.02529.x PMID:16487217

Peterson, A. M., Takiya, L., & Finley, R. (2003). Meta-analysis of trials of interventions to improve medication adherence. *American Journal of Health-System Pharmacy*, *60*(7), 657–665. doi:10.1093/ajhp/60.7.657 PMID:12701547

Pharmaceutical Care Network Europe. (2019, Jun). *Classification for drug related problems v9.00.* Retrieved 7 Apr, 2020, from https://www.pcne.org/upload/files/334_PCNE_classification_V9-0.pdf

Puts, M. T., Tu, H. A., Tourangeau, A., Howell, D., Fitch, M., Springall, E., & Alibhai, S. M. (2014). Factors influencing adherence to cancer treatment in older adults with cancer: A systematic review. *Annals of Oncology*, *25*(3), 564–577. doi:10.1093/annonc/mdt433 PMID:24285020

Rickles, N. M. (2010). A multi-theoretical approach to linking medication adherence levels and the comparison of outcomes. *Research in Social & Administrative Pharmacy*, *6*(1), 49–62. doi:10.1016/j.sapharm.2009.02.006 PMID:20188328

Riechelmann, R. P., & Saad, E. D. (2006). A systematic review on drug interactions in oncology. *Cancer Investigation*, *24*(7), 704–712. doi:10.1080/07357900601063766 PMID:17118781

Riechelmann, R. P., Tannock, I. F., Wang, L., Saad, E. D., Taback, N. A., & Krzyzanowska, M. K. (2007). Potential drug interactions and duplicate prescriptions among cancer patients. *Journal of the National Cancer Institute*, *99*(8), 592–600. doi:10.1093/jnci/djk130 PMID:17440160

Rosen, O. Z., Fridman, R., Rosen, B. T., Shane, R., & Pevnick, J. M. (2017). Medication adherence as a predictor of 30-day hospital readmissions. *Patient Preference and Adherence*, *11*, 801–810. doi:10.2147/PPA.S125672 PMID:28461742

Rosenbaum, M., & Ben-Ari Smira, K. (1986). Cognitive and personality factors in the delay of gratification of hemodialysis patients. *Journal of Personality and Social Psychology*, *51*(2), 357–364. doi:10.1037/0022-3514.51.2.357 PMID:3746617

Ruddy, K., Mayer, E., & Partridge, A. (2009). Patient adherence and persistence with oral anticancer treatment. *CA: A Cancer Journal for Clinicians*, *59*(1), 56–66. doi:10.3322/caac.20004 PMID:19147869

Sabaté, E., & Sabaté, E. (2003). *Adherence to long-term therapies: Evidence for action*. World Health Organization.

Scheel, J., Reber, S., Stoessel, L., Waldmann, E., Jank, S., Eckardt, K.-U., ... Erim, Y. (2017). Patient-reported non-adherence and immunosuppressant trough levels are associated with rejection after renal transplantation. *BMC Nephrology*, *18*(1), 107. doi:10.118612882-017-0517-6 PMID:28356080

Schneider, S. M., Adams, D. B., & Gosselin, T. (2014). A tailored nurse coaching intervention for oral chemotherapy adherence. *Journal of the Advanced Practitioner in Oncology*, *5*(3), 163–172. PMID:25089216

Schneider, S. M., Hess, K., & Gosselin, T. (2011). Interventions to promote adherence with oral agents. *Seminars in Oncology Nursing*, *27*(2), 133–141. doi:10.1016/j.soncn.2011.02.005 PMID:21514482

Scripture, C. D., & Figg, W. D. (2006). Drug interactions in cancer therapy. *Nature Reviews. Cancer*, *6*(7), 546–558. doi:10.1038/nrc1887 PMID:16794637

Seal, B. S., Anderson, S., & Shermock, K. M. (2016). Factors associated with adherence rates for oral and intravenous anticancer therapy in commercially insured patients with metastatic colon cancer. *Journal of Managed Care & Specialty Pharmacy*, *22*(3), 227–235. doi:10.18553/jmcp.2016.22.3.227 PMID:27003552

Seal, F., Cave, A. J., & Atkinson, L. L. (2017). Primary non-adherence of prescribed pharmaceutical treatments and interventions: An investigative review to improve quality in primary care. *Quality in Primary Care*, *25*(5), 344–359.

Shafrin, J., Sullivan, J., Chou, J. W., Neely, M. N., Doan, J. F., & Maclean, J. R. (2017). The effect of medication nonadherence on progression-free survival among patients with renal cell carcinoma. *Cancer Management and Research*, *9*, 731–739. doi:10.2147/CMAR.S148199 PMID:29238223

Shih, V., Chiang, J. Y., & Chan, A. (2009). Complementary and alternative medicine (CAM) usage in Singaporean adult cancer patients. *Annals of Oncology*, *20*(4), 752–757. doi:10.1093/annonc/mdn659 PMID:19150956

Simons, S., Ringsdorf, S., Braun, M., Mey, U. J., Schwindt, P. F., Ko, Y. D., ... Jaehde, U. (2011). Enhancing adherence to capecitabine chemotherapy by means of multidisciplinary pharmaceutical care. *Supportive Care in Cancer, 19*(7), 1009–1018. doi:10.100700520-010-0927-5 PMID:20552377

Solomon, M. D., & Majumdar, S. R. (2010). Primary non-adherence of medications: Lifting the veil on prescription-filling behaviors. *Journal of General Internal Medicine, 25*(4), 280–281. doi:10.100711606-010-1286-0 PMID:20195783

Sommers, R. M., Miller, K., & Berry, D. L. (2012). Feasibility pilot on medication adherence and knowledge in ambulatory patients with gastrointestinal cancer. *Oncology Nursing Forum, 39*(4), E373–E379. doi:10.1188/12.ONF.E373-E379 PMID:22750908

Spoelstra, S. L., Given, B. A., Given, C. W., Grant, M., Sikorskii, A., You, M., & Decker, V. (2013). An intervention to improve adherence and management of symptoms for patients prescribed oral chemotherapy agents: An exploratory study. *Cancer Nursing, 36*(1), 18–28. doi:10.1097/NCC.0b013e3182551587 PMID:23235499

Spoelstra, S. L., Given, C. W., Sikorskii, A., Coursaris, C. K., Majumder, A., DeKoekkoek, T., ... Given, B. A. (2016). Proof of concept of a mobile health short message service text message intervention that promotes adherence to oral anticancer agent medications: A randomized controlled trial. *Telemedicine Journal and e-Health, 22*(6), 497–506. doi:10.1089/tmj.2015.0126 PMID:26716365

Stedman, T. L. (2005). *Stedman's Medical Dictionary* (28th ed.). Baltimore, MD: Lippincott Williams & Wilkins.

Stiefel, F. C., Kornblith, A. B., & Holland, J. C. (1990). Changes in the prescription patterns of psychotropic drugs for cancer patients during a 10-year period. *Cancer, 65*(4), 1048–1053. doi:10.1002/1097-0142(19900215)65:4<1048::AID-CNCR2820650434>3.0.CO;2-N PMID:1967546

Subramani, R., & Lakshmanaswamy, R. (2017). Complementary and alternative medicine and breast cancer. *Progress in Molecular Biology and Translational Science, 151*, 231–274. doi:10.1016/bs.pmbts.2017.07.008 PMID:29096896

Sun, L., Mao, J. J., Vertosick, E., Seluzicki, C., & Yang, Y. (2018). Evaluating cancer patients' expectations and barriers toward traditional Chinese medicine utilization in China: A patient-support group-based cross-sectional survey. *Integrative Cancer Therapies*, *17*(3), 885–893. doi:10.1177/1534735418777117 PMID:29888609

Tabish, S. A. (2008). Complementary and alternative healthcare: Is it evidence-based? *International Journal of Health Sciences*, *2*(1), V–IX. PMID:21475465

Tasaki, K., Maskarinec, G., Shumay, D. M., Tatsumura, Y., & Kakai, H. (2002). Communication between physicians and cancer patients about complementary and alternative medicine: Exploring patients' perspectives. *Psycho-Oncology*, *11*(3), 212–220. doi:10.1002/pon.552 PMID:12112481

Taylor, K. L., Davis, J. L. III, Turner, R. O., Johnson, L., Schwartz, M. D., Kerner, J. F., & Leak, C. (2006). Educating African American men about the prostate cancer screening dilemma: A randomized intervention. *Cancer Epidemiology, Biomarkers & Prevention*, *15*(11), 2179–2188. doi:10.1158/1055-9965.EPI-05-0417 PMID:17119044

Timmers, L., Boons, C. C., Kropff, F., van de Ven, P. M., Swart, E. L., Smit, E. F., ... Hugtenburg, J. G. (2014). Adherence and patients' experiences with the use of oral anticancer agents. *Acta Oncologica*, *53*(2), 259–267. doi:10.3109/0284186X.2013.844353 PMID:24266637

Tschida, S. J., Aslam, S., Lal, L. S., Khan, T. T., Shrank, W. H., Bhattarai, G. R., ... Newcomer, L. N. (2012). Outcomes of a specialty pharmacy program for oral oncology medications. *The American Journal of Pharmacy Benefits*, *4*(4), 165–174.

U.S. National Institutes of Health. (n.d.). *National Cancer Institute (NCI)*. Retrieved 17 Feb, 2020, from https://www.cancer.gov/

van Boven, J. F., Chavannes, N. H., van der Molen, T., Rutten-van Molken, M. P., Postma, M. J., & Vegter, S. (2014). Clinical and economic impact of non-adherence in COPD: A systematic review. *Respiratory Medicine*, *108*(1), 103–113. doi:10.1016/j.rmed.2013.08.044 PMID:24070566

Veronin, M. A., & Nguyen, N. T. (2008). Comparison of simvastatin tablets from the US and international markets obtained via the Internet. *The Annals of Pharmacotherapy*, *42*(5), 613–620. doi:10.1345/aph.1K560 PMID:18413690

Viswanathan, M., Golin, C. E., Jones, C. D., Ashok, M., Blalock, S. J., Wines, R. C. M., ... Lohr, K. N. (2012). Interventions to improve adherence to self-administered medications for chronic diseases in the United States: A systematic review. *Annals of Internal Medicine*, *157*(11), 785–795. doi:10.7326/0003-4819-157-11-201212040-00538 PMID:22964778

Vrijens, B., De Geest, S., Hughes, D. A., Przemyslaw, K., Demonceau, J., Ruppar, T., ... Team, A. B. C. P. (2012). A new taxonomy for describing and defining adherence to medications. *British Journal of Clinical Pharmacology*, *73*(5), 691–705. doi:10.1111/j.1365-2125.2012.04167.x PMID:22486599

Wallston, K. A., Stein, M. J., & Smith, C. A. (1994). Form C of the MHLC scales: A condition-specific measure of locus of control. *Journal of Personality Assessment*, *63*(3), 534–553. doi:10.120715327752jpa6303_10 PMID:7844739

Walsh, K. E., Dodd, K. S., Seetharaman, K., Roblin, D. W., Herrinton, L. J., Von Worley, A., ... Gurwitz, J. H. (2009). Medication errors among adults and children with cancer in the outpatient setting. *Journal of Clinical Oncology*, *27*(6), 891–896. doi:10.1200/JCO.2008.18.6072 PMID:19114695

Walter, C., Mellor, J. D., Rice, C., Kirsa, S., Ball, D., Duffy, M., ... Mileshkin, L. (2016). Impact of a specialist clinical cancer pharmacist at a multidisciplinary lung cancer clinic. *Asia Pacific Journal of Clinical Oncology*, *12*(3), e367–e374. doi:10.1111/ajco.12267 PMID:25227909

Weingart, S. N., Brown, E., Bach, P. B., Eng, K., Johnson, S. A., Kuzel, T. M., ... Walters, R. S. (2008). NCCN task force report: Oral chemotherapy. *Journal of the National Comprehensive Cancer Network: JNCCN*, *6*(Suppl 3), S1–S14. PMID:18377852

Winterhalder, R., Hoesli, P., Delmore, G., Pederiva, S., Bressoud, A., Hermann, F., & von Moos, R. (2011). Self-reported compliance with capecitabine: Findings from a prospective cohort analysis. *Oncology*, *80*(1-2), 29–33. doi:10.1159/000328317 PMID:21606661

World Health Organization. (2003). *Failure to take prescribed medicine for chronic diseases is a massive, world-wide problem*. Retrieved 7 Apr, 2020, from https://www.who.int/mediacentre/news/releases/2003/pr54/en/

Yagasaki, K., Komatsu, H., & Takahashi, T. (2015). Inner conflict in patients receiving oral anticancer agents: A qualitative study. *BMJ Open*, *5*(4), e006699. doi:10.1136/bmjopen-2014-006699 PMID:25872938

Yap, K. Y., Chan, A., & Chui, W. K. (2009). Improving pharmaceutical care in oncology by pharmacoinformatics: The evolving role of informatics and the internet for drug therapy. *Lancet Oncology*, *10*(10), 1011–1019. doi:10.1016/S1470-2045(09)70104-4 PMID:19796753

Yap, K. Y., Chui, W. K., & Chan, A. (2008). Drug interactions between chemotherapeutic regimens and antiepileptics. *Clinical Therapeutics*, *30*(8), 1385–1407. doi:10.1016/j.clinthera.2008.08.011 PMID:18803983

Yap, K. Y., Chui, W. K., & Chan, A. (2011). Development of a chemotherapy regimen interaction database for the mobile internet: Detecting interactions with psychotropics through OncoRx-MI. *Informatics for Health & Social Care*, *36*(3), 132–146. doi:10.3109/17538157.2011.584996 PMID:21848450

Yap, K. Y., See, C. S., & Chan, A. (2010). Clinically-relevant chemotherapy interactions with complementary and alternative medicines in patients with cancer. *Recent Patents on Food, Nutrition & Agriculture*, *2*(1), 12–55. doi:10.2174/2212798411002010012 PMID:20653549

Yap, K. Y., See, C. S., Kuo, E. Y., Chui, W. K., & Chan, A. (2012). Utilizing mobile networks for the detection of clinically relevant interactions between chemotherapy regimens and complementary and alternative medicines. *Journal of Alternative and Complementary Medicine (New York, N.Y.)*, *18*(2), 165–174. doi:10.1089/acm.2010.0846 PMID:22320169

Yen, H. R., Lai, W. Y., Muo, C. H., & Sun, M. F. (2017). Characteristics of traditional Chinese medicine use in pediatric cancer patients: A nationwide, retrospective, Taiwanese-registry, population-based study. *Integrative Cancer Therapies*, *16*(2), 147–155. doi:10.1177/1534735416659357 PMID:27405933

Zabora, J., BrintzenhofeSzoc, K., Curbow, B., Hooker, C., & Piantadosi, S. (2001). The prevalence of psychological distress by cancer site. *Psycho-Oncology*, *10*(1), 19–28. doi:10.1002/1099-1611(200101/02)10:1<19::AID-PON501>3.0.CO;2-6 PMID:11180574

Zullig, L. L., & Bosworth, H. (2017, May 14). Engaging patients to optimize medication adherence. *NEJM Catalyst.* Retrieved 18 May, 2018, from https://catalyst.nejm.org/optimize-patients-medication-adherence/

Chapter 2
The Role of mHealth in Improving Health and Medication Management

ABSTRACT

Mobile health (mHealth) involves the application of mobile devices and their related technologies in the provision of healthcare. In recent years, mHealth has become one of the most promising fields in improving healthcare quality and outcomes. There were over 325,000 mHealth apps in 2017, and this number is expected to grow tremendously due to continued investments in health apps. With advancements in mobile technologies and connectivity, mobile app developers now have the flexibility to develop and implement various mHealth-based interventions for medication management. Through improved functionalities and integration with electronic medical records, mHealth can potentially enable the provision of macro-, meso-, micro- and patient-level interventions in a more efficient manner. Chapter 2 provides an overview of the various mHealth interventions that have targeted medication management and medication non-adherence throughout the years, such as short-messaging services (SMSes) and smartphone apps. The functionalities that are useful in mHealth apps will also be discussed.

DOI: 10.4018/978-1-7998-3832-6.ch002

INTRODUCTION

Mobile health (mHealth) is a domain that involves the application of mobile devices and related technologies, such as mobile/ smartphones, patient monitoring devices, personal digital assistants (PDAs), portable media players, tablet personal computers (PCs) and other wireless devices, in the provision of healthcare or for medical and public health practices (Bashshur, Shannon, Krupinski, & Grigsby, 2011; Free et al., 2013; WHO Global Observatory for eHealth, 2011). Some of the functionalities of mobile devices with healthcare applications include mobile apps, short message services (SMSes), paging, automated sensing, media capabilities and video conferencing (Free, et al., 2013; Klasnja & Pratt, 2012; O'Shea, McGavigan, Clark, Chew, & Ganesan, 2017). Over the years, the evolution of mobile devices has led to an expansion of mHealth uses, from supporting health services (e.g. clinical decision support systems, drug information sources and systems to augment documentation of patient medical records) to more diversified purposes, including preventive care, health promotion, diagnosis, treatment and monitoring (Eskinder Eshetu Ali, Chew, & Yap, 2016).

The focus of mHealth research has also shifted from communicable diseases (e.g. AIDS), which had relatively few publications, to non-communicable diseases such as mood disorders. From 2008-2015, there was an average of 29 mHealth articles published each year (total of 235 articles over the 8 years) on mood disorders and this number increased to 175 (11.7%) articles in 2018. In contrast, research targeting neoplasms and infections steadily decreased from prior 2015 to 2018 by 5.0% and 6.3% respectively (H. Park & Park, 2019) (Table 1).

Table 1. Trends in the focus of medical conditions in mHealth research between 2008-2018

mHealth Trends on Medical Conditions	Number of Publications (%)				
	2008-2015 (%)	2016 (%)	2017 (%)	2018 (%)	Total (%)
Mood disorders	235 (10.1)	63 (11.2)	71 (9.3)	175 (11.7)	544 (9.7)
Infections	277 (11.9)	55 (9.8)	58 (7.6)	84 (5.6)	474 (8.5)
Neoplasms	266 (11.5)	53 (9.4)	55 (7.2)	97 (6.5)	471 (8.4)
AIDS	192 (8.3)	43 (7.7)	60 (7.9)	121 (8.1)	416 (7.4)
Total for all medical conditions in study	2322	561	764	1497	5600

(Adapted from Park et al.(H. Park & Park, 2019))

Similarly, distinct trends were also observed in mHealth research as the type of mobile devices evolved (Figure 1A). Before 2007, when PDAs had a widespread popularity, especially with the young medical professionals in developed nations of the early 2000s (Martin, 2003), the number of research articles reporting on the use of PDAs was predominant. After the mid-2000s, mHealth research started to focus on the ever-increasing ownership of mobile phones in the general population (Tuckel & O'Neill, 2006). From 2013, the direction of mHealth research geared more towards the use of smart devices such as smartphones, tablet PCs, iPod touch or a combination of any of these devices (Eskinder Eshetu Ali, et al., 2016).

Mobile device functionality used in mHealth research also followed the trends in devices (Figure 1B). Apps were the ever increasingly used mobile device functionality in mHealth research from 2012 to 2014. The ease of installing apps in the different kinds of mobile devices could have caused this increase in app research (Fling, 2009). An increasing amount of research during those years also reported the use of SMS-based, automated sensing and media-based interventions (Eskinder Eshetu Ali, et al., 2016). The limited

*Figure 1. Trends in mHealth research over the years. (A) Trends in mobile devices (MDs). *Smart devices included: smartphones, tablet PCs, iPod touch and a combination of any of the three. ** Other devices included: a combination of mobile devices, pagers, devices with wireless communication capabilities, a mobile phone with inbuilt glucometer, and wearable devices. (B) Trends in mobile device (MD) functionalities. *Other functionalities included: beep and alphanumeric text, web-based intervention, missed call (buzzing), central mobile locating system, phone vibration, alarm and a combination of mobile device functionalities*
(Adopted from Ali et al. (Eskinder Eshetu Ali, et al., 2016))

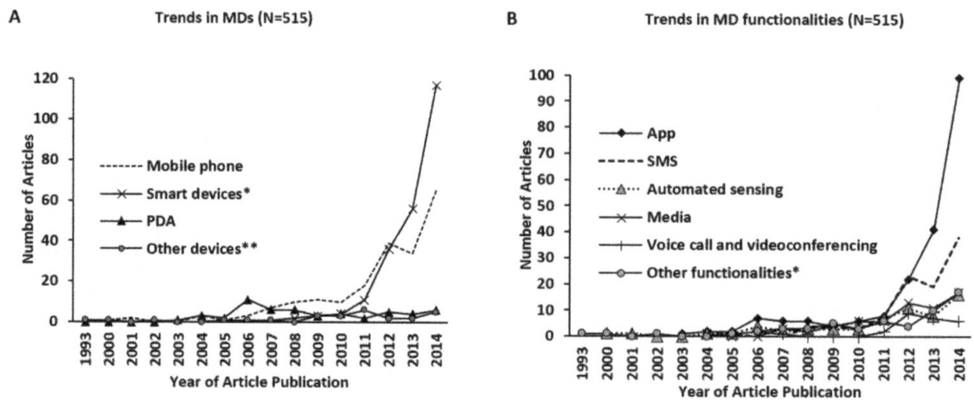

use of SMS-based interventions in the early 2000s was due to the fact that SMSes were not very popular during that time (Wilson & Stimpson, 2010).

In the years before 2007, PDA apps were the most common for the purposes of supporting health services (Buck, Rochon, & Turley, 2005; Diero et al., 2006; Nagykaldi & Mold, 2003) and for monitoring different aspects of health (Glanz, Murphy, Moylan, Evensen, & Curb, 2006; Kvien et al., 2005). However, there were emerging mHealth trends for certain features of mobile devices, such as the early use of camera phones and smartphones. In 2004, a 0.11-megapixel camera phone was used for the assessment of finger injuries in the emergency room (Hsieh et al., 2004). The first smartphone-based mHealth study had used a Nokia 7650 Symbian smartphone connected to a child's glucometer via Bluetooth to automatically SMS the child's glucose readings to the parents (Gammon et al., 2005). Similarly, the only wearable device that was used before 2007 was a small pager-sized device worn by the elderly on the waist or chest for falls detection (Doughty, Lewis, & McIntosh, 2000). This device triggered a radio signal to a community alarm system when a fall was detected.

From 2007 to 2012, notable mHealth interventions included the use of smart device-based videoconferencing (Demaerschalk et al., 2012; Luxton, Mishkind, Crumpton, Ayers, & Mysliwiec, 2012), and camera phones mounted on microscope eyepieces to facilitate the diagnosis of different medical conditions (Bellina & Missoni, 2009; Breslauer, Maamari, Switz, Lam, & Fletcher, 2009). During this period, tablet PCs and iPod touch were also reported for the first time in mHealth (Hudson et al., 2012; Krogh, Rough, & Thomley, 2008). Other unique devices included the use of an inbuilt device in a mobile phone for self-monitoring of diabetes (Cho, Lee, Lim, Kwon, & Yoon, 2009), and a PDA-type glucometer that could transfer data to a server wirelessly (Cho, Kwon, Kim, Oh, & Yoon, 2011).

In the years after 2012, apps and SMSes were the most widely used mHealth interventions (Table 2). The proportion of SMSes and mobile app publications increased from 8.9-20.7% and 0-21.6% respectively from 2012 to 2018. The proportion of internet-based intervention studies also increased steadily from 5.5% to 18.5% (H. Park & Park, 2019). Examples of smartphone and mobile phone functionalities used in the mHealth domain included the use of WhatsApp, the instant messaging app, to facilitate communication between surgeons at a tertiary care health facility (Wani, Rabah, Alfadil, Dewanjee, & Najmi, 2013); smartphone-based test reader platforms for the diagnosis of leprosy in blood samples (Duthie et al., 2014); and the use of a missed call/buzzing functionality to remind newly diagnosed HIV patients

Table 2. Most frequent mHealth research interventions between 2012 to 2018.

mHealth Intervention	Number of Publications (%)							
	2012 (%)	2013 (%)	2014 (%)	2015 (%)	2016 (%)	2017 (%)	2018 (%)	No. of Articles (%)
SMS	29 (8.9)	32 (10.1)	49 (12.8)	82 (16.3)	110 (19.6)	150 (19.6)	310 (20.7)	762 (17.6)
Internet-based	18 (5.5)	28 (8.8)	40 (10.4)	74 (14.7)	92 (16.4)	122 (16.0)	277 (18.5)	651 (15.0)
App application	0 (0)	4 (1.3)	4 (1.0)	16 (3.2)	45 (8.0)	107 (14.0)	324 (21.6)	500 (11.5)
Telephone	21 (6.5)	21 (6.6)	30 (7.8)	46 (9.2)	57 (10.2)	85 (11.1)	156 (10.4)	416 (9.6)
Face-to-face	7 (2.2)	4 (1.3)	8 (2.1)	20 (4.0)	27 (4.8)	44 (5.8)	79 (5.3)	189 (4.4)
Total number of articles by year	325	318	384	502	561	764	1497	4351

(Adapted from Park et al. (H. Park & Park, 2019))

about their follow-up appointments (Kliner, Knight, Mamvura, Wright, & Walley, 2013).

In recent years, mHealth has become one of the most promising domains that are directed at the improvement of healthcare quality and outcomes (Eskinder Eshetu Ali, et al., 2016). Mobile devices are becoming ubiquitous and have significant contributions in day-to-day life (GSM Association, 2020). In 2017, there were ~325,000 mHealth apps listed in the major app stores, and this number is expected to rise due to the continued increase in investments in health apps (Research2Guidance, 2017). According to market forecasts, the mHealth app market revenue is expected reach $31 billion by 2020 (Jahns). Furthermore, advancements in mobile technologies are expected to provide more flexibility in the use of mobile devices for healthcare by way of functionalities embedded in the devices or connectivity to external devices (Daponte P, Vito LD, Picariello F, & M., 2013).

With the ubiquity of mobile devices and their multiple functionalities, there is a considerable potential for the development and implementation of mHealth-based adherence interventions at a more personal level for patients (Car, Tan, Huang, Sloot, & Franklin, 2017; L. Dayer, Heldenbrand, Anderson, Gubbins, & Martin, 2013; L. E. Dayer et al., 2017; L. G. Park, Howie-Esquivel, & Dracup, 2014). These interventions can range from simple SMS reminders to more complex smartphone apps that can link to patient monitoring devices (Gandapur et al., 2016). Through integration with electronic medical records

(EMRs), mHealth can potentially enable the provision of macro-, meso-, micro- and patient-level interventions in an efficient manner (Badawy, Thompson, & Kuhns, 2017; O'Shea, et al., 2017), through mHealth-based delivery of financial information (macro-level), continuing education to healthcare professionals (meso-level), a platform for communication between patients and healthcare professionals (micro-level) and medication reminders to patients (patient-level) (Badawy, et al., 2017; Bestvina et al., 2014; O'Rourke, 2016; O'Shea, et al., 2017; Walter et al., 2016).

However, mHealth interventions aimed at improving medication adherence have mainly targeted patient- and micro-level determinants of non-adherence. One of the most widely evaluated functionalities in the medication adherence literature is SMS texting (Anglada-Martinez et al., 2015; DeKoekkoek et al., 2015; Nieuwlaat et al., 2014; L. G. Park, et al., 2014; Thakkar, Kurup, Laba, & et al., 2016), which can range from simple reminders for taking medications to those that enable personalized monitoring and management of side-effects (Anglada-Martinez, et al., 2015; H.-L. Huang et al., 2013; King et al., 2017; Lester et al., 2010). In some cases, SMS reminders also incorporate requests for patients to confirm their medication administration, which enables monitoring of their adherence behavior (Pandey, Krumme, Patel, & Choudhry, 2017). Despite their advantages, SMS-based interventions are limited by the number of determinants of non-adherence that they can address in a single program and options available to maximize user experience (Ainsworth et al., 2013).

In this regard, smartphone apps have an advantage because of their ability to maximize user experience streamlining graphical user interfaces (L. Dayer, et al., 2013; Hilliard, Hahn, Ridge, Eakin, & Riekert, 2014; Morrissey, Corbett, Walsh, & Molloy, 2016). The high market penetration of smartphones further enhances the potential utility of apps for improving medication adherence. For example, 72% and 60% of the adult population in the US and Europe own smartphones respectively (Pew Research Center, 2016). In addition, the smartphone penetration rate is as high as 90% in some countries (Goeres & Wuppermann, 2015). Moreover, studies show that patients are generally receptive to mHealth and app-based interventions to improve medication management (E. E. Ali, Leow, Chew, & Yap, 2018; Sankaranarayanan & Sallach, 2014).

Smartphone functionalities, such as the camera, Bluetooth and near-field communication (NFC) sensors, can also provide benefits in terms of enhancing medication adherence. For example, studies have shown that smartphone apps can be used to improve the efficiency of adherence monitoring through directly observed treatment (DOT) programs for tuberculosis (TB) patients (Story et al., 2016). The use of the video functionality in video/virtually observed therapy (VOT) systems for monitoring the patient's adherence patterns in TB are generally considered to be more convenient and confidential than DOT. VOT-based programs also have a significant potential for cost savings (Garfein et al., 2015; Holzman, Zenilman, & Shah, 2018). The advancement in digital therapeutics has also led to the development of the Proteus' digital medicine system, which consists of ingestible sensors embedded in oral dosage forms, and can enable adherence monitoring through the use of a smartphone app and a wearable patch (Muoio, 2018; Peters-Strickland et al., 2016). Other sensors that have been developed for adherence tracking can be embedded into pill bottles and inhaler devices, which use Bluetooth technology to transfer adherence data to a smartphone app that is capable of generating reminders and adherence reports (Ahmed et al., 2018; Cushing, Manice, Ting, & Parides, 2016; Fallahzadeh, Minor, Evangelista, Cook, & Ghasemzadeh, 2017).

The integration of image and motion sensors in mobile phones has allowed researchers to harness these functionalities as diagnosis tools. Smartphone cameras have been used to monitor various health issues (Majumder & Deen, 2019), such as skin health (Hubiche et al., 2016), heart rate (Siddiqui, Zhang, Feng, & Kos, 2016) and blood pressure (Luo et al., 2019). However, these analyses have been performed based on different camera settings on various mobile phones, which can potentially impact the data accuracy if proper camera calibration is not done (Otero, Garcia-Porta, Tabernero, & Pardhan, 2020). Furthermore, the microphone functionality can also be used to monitor cough symptoms in people at high risk for chronic pulmonary diseases (Larson, Lee, Liu, Rosenfeld, & Patel, 2011). Similarly, the integration of accelerometers, gyroscopes, magnetometers, and global positioning system (GPS) trackers have also been used to detect activities such as sleep patterns (Natale et al., 2012) and falls detection (Luque, Casilari, Morón, & Redondo, 2014).

The use of mobile apps and SMSes for medication management in chronic diseases, such as diabetes and cardiovascular diseases, is not uncommon (Armitage, Kassavou, & Sutton, 2020; Kannisto, Koivunen, & Valimaki, 2014; Krishna & Boren, 2008; Osborn, Mayberry, Mulvaney, & Hess, 2010; Santo et al., 2019). However, due to lack of design considerations and user involvement, many of the apps lack features for medication adherence and medication safety (Z. Huang et al., 2019; Martinez et al., 2017). Huang and colleagues evaluated a total of 143 diabetes apps and found that only 9 apps (11%) had medication refill reminders, while only 8 apps (6%) had a feature to reinforce the importance of medication adherence (Z. Huang, et al., 2019). In addition, majority of the apps lacked a good communication system with the healthcare provider or caregiver. For example, there were only 16 apps (11%) that allowed the user to communicate with a healthcare professional and only 9 apps (6%) that allowed data synchronization with a caregiver's phone (Z. Huang, et al., 2019). In a systematic review of 23 randomized control trials of 22 mHealth apps, there were only 11 trials that had positive outcomes (Byambasuren, Sanders, Beller, & Glasziou, 2018). Furthermore, only 1 pilot trial managed to progress to large clinical trial (Byambasuren, et al., 2018). This showed that there is a low quality of evidence for mHealth apps, which may greatly impact the prescribability of such apps in clinical practice (Byambasuren, et al., 2018; Marcolino et al., 2018).

In the attempt to tackle these challenges, government bodies such as the United States Food and Drug And Administration (US FDA) have started to move away from evaluation of individual apps, but rather, focusing its regulatory efforts on app makers (Torous et al., 2019). For example, the FDA released a policy and guide for app makers on device software function and the development of medical apps (Shuren, Patel, & Gottlieb, 2018). Similarly, the UK National Health Service and the National Institute of Health and Care Excellence (NICE) in the European Union have also started to provide recommendations and standards for mHealth apps across a range of medical conditions (Torous, et al., 2019). Recently, several mHealth apps that have shown a positive impact on disease and medication management, such as Alivecor KardiaMobile, BlueStar from Welldoc and reSET-O from Pear Therapeutic, have made it to the list of FDA-approved apps. BlueStar, which is a mobile diabetes management platform from Welldoc, has been approved by FDA to support individuals with Type 1 diabetes (Muoio, 2019; Welldoc, 2019). On the other hand, the Alivecor KardiaMobile has also shown to be effective in a mHealth telemonitoring program for patients with congenital heart disease (Shuren, et al., 2018). Similarly, Pear Therapeutic's reSET-O™ app, which is a digital therapeutic that delivers cognitive behavioral therapy and contingency management via a mobile app, showed improvements in abstinence and treatment retention in a randomized controlled trial of patients with opioid use disorder (Lowry, 2018; Walsh, 2018).

As can be seen, the trend in mobile technologies points towards providing more flexibility in mHealth by way of functionalities embedded in mobile devices or through connectivity to other external devices. Improvements in smartphone operating systems and cloud computing systems are also expected to fuel a wider range of mHealth applications and research (Eskinder Eshetu

Ali, et al., 2016). Furthermore, the increasing availability of smartphones in many parts of the developing world, and the increased penetration of mobile networks in previously unreachable areas will provide greater opportunities for collaborative mHealth research to be conducted, so that quality healthcare can be accessible to all.

REFERENCES

Ahmed, I., Ahmad, N. S., Ali, S., Ali, S., George, A., Saleem Danish, H., ... Darzi, A. (2018). Medication adherence apps: Review and content analysis. *JMIR mHealth and uHealth*, *6*(3), e62. doi:10.2196/mhealth.6432 PMID:29549075

Ainsworth, J., Palmier-Claus, J. E., Machin, M., Barrowclough, C., Dunn, G., Rogers, A., ... Lewis, S. (2013). A comparison of two delivery modalities of a mobile phone-based assessment for serious mental illness: Native smartphone application vs text-messaging only implementations. *Journal of Medical Internet Research*, *15*(4), e60. doi:10.2196/jmir.2328 PMID:23563184

Ali, E. E., Chew, L., & Yap, K. Y.-L. (2016). Evolution and current status of mhealth research: A systematic review. *BMJ Innovations*, *2*(1), 33–40. doi:10.1136/bmjinnov-2015-000096

Ali, E. E., Leow, J. L., Chew, L., & Yap, K. Y. (2018). Patients' perception of app-based educational and behavioural interventions for enhancing oral anticancer medication adherence. *Journal of Cancer Education*, *33*(6), 1306–1313. doi:10.100713187-017-1248-x PMID:28707206

Anglada-Martinez, H., Riu-Viladoms, G., Martin-Conde, M., Rovira-Illamola, M., Sotoca-Momblona, J. M., & Codina-Jane, C. (2015). Does mHealth increase adherence to medication? Results of a systematic review. *International Journal of Clinical Practice*, *69*(1), 9–32. doi:10.1111/ijcp.12582 PMID:25472682

Armitage, L. C., Kassavou, A., & Sutton, S. (2020). Do mobile device apps designed to support medication adherence demonstrate efficacy? A systematic review of randomised controlled trials, with meta-analysis. *BMJ Open*, *10*(1), e032045. doi:10.1136/bmjopen-2019-032045 PMID:32005778

GSM Association (2020). *The mobile economy 2020*. Retrieved 10 Jan, 2020, from https://www.gsma.com/mobileeconomy/

Badawy, S. M., Thompson, A. A., & Kuhns, L. M. (2017). Medication adherence and technology-based interventions for adolescents with chronic health conditions: A few key considerations. *JMIR mHealth and uHealth, 5*(12), e202. doi:10.2196/mhealth.8310 PMID:29273573

Bashshur, R., Shannon, G., Krupinski, E., & Grigsby, J. (2011). The taxonomy of telemedicine. *Telemedicine Journal and e-Health, 17*(6), 484–494. doi:10.1089/tmj.2011.0103 PMID:21718114

Bellina, L., & Missoni, E. (2009). Mobile cell-phones (M-phones) in telemicroscopy: Increasing connectivity of isolated laboratories. *Diagnostic Pathology, 4*(1), 19. doi:10.1186/1746-1596-4-19 PMID:19545373

Bestvina, C. M., Zullig, L. L., Rushing, C., Chino, F., Samsa, G. P., Altomare, I., ... Zafar, S. Y. (2014). Patient-oncologist cost communication, financial distress, and medication adherence. *Journal of Oncology Practice / American Society of Clinical Oncology, 10*(3), 162–167. doi:10.1200/JOP.2014.001406 PMID:24839274

Breslauer, D. N., Maamari, R. N., Switz, N. A., Lam, W. A., & Fletcher, D. A. (2009). Mobile phone based clinical microscopy for global health applications. *PLoS One, 4*(7), e6320. doi:10.1371/journal.pone.0006320 PMID:19623251

Buck, D. S., Rochon, D., & Turley, J. P. (2005). Taking it to the streets: Recording medical outreach data on personal digital assistants. *Computers, Informatics, Nursing, 23*(5), 250–255. doi:10.1097/00024665-200509000-00008 PMID:16166826

Byambasuren, O., Sanders, S., Beller, E., & Glasziou, P. (2018). Prescribable mHealth apps identified from an overview of systematic reviews. *NPJ Digital Medicine, 1*(1), 12. doi:10.103841746-018-0021-9 PMID:31304297

Car, J., Tan, W. S., Huang, Z., Sloot, P., & Franklin, B. D. (2017). eHealth in the future of medications management: Personalisation, monitoring and adherence. *BMC Medicine, 15*(1), 73. doi:10.118612916-017-0838-0 PMID:28376771

Cho, J. H., Kwon, H. S., Kim, H. S., Oh, J. A., & Yoon, K. H. (2011). Effects on diabetes management of a health-care provider mediated, remote coaching system via a PDA-type glucometer and the Internet. *Journal of Telemedicine and Telecare, 17*(7), 365–370. doi:10.1258/jtt.2011.100913 PMID:21933896

Cho, J. H., Lee, H. C., Lim, D. J., Kwon, H. S., & Yoon, K. H. (2009). Mobile communication using a mobile phone with a glucometer for glucose control in Type 2 patients with diabetes: As effective as an Internet-based glucose monitoring system. *Journal of Telemedicine and Telecare*, *15*(2), 77–82. doi:10.1258/jtt.2008.080412 PMID:19246607

Cushing, A., Manice, M. P., Ting, A., & Parides, M. K. (2016). Feasibility of a novel mHealth management system to capture and improve medication adherence among adolescents with asthma. *Patient Preference and Adherence*, *10*, 2271–2275. doi:10.2147/PPA.S115713 PMID:27853357

Daponte, P., Vito, L. D., & Picariello, F. (2013). State of the art and future developments of measurement applications on smartphones. *Measurement*, *46*(9), 3291–3307. doi:10.1016/j.measurement.2013.05.006

Dayer, L., Heldenbrand, S., Anderson, P., Gubbins, P., & Martin, B. (2013). Smartphone medication adherence apps: Potential benefits to patients and providers. *Journal of the American Pharmacists Association*, *53*(2), 172–181. doi:10.1331/JAPhA.2013.12202 PMID:23571625

Dayer, L. E., Shilling, R., Van Valkenburg, M., Martin, B. C., Gubbins, P. O., Hadden, K., & Heldenbrand, S. (2017). Assessing the medication adherence app marketplace from the health professional and consumer vantage points. *JMIR mHealth and uHealth*, *5*(4), e45. doi:10.2196/mhealth.6582 PMID:28428169

DeKoekkoek, T., Given, B., Given, C. W., Ridenour, K., Schueller, M., & Spoelstra, S. L. (2015). mHealth SMS text messaging interventions and to promote medication adherence: An integrative review. *Journal of Clinical Nursing*, *24*(19-20), 2722–2735. doi:10.1111/jocn.12918 PMID:26216256

Demaerschalk, B. M., Vegunta, S., Vargas, B. B., Wu, Q., Channer, D. D., & Hentz, J. G. (2012). Reliability of real-time video smartphone for assessing National Institutes of Health Stroke Scale scores in acute stroke patients. *Stroke*, *43*(12), 3271–3277. doi:10.1161/STROKEAHA.112.669150 PMID:23160878

Diero, L., Rotich, J. K., Bii, J., Mamlin, B. W., Einterz, R. M., Kalamai, I. Z., & Tierney, W. M. (2006). A computer-based medical record system and personal digital assistants to assess and follow patients with respiratory tract infections visiting a rural Kenyan health centre. *BMC Medical Informatics and Decision Making*, *6*(1), 21. doi:10.1186/1472-6947-6-21 PMID:16606466

Doughty, K., Lewis, R., & McIntosh, A. (2000). The design of a practical and reliable fall detector for community and institutional telecare. *Journal of Telemedicine and Telecare*, *6*(Suppl 1), S150–S154. doi:10.1258/1357633001934483 PMID:10794003

Duthie, M. S., Balagon, M. F., Maghanoy, A., Orcullo, F. M., Cang, M., Dias, R. F., ... Reed, S. G. (2014). Rapid quantitative serological test for detection of infection with Mycobacterium leprae, the causative agent of leprosy. *Journal of Clinical Microbiology*, *52*(2), 613–619. doi:10.1128/JCM.02085-13 PMID:24478496

Fallahzadeh, R., Minor, B., Evangelista, L. S., Cook, D. J., & Ghasemzadeh, H. (2017, April). Mobile sensing to improve medication adherence: Demo abstract. *IPSN'17: Proceedings of the 16th ACM/IEEE International Conference on Information Processing in Sensor Networks*. 10.1145/3055031.3055045

Fling, B. (2009). *Mobile Design and Development: Practical Concepts and Techniques for Creating Mobile Sites and Web Apps* (1st ed.). O'Reilly Media, Inc.

Free, C., Phillips, G., Watson, L., Galli, L., Felix, L., Edwards, P., ... Haines, A. (2013). The effectiveness of mobile-health technologies to improve health care service delivery processes: A systematic review and meta-analysis. *PLoS Medicine*, *10*(1), e1001363. doi:10.1371/journal.pmed.1001363 PMID:23458994

Gammon, D., Arsand, E., Walseth, O. A., Andersson, N., Jenssen, M., & Taylor, T. (2005). Parent-child interaction using a mobile and wireless system for blood glucose monitoring. *Journal of Medical Internet Research*, *7*(5), e57. doi:10.2196/jmir.7.5.e57 PMID:16403721

Gandapur, Y., Kianoush, S., Kelli, H. M., Misra, S., Urrea, B., Blaha, M. J., ... Martin, S. S. (2016). The role of mHealth for improving medication adherence in patients with cardiovascular disease: A systematic review. *European Heart Journal Quality of Care & Clinical Outcomes*, *2*(4), 237–244. doi:10.1093/ehjqcco/qcw018 PMID:29474713

Garfein, R. S., Collins, K., Munoz, F., Moser, K., Cerecer-Callu, P., Raab, F., ... Patrick, K. (2015). Feasibility of tuberculosis treatment monitoring by video directly observed therapy: A binational pilot study. *The International Journal of Tuberculosis and Lung Disease*, *19*(9), 1057–1064. doi:10.5588/ijtld.14.0923 PMID:26260824

Glanz, K., Murphy, S., Moylan, J., Evensen, D., & Curb, J. D. (2006). Improving dietary self-monitoring and adherence with hand-held computers: A pilot study. *American Journal of Health Promotion, 20*(3), 165–170. doi:10.4278/0890-1171-20.3.165 PMID:16422134

Goeres, J., & Wuppermann, J. (2015). *Mobile multiplies: Global mobile consumer survey*. Retrieved 24 May, 2018, from https://goo.gl/D98jEH

Hilliard, M. E., Hahn, A., Ridge, A. K., Eakin, M. N., & Riekert, K. A. (2014). User preferences and design recommendations for an mHealth app to promote cystic fibrosis self-management. *JMIR mHealth and uHealth, 2*(4), e44. doi:10.2196/mhealth.3599 PMID:25344616

Holzman, S. B., Zenilman, A., & Shah, M. (2018). Advancing patient-centered care in tuberculosis management: A mixed-methods appraisal of video directly observed therapy. *Open Forum Infectious Diseases, 5*(4), ofy046. doi:10.1093/ofid/ofy046 PMID:29732378

Hsieh, C. H., Tsai, H. H., Yin, J. W., Chen, C. Y., Yang, J. C., & Jeng, S. F. (2004). Teleconsultation with the mobile camera-phone in digital soft-tissue injury: A feasibility study. *Plastic and Reconstructive Surgery, 114*(7), 1776–1782. doi:10.1097/01.PRS.0000142402.07896.21 PMID:15577348

Huang, H.-L., Li, Y.-C. J., Chou, Y.-C., Hsieh, Y.-W., Kuo, F., Tsai, W.-C., ... Chuang, C.-J. (2013). Effects of and satisfaction with short message service reminders for patient medication adherence: A randomized controlled study. *BMC Medical Informatics and Decision Making, 13*(1), 127. doi:10.1186/1472-6947-13-127 PMID:24238397

Huang, Z., Lum, E., Jimenez, G., Semwal, M., Sloot, P., & Car, J. (2019). Medication management support in diabetes: A systematic assessment of diabetes self-management apps. *BMC Medicine, 17*(1), 127. doi:10.118612916-019-1362-1 PMID:31311573

Hubiche, T., Valerio, L., Boralevi, F., Mahe, E., Bodemer Skandalis, C., Phan, A., & del Giudice, P. (2016). Visualization of patients' skin lesions on their smartphones: A new step during dermatology visits. *JAMA Dermatology, 152*(1), 95–97. doi:10.1001/jamadermatol.2015.2977 PMID:26443967

Hudson, J., Nguku, S. M., Sleiman, J., Karlen, W., Dumont, G. A., Petersen, C. L., ... Ansermino, J. M. (2012). Usability testing of a prototype phone oximeter with healthcare providers in high- and low-medical resource environments. *Anaesthesia, 67*(9), 957–967. doi:10.1111/j.1365-2044.2012.07196.x PMID:22861503

Jahns, R.-G. (n.d.). *The mHealth app market will grow by 15% to reach $31 billion by 2020.* Retrieved 20 Feb, 2020, from https://research2guidance.com/the-mhealth-app-market-reaches-31-billion-by-2020/

Kannisto, K. A., Koivunen, M. H., & Valimaki, M. A. (2014). Use of mobile phone text message reminders in health care services: A narrative literature review. *Journal of Medical Internet Research, 16*(10), e222. doi:10.2196/jmir.3442 PMID:25326646

King, E., Kinvig, K., Steif, J., Qiu, Q. A., Maan, J. E., Albert, Y. K. A., ... Murray, M. M. C. (2017). Mobile text messaging to improve medication adherence and viral load in a vulnerable Canadian population living with human immunodeficiency virus: A repeated measures study. *Journal of Medical Internet Research, 19*(6), e190. doi:10.2196/jmir.6631 PMID:28572079

Klasnja, P., & Pratt, W. (2012). Healthcare in the pocket: Mapping the space of mobile-phone health interventions. *Journal of Biomedical Informatics, 45*(1), 184–198. doi:10.1016/j.jbi.2011.08.017 PMID:21925288

Kliner, M., Knight, A., Mamvura, C., Wright, J., & Walley, J. (2013). Using no-cost mobile phone reminders to improve attendance for HIV test results: A pilot study in rural Swaziland. *Infectious Diseases of Poverty, 2*(1), 12. doi:10.1186/2049-9957-2-12 PMID:23849508

Krishna, S., & Boren, S. A. (2008). Diabetes self-management care via cell phone: A systematic review. *Journal of Diabetes Science and Technology, 2*(3), 509–517. doi:10.1177/193229680800200324 PMID:19885219

Krogh, P. R., Rough, S., & Thomley, S. (2008). Comparison of two personal-computer-based mobile devices to support pharmacists' clinical documentation. *American Journal of Health-System Pharmacy, 65*(2), 154–157. doi:10.2146/ajhp070177 PMID:18192262

Kvien, T. K., Mowinckel, P., Heiberg, T., Dammann, K. L., Dale, O., Aanerud, G. J., ... Uhlig, T. (2005). Performance of health status measures with a pen based personal digital assistant. *Annals of the Rheumatic Diseases, 64*(10), 1480–1484. doi:10.1136/ard.2004.030437 PMID:15843456

Larson, E. C., Lee, T., Liu, S., Rosenfeld, M., & Patel, S. N. (2011, Sep). Accurate and privacy preserving cough sensing using a low-cost microphone. *UbiComp'11: Proceedings of the 13th International Conference on Ubiquitous Computing*. 10.1145/2030112.2030163

Lester, R. T., Ritvo, P., Mills, E. J., Kariri, A., Karanja, S., Chung, M. H., ... Plummer, F. A. (2010). Effects of a mobile phone short message service on antiretroviral treatment adherence in Kenya (WelTel Kenya1): A randomised trial. *Lancet*, *376*(9755), 1838–1845. doi:10.1016/S0140-6736(10)61997-6 PMID:21071074

Lowry, F. (2018). *New digital therapeutic shows promise for opioid addiction*. Retrieved 20 Feb, 2020, from https://www.medscape.com/viewarticle/906260

Luo, H., Yang, D., Barszczyk, A., Vempala, N., Wei, J., Wu, S. J., ... Feng, Z. P. (2019). Smartphone-based blood pressure measurement using transdermal optical imaging technology. *Circulation: Cardiovascular Imaging*, *12*(8), e008857. doi:10.1161/CIRCIMAGING.119.008857 PMID:31382766

Luque, R., Casilari, E., Morón, M.-J., & Redondo, G. (2014). Comparison and characterization of android-based fall detection systems. *Sensors (Basel)*, *14*(10), 18543–18574. doi:10.3390141018543 PMID:25299953

Luxton, D. D., Mishkind, M. C., Crumpton, R. M., Ayers, T. D., & Mysliwiec, V. (2012). Usability and feasibility of smartphone video capabilities for telehealth care in the U.S. military. *Telemedicine Journal and e-Health*, *18*(6), 409–412. doi:10.1089/tmj.2011.0219 PMID:22650351

Majumder, S., & Deen, M. J. (2019). Smartphone sensors for health monitoring and diagnosis. *Sensors (Basel)*, *19*(9), 2164. doi:10.339019092164 PMID:31075985

Marcolino, M. S., Oliveira, J. A. Q., D'Agostino, M., Ribeiro, A. L., Alkmim, M. B. M., & Novillo-Ortiz, D. (2018). The impact of mHealth interventions: Systematic review of systematic reviews. *JMIR mHealth and uHealth*, *6*(1), e23. doi:10.2196/mhealth.8873 PMID:29343463

Martin, S. (2003). More than half of MDs under age 35 now using PDAs. *Canadian Medical Association Journal*, *169*(9), 952. PMID:14581327

Martinez, M., Park, S. B., Maison, I., Mody, V., Soh, L. S., & Parihar, H. S. (2017). iOS appstore-based phone apps for diabetes management: Potential for use in medication adherence. *JMIR Diabetes*, *2*(2), e12. doi:10.2196/diabetes.6468 PMID:30291096

Morrissey, E. C., Corbett, T. K., Walsh, J. C., & Molloy, G. J. (2016). Behavior change techniques in apps for medication adherence: A content analysis. *American Journal of Preventive Medicine*, *50*(5), e143–e146. doi:10.1016/j.amepre.2015.09.034 PMID:26597504

Muoio, D. (2018). *Proteus CMO talks regulation hurdles, future plans for digital pill*. Retrieved 24 May, 2018, from https://goo.gl/r6RVTi

Muoio, D. (2019). *WellDoc's BlueStar cleared for Type 1 diabetes management, CGM integrations*. Retrieved 20 Feb, 2020, from https://www.mobihealthnews.com/news/north-america/welldocs-bluestar-cleared-type-1-diabetes-management-cgm-integrations

Nagykaldi, Z., & Mold, J. W. (2003). Diabetes Patient Tracker, a personal digital assistant-based diabetes management system for primary care practices in Oklahoma. *Diabetes Technology & Therapeutics*, *5*(6), 997–1001. doi:10.1089/152091503322641051 PMID:14709203

Natale, V., Drejak, M., Erbacci, A., Tonetti, L., Fabbri, M., & Martoni, M. (2012). Monitoring sleep with a smartphone accelerometer. *Sleep and Biological Rhythms*, *10*(4), 287–292. doi:10.1111/j.1479-8425.2012.00575.x

Nieuwlaat, R., Wilczynski, N., Navarro, T., Hobson, N., Jeffery, R., Keepanasseril, A., ... Haynes, R. B. (2014). Interventions for enhancing medication adherence. *Cochrane Database of Systematic Reviews*, *11*, CD000011. doi:10.1002/14651858.CD000011.pub4 PMID:25412402

O'Rourke, K. M. (2016). *'Nonadherence may be the norm': Why cancer patients don't take their medications*. Retrieved 28 May, 2018, from https://wb.md/2sgC9Bf

O'Shea, C. J., McGavigan, A. D., Clark, R. A., Chew, D. P. B., & Ganesan, A. (2017). Mobile health- an emerging technology with implications for global internal medicine. *Internal Medicine Journal*, *47*(6), 616–618. doi:10.1111/imj.13440 PMID:28580749

Osborn, C. Y., Mayberry, L. S., Mulvaney, S. A., & Hess, R. (2010). Patient web portals to improve diabetes outcomes: A systematic review. *Current Diabetes Reports, 10*(6), 422–435. doi:10.100711892-010-0151-1 PMID:20890688

Otero, C., Garcia-Porta, N., Tabernero, J., & Pardhan, S. (2020). Author Correction: Comparison of different smartphone cameras to evaluate conjunctival hyperaemia in normal subjects. *Scientific Reports, 10*(1), 3331. doi:10.103841598-020-60004-7 PMID:32071386

Pandey, A., Krumme, A., Patel, T., & Choudhry, N. (2017). The impact of text messaging on medication adherence and exercise among postmyocardial infarction patients: Randomized controlled pilot trial. *JMIR mHealth and uHealth, 5*(8), e110. doi:10.2196/mhealth.7144 PMID:28778843

Park, H., & Park, M. S. (2019). Capturing the trend of mHealth research using text mining. *mHealth, 5*, 48. doi:10.21037/mhealth.2019.09.06 PMID:31728383

Park, L. G., Howie-Esquivel, J., & Dracup, K. (2014). A quantitative systematic review of the efficacy of mobile phone interventions to improve medication adherence. *Journal of Advanced Nursing, 70*(9), 1932–1953. doi:10.1111/jan.12400 PMID:24689978

Peters-Strickland, T., Pestreich, L., Hatch, A., Rohatagi, S., Baker, R. A., Docherty, J. P., ... Walling, D. P. (2016). Usability of a novel digital medicine system in adults with schizophrenia treated with sensor-embedded tablets of aripiprazole. *Neuropsychiatric Disease and Treatment, 12*, 2587–2594. doi:10.2147/NDT.S116029 PMID:27785036

Pew Research Center. (2016). *Smartphone ownership and Internet usage continues to climb in emerging economies.* Retrieved 7 Sep, 2019, from https://www.pewresearch.org/global/2016/02/22/smartphone-ownership-and-internet-usage-continues-to-climb-in-emerging-economies/technology-report-01-03/

Research2Guidance. (2017). *mHealth economics 2017: Current status and future trends in mobile health.* Retrieved from https://research2guidance.com/product/mhealth-economics-2017-current-status-and-future-trends-in-mobile-health/

Sankaranarayanan, J., & Sallach, R. E. (2014). Rural patients' access to mobile phones and willingness to receive mobile phone-based pharmacy and other health technology services: A pilot study. *Telemedicine Journal and e-Health, 20*(2), 182–185. doi:10.1089/tmj.2013.0150 PMID:24205837

Santo, K., Singleton, A., Rogers, K., Thiagalingam, A., Chalmers, J., Chow, C. K., & Redfern, J. (2019). Medication reminder applications to improve adherence in coronary heart disease: A randomised clinical trial. *Heart (British Cardiac Society), 105*(4), 323–329. doi:10.1136/heartjnl-2018-313479 PMID:30150326

Shuren, J., Patel, B., & Gottlieb, S. (2018). FDA Regulation of Mobile Medical Apps. *Journal of the American Medical Association, 320*(4), 337–338. doi:10.1001/jama.2018.8832 PMID:29971339

Siddiqui, S. A., Zhang, Y., Feng, Z., & Kos, A. (2016). A pulse rate estimation algorithm using PPG and smartphone camera. *Journal of Medical Systems, 40*(5), 126. doi:10.100710916-016-0485-6 PMID:27067432

Story, A., Garfein, R. S., Hayward, A., Rusovich, V., Dadu, A., Soltan, V., ... Falzon, D. (2016). Monitoring therapy adherence of tuberculosis patients by using video-enabled electronic devices. *Emerging Infectious Diseases, 22*(3), 538–540. doi:10.3201/eid2203.151620 PMID:26891363

Thakkar, J., Kurup, R., Laba, T., Santo, K., Thiagalingam, A., Rodgers, A., ... Chow, C. K. (2016). Mobile telephone text messaging for medication adherence in chronic disease: A meta-analysis. *JAMA Internal Medicine, 176*(3), 340–349. doi:10.1001/jamainternmed.2015.7667 PMID:26831740

Torous, J., Andersson, G., Bertagnoli, A., Christensen, H., Cuijpers, P., Firth, J., ... Arean, P. A. (2019). Towards a consensus around standards for smartphone apps and digital mental health. *World Psychiatry; Official Journal of the World Psychiatric Association (WPA), 18*(1), 97–98. doi:10.1002/wps.20592 PMID:30600619

Tuckel, P., & O'Neill, H. (2006). *Ownership and usage patterns of cell phones: 2000–2005.* Paper presented at the Second International Conference on Telephone Survey Methodology, Miami, FL.

Walsh, S. (2018). *FDA clears mobile medical app to help those with opioid use disorder stay in recovery programs.* Retrieved 20 Feb, 2020, from https://www.fda.gov/news-events/press-announcements/fda-clears-mobile-medical-app-help-those-opioid-use-disorder-stay-recovery-programs

Walter, C., Mellor, J. D., Rice, C., Kirsa, S., Ball, D., Duffy, M., ... Mileshkin, L. (2016). Impact of a specialist clinical cancer pharmacist at a multidisciplinary lung cancer clinic. *Asia Pacific Journal of Clinical Oncology, 12*(3), e367–e374. doi:10.1111/ajco.12267 PMID:25227909

Wani, S. A., Rabah, S. M., Alfadil, S., Dewanjee, N., & Najmi, Y. (2013). Efficacy of communication amongst staff members at plastic and reconstructive surgery section using smartphone and mobile WhatsApp. *Indian Journal of Plastic Surgery: Official Publication of the Association of Plastic Surgeons of India, 46*(3), 502–505. doi:10.4103/0970-0358.121990 PMID:24459338

Welldoc. (2019). *Welldoc's Award-winning Digital Health Solution BlueStar Adds FDA-Clearance for Use in Type 1 Diabetes.* Retrieved 02 Feb, 2020, from https://www.welldoc.com/news/fda-clearance-for-use-in-type-1-diabetes/

WHO Global Observatory for eHealth. (2011). *mHealth: New horizons for health through mobile technologies: Second global survey on eHealth.* Retrieved from https://apps.who.int/iris/handle/10665/44607

Wilson, F. A., & Stimpson, J. P. (2010). Trends in fatalities from distracted driving in the United States, 1999 to 2008. *American Journal of Public Health, 100*(11), 2213–2219. doi:10.2105/AJPH.2009.187179 PMID:20864709

Chapter 3
Design Principles in the Development of Digital Health Applications

ABSTRACT

The roles of patients and healthcare professionals have evolved with the digital age. The convergence of digital technologies with health and healthcare services has led to the birth of disciplines such as digital health and pharmaco-cybernetics. Development of digital health innovations and mHealth applications need to be useful and user-friendly. For example, ease-of-use associated with mobile app interfaces can be more important to patients than the number and type of functionalities. Therefore, the application of health behavior theories and patient-centered approaches is needed to develop clinically relevant digital health systems and mHealth apps. This chapter introduces the pharmaco-cybernetic frameworks that are relevant for designing digital health innovations and an Intervention Mapping (IM) framework that can help inform behavioral change techniques. Concepts such as the Pharmaco-cybernetic Maxims, user-centered (UCD), experience-centered (ECD) and activity-centered designs (ACD), and the Ecological Systems Theory applied to technological and mHealth systems will be described. In addition, the consideration factors for technological product design based on UCD, ECD and ACD, as well as for iOS and Android platforms will be discussed.

DOI: 10.4018/978-1-7998-3832-6.ch003

INTRODUCTION

In traditional medical practice, healthcare professionals have always played active roles in the care of patients. Doctors tell their patients what is wrong and how to get better, while pharmacists dispense and counsel patients with regards to their medications. In addition, patients are usually given supplementary materials such as pamphlets as part of their education. However, the patients' understanding of their medication therapies is limited to the time during each counseling session, and the frequency in which they re-visit the clinic for follow-up. Thus, their knowledge on their medications may be limited, particularly for those who are on their medications for the first time or if they are on complex regimens. The lack of knowledge or misinterpretation of information about the drug or its use can affect patients' compliance to their medication, which may consequently lead to the patients suffering from drug-related problems (DRPs) such as under- or overdosing, or potential drug-drug, drug-food or drug-herb interactions (American Society of Hospital Pharmacists, 1993).

The roles of patients and healthcare professionals have evolved with the digital age. Internet and informatics technologies brought about by the cyber era have been critical in transforming the public's attitudes towards healthcare and medicine. The advent of the World Wide Web has led to the creation of many web publishing platforms. Patients are becoming more well-informed about health-related and drug-related information over the internet. In recent years, the internet connectivity of mobile phones has also become popular. Nowadays, it is not uncommon for patients to search for online health-related information using their mobile phones. However, operational and technical problems experienced by internet users have led to the need to develop common standards for data, information and software applications for the World Wide Web (Internet Society; Jean-Guilhem). Through these standards, users are able to navigate through vast amounts of health-related information on cross-platform mobile browsers and interact with complex web documents through features such as buttons, tables, scroll lists and pop-up menus. The integration of interactive media technologies has further enhanced the communication and interaction among internet users. Users can now learn about health-related and medication management information and gain knowledge through a variety of digital media channels – including text, audio, video, graphics, images, animations and even games (Liaskos & Diomidus, 2002). For example, WarfarINT (Kevin Y. Yap et al., 2009) was a game that educated users about the different strengths of warfarin tablets (an anticoagulant), as well as its interaction with drugs, herbs and food. Similarly, Herbopolis (Ee, Yap, & Yap, 2018) was a mobile game that educated players on herbal medicines.

The digital revolution has also led to an evolution of patients in the digital age who are connected to technologies, internet and the World Wide Web. Known as the "Generation Cs", this group originally referred to patients belonging to the 25 to 41-year-olds, known as the Generation Ys (The Nielsen Company (US) LLC, 2012). This group of patients are digitally connected to technologies, the internet and are web-savvy; and they tend to communicate more quickly and effectively by email, social media and text messaging, compared to the traditional ways of communication. The characteristic that defines them is that they gravitate towards social media and online communities to participate in discussions and connect with people with shared interests. However, a new school of thought has now classified the "Gen Cs" as not being bound by any demographic age group, but by their "psychographics" of similar values, interests, attitudes and behavior (Energy Resourcing, n.d.; Pickett, 2019). Therefore, the Gen Cs can encompass the Generations X and Y, or even the Millennials (Energy Resourcing, n.d.; Pickett, 2019), who are also known as the "Generation Z", "digital natives", "net generation" or "Google generation" (Cut, 2017). The Millennials are generally more comfortable around technologies and more positively inclined towards using the internet and social media to find out about health-related and drug-related information. Although most Millennials enjoy technology and gadgets (i.e. the enthusiasts), a small proportion tend to use technology minimally (i.e. the minimalists) or do not have an affinity for technology (i.e. the avoiders). Interestingly, all 3 groups of Millennials have the same thing in common – they all own mobile phones. In addition, another category of patients who are fast catching up in digital technologies is the growing elderly population known as the "Silver Tsunami". The US Census Bureau estimates that ~78 million people will be over the age of 65 in the year 2035 (Sullivan, 2019). Associated with this group are patients with multiple chronic diseases and comorbidities, among which, many are on multiple medications or polypharmacy. These patients can be overwhelmed by concerns regarding their treatment options or the disease itself. For example, patients who are on new medications will want to know more about their medications, while those on chronic medications will want reassurance that they still need their medications and that their medications are still effective. As such, many of them tend to surf the internet (or mobile internet) and use digital technologies to help them understand their medications and conditions – hence earning them the term "Silver Surfers" (Dailey, Kalis, & Sather, 2015; Manovel & Sather, 2017).

The convergence of digital technologies with health and healthcare services has led to the birth of digital health – a discipline that involves the use of information and communication technologies to help manage diseases and health risks, and promote health and wellbeing (Bhavnani, Narula, & Sengupta, 2016; US Food and Drug Administration, 2020). Its ultimate goal is to improve the healthcare of patients. Pharmaco-cybernetics, also known as cybernetics pharmacy or cyber-pharmacy, is an upcoming discipline within digital health that describes the science of supporting medication and drug use through the application and evaluation of informatics and internet technologies, so as to improve the pharmaceutical care of patients (Kevin Y. Yap, et al., 2009). It involves communication and feedback with users and takes into account the flow of drug information and knowledge between the user and the cybernetic system or environment, user interactivity and the actions taken by users to achieve their goals (Kevin Y. Yap, et al., 2009). In contrast to the field of pharmaco-informatics, which utilizes informatics and internet technologies to target drug-related problems (DRPs) (K. Y. Yap, Chan, & Chui, 2009); pharmaco-cybernetics goes a step further by merging the science of technology with human-computer-environment interactions, so that technological innovations targeted at medication management and drug use, and preventing or reducing DRPs, can be designed, developed, applied and evaluated in clinical practices and patient populations (Kevin Y. Yap, et al., 2009). Clinical knowledge and experience, as well as skills in technologies and human-computer-environment interactions are essential to the success of implementing such technological innovations in practice.

PHARMACO-CYBERNETIC FRAMEWORKS FOR DESIGNING DIGITAL HEALTH INNOVATIONS

While pharmaco-cybernetics is largely focused on improving pharmaceutical care and supporting medicines and drugs use, its approaches target the digital health innovation process for technological innovations that aim to address DRPs. This process is an iterative cycle that comprises of 5 main activities (Wikipedia, 2019) – beginning from identification of the healthcare problem, conducting research through engagement with stakeholders, co-designing and

Figure 1. The 5 main activities in the digital health innovation process cycle.

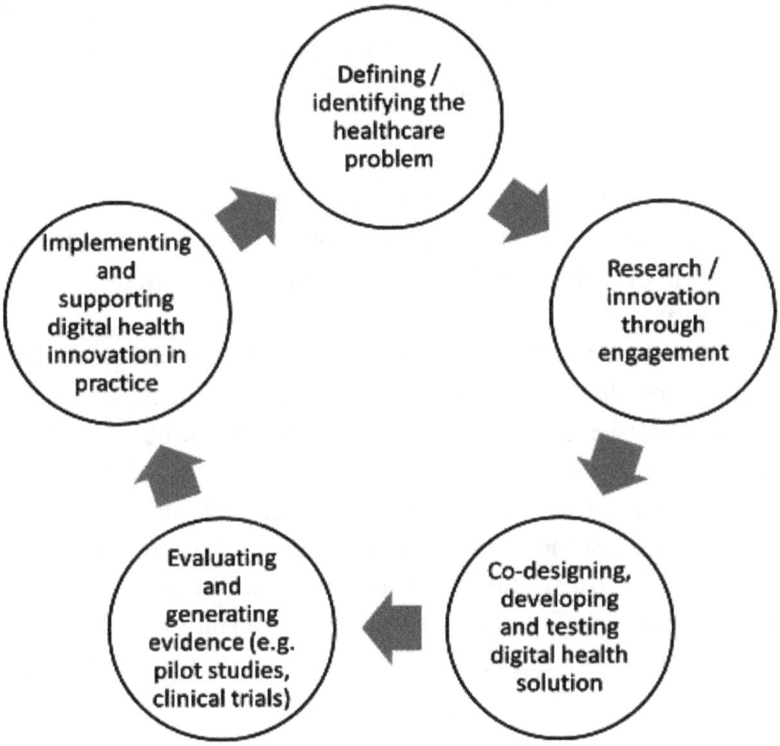

developing the digital health solution, evaluating the solution and generating an evidence base, and lastly, implementation in clinical practices (Figure 1).

There are several frameworks that are relevant to the pharmaco-cybernetic approaches to designing digital health innovations. The rest of this chapter describes these frameworks in the context of designing such technological systems and applications. Core to the frameworks are the Pharmaco-cybernetics Maxims, and the types of environments that are related to the user of these applications (e.g. the patient). In addition, many of these technological innovations are based on user-centered (UCD), experience-centered (ECD) or activity-centered designs (ACD).

The Pharmaco-cybernetic Maxims

The 4 pharmaco-cybernetic maxims are design principles that are useful for designers and developers of digital health innovations that provide health-related and drug-related information to various audiences, such as clinicians and patients (Chan & Yap, 2010; Kevin Y. Yap, et al., 2009; K.Y. Yap & Lim, 2012). Originally adapted for use in the development of a medication information application that aimed to educate patients on warfarin, an anticoagulant drug (Kevin Y. Yap, et al., 2009), these maxims are in relation to the:

1. *Quality of health/ drug information:* The content provided by the innovation should be accurate and follow evidence-based resources, e.g. journal articles, established databases and medication package information;
2. *Quantity of health/ drug information:* The content provided by the innovation should be adequate enough for users to know how to minimize the risk of DRPs, e.g. overdose, adverse drug reactions, drug interactions;
3. *Relation to target audiences:* The content provided by the innovation should be catered towards what the target audience(s) need to know without confusing them, but instead, clarifying their doubts; and
4. *Manner of data presentation:* The content provided by the innovation should be presented in a clear and appropriate manner that avoids ambiguity and misinterpretation, e.g. the use of non-medical jargon for layman users.

Developers of digital health innovations that are designed for the purpose of providing health-related and drug-related information should abide by these principles, so that the technological system or application can be successfully implemented in its target population.

Types of Environments in Pharmaco-cybernetic Approaches

From a pharmaco-cybernetics perspective, the environment that a patient interacts with can be categorized into many types based on the Ecological Systems Theory (The Psychology Notes HQ, 2019; Kevin Y. Yap, et al., 2009). We are all intertwined with the technologies that we use and the environment in which we live. Our interactions and social experiences of sharing information and exchanging ideas are important in order for technological systems and applications to be successful, which in turn are affected by the environment at various different levels. The Ecological Systems Theory describes how users interact with their immediate environments (micro, meso, exo, macro, chrono), and how these environments affect the user in a wider context (The Psychology Notes HQ, 2019). As an example, when a female patient who is diagnosed with breast cancer searches the internet for information regarding her condition, therapeutic options and supportive care, her interactions with her environments are as follows (Figure 2):

1. *Microsystem (her immediate environment):* This refers to the physical characteristics of the technologies that she is in contact with when conducting her searches on the internet, such as whether it is on a desktop or laptop, smartphone or tablet, the level of mouse or touch sensitivity, the screen size and/or contact surface that she uses, and the hardware or software faults that she may experience.
2. *Mesosystem (the relation between her immediate environments):* Her experiences, psychological state and behavior will be affected by whether she carries out her searches alone or in the company of other people.
3. *Exosystem (the external settings that indirectly affects, but do not include her):* When her family understands her condition and provides support and encouragement to her, the sense of closeness experienced by her may lead to improved compliance to her medication therapies.
4. *Macrosystem (larger cultural context related to her):* Seeking comfort and sharing her experiences with other similar patients on social media or online patient network portals may alleviate the stigma that she feels in relation to losing a breast, and can positively improve her experiences as she goes through her breast surgery, chemotherapy and supportive care.
5. *Chronosystem (the time-space dimension over her course of life as a cancer survivor):* The moral support that she gains as time goes by can enable her to better adapt to life as a cancer survivor, and she may even be motivated to improve her lifestyle so as to maintain a higher standard for her quality of life.

Hence, as demonstrated by the above-mentioned example, the environments associated with the pharmaco-cybernetic approaches can empower patients with the appropriate knowledge regarding their medical conditions and medication therapies, so that they can better participate in the management of their own health. This can potentially help them to adapt to any changes in their dietary habits and lifestyles, as well as improve compliance, and ultimately, improve the pharmaceutical care of patients. Healthcare providers, patients and developers of digital health systems and applications should realize the

Figure 2. Application example of how a breast cancer patient is intertwined with the different levels of her environment when she searches for information about her condition.

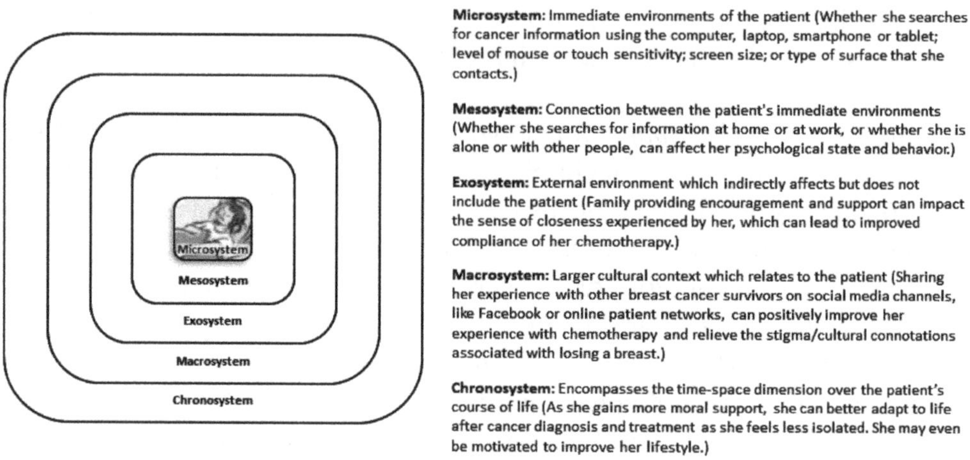

importance of these principles when designing for pharmaco-cybernetics applications. Understanding how users structure their individual experiences, immediate environments, and tasks is just the beginning when designing such products. Designers should also consider how external forces such as socio-cultural and inter-personal factors shape the user's overall experience, attitude and goals when using the applications through an ecological perspective, so that the digital health innovations can be catered for a wider target audience.

User-Centered Design (UCD) Approach

User-centered design (UCD) is a term used to describe the design processes in which end-users play a role in influencing how the technological solution's design takes shape throughout the planning, creation and development phases of the product. The concept of the UCD approach is that there is a need to involve potential users in the environment in which the product will be used, so as to increase its effectiveness, acceptance and success – thus, visibility, mapping and feedback are crucial (Donald A Norman, 2002b). In the principle of visibility, users figure out the use of a product based on the visibility of its components. In order to understand this principle, the concepts of affordance, signifiers and constraints are needed (D. Norman, 2013). Affordance refers to the relationship between the properties of an object (e.g. mobile phone) to a person's capabilities (i.e. talking and listening), in order to determine how the object can possibly be used (i.e. person using the mobile phone to call and talk). Signifiers, on the other hand, communicate where and how an action should occur – for example, whether a button on the smartphone screen should be tapped, or slide upwards, downwards or sideways using a stylus or fingers. A good signifier will communicate the purpose, structure and operation of the technology to its users. In contrast, constraints refer to the ways that restrict the user's possible actions and the kind of user interaction that can take place at a given moment. There are four types of constraints: physical, cultural, semantic and logical. When designed appropriately, constraints can enable users to easily determine the proper course of action. Therefore, from a holistic viewpoint, the product's parts or components should convey a correct message regarding its usage (Donald A Norman, 2002b). The features of the technical product should not distract users' attention from salient information, but rather, convey its intended message across to its users. The product should be designed such that users can focus on its essential features and/or relevant aspects. The intended information to be conveyed to users should generally be in the middle of the graphical user interface (GUI) of the product so that the user's attention will be focused on the relevant details. Sometimes, contrasting backgrounds can be used for emphasis. On the other hand, titles and instructions should be kept short and simple, concise and self-explanatory, so that first-time users know what to expect of the product. The use of 'backup' text to provide additional details regarding a product feature can help users understand the use or rationale better if it is used sparingly. Similarly, sounds can also help reduce ambiguity in interpretation by users, when used appropriately. When used inappropriately, sounds can cause distractions and confuse the user instead of enhancing their product experience.

Humans have limited visual processing capability. When faced with a visually cluttered display, users tend to ignore some components in their perceptual field, and this often impedes the delivery of the intended message. Therefore, it is important that clutter is avoided in the GUI of the product, especially if its screen size is small (e.g. smartphone screens). One way to declutter the screen is to classify the health-related or drug-related information into appropriate categories so that users can expand or collapse these categories as needed. In addition, the use of appropriate colors and adherence to color conventions are also important, as they not only help convey the appropriate messages to users, but also affect the users' perceptions of depth and space. Irrelevant color differences can distract and mislead users of the product. For example, green can give a sense of calm to the user, since green is often associated with safety (e.g. traffic lights) or nature (e.g. trees). In contrast, red often associated with warning.

The second principle is mapping (Donald A Norman, 2002b), which describes the link between the user's intended actions (what one wants to do) to actual operations (what appears to be possible). This principle is important in the design and layout of displays and controls (D. Norman, 2013). Here, the insight of semiotics is useful – users are more inclined to products that are mapped to processes or objects that are known or familiar to them. For example, proper positioning and organization of features in the product design can help users understand how to use the product. The natural mapping of the left to right clicks on the product controls should be familiar to users, such as the clicks of a mouse when searching for health and drug information. This leads to an immediate understanding of how to use these controls. Gestalt's law of proximity should also be applied (Soegaard, 2019)– the law states that 'related items should be placed closer together than non-related items'. Similarly, features or information deemed to be of greater importance to users should appear in positions of greater importance from the user's perspective. Related items are also grouped together in time, space and shape. For products involving animations, the duration of exposure affects users' ability to interpret and understand information about the product. If the exposure time is too long, it can lead to fatigue and boredom; and if it is too short, it can leave the user confused. In general, if the correct amount of information exposure cannot be determined, one should remember that "too-much is better than too-little".

The third principle is feedback, which is a crucial component that reflects to the user about what action has been done and what result is achieved (Donald A Norman, 2002b). Feedback from the technological product should be informative, immediate and as realistic as possible. "Unreal" aspects of the product behavior can hinder users from interpreting the correct message. Furthermore, feedback should also be prioritized so that important signals are able to capture the attention of the user, while less important information can be presented in an unobtrusive way (D. Norman, 2013). Sometimes, poor feedback from the technological product can be worse than having no feedback, since it is not only uninformative and distracting, but it can also annoy and cause anxiety in the user. As much as UCD is about engineering usability, it is also important to consider environmental and socio-cultural factors, for example, varying educational levels or the settings and/or situations in which potential users will be using the product. "Design myopia" describes the short-sightedness of the product designer. The product may appear suitable, or even ideal, to the designer; but this same product may seem unobvious and obscure to the common layman. This can lead to an "adverse outcome" of hindering the user from using the product properly. An approach to circumvent this problem is through user-testing to seek "fresh eyes" on the product, so that the product can be ensured to be fit for its intended purpose, and is also effective and efficient during its development (Preece, Sharp, & Rogers, 2015).

Perhaps the most important principle of UCD is the conceptual model of the system (D. Norman, 2013). A conceptual model is simply put, a simplified explanation of how a technological product works. In technology design, the models are usually "mental models" that represent the designer's understanding of how the product and its features work, so that users will be able to infer from the product itself. In particular, how the product works will come from the perceived structure from the user, who should be able to infer from the affordances, signifiers, constraints and mappings of the product design. A good conceptual model is able to facilitate the user to predict the effects of their actions on the product. If the product does not have a good conceptual model, for example, if the user is not able to tell the relationship between the operating controls and the functions of the product, or if a function can only be activated through complex operations (e.g. simultaneous pressing of several buttons), the user will not be able to remember all the functions and the only way is to read the technical manual over and over again. This will cause frustration to the user, who may ultimately abandon the product or its features. Thus, the key to understandable and usable technological products are good conceptual models, which relies on good communication between the product designer and users.

Experience-Centered Design (ECD) Approach

The experience-centered design (ECD) approach is based on Norman's principles on emotional design, which stems from our varied responses towards everyday things. The variables that deliver a positive emotional experience can vary greatly with the appearance or functioning of a tool (Donald A Norman, 2002a), and can be matched with the visceral, behavioral and reflective levels of design (Komninos, 2019; D.A. Norman, 2004). The visceral level is concerned with how the appearances or perceptible qualities of the product make the user feel. A product with better physical features (e.g. look, feel, sound) can dominate the emotional responses of its user over an otherwise usable but plain looking product. While most products within a particular group have a similar set of features or functions, this concept essentially refers to distinguishing one's product from others by tapping into the user's attitudes, beliefs and feelings, so as to evoke particular emotional responses through colors, shapes and styles, so as to improve the product's visual appeal or serve some business interest.

The behavioral level sees functionality as being paramount (Komninos, 2019; D.A. Norman, 2004). It is concerned with how users use the product to carry out their activities, how accurately or quickly users can achieve their aims and objectives, and how well the product is catered to both skilled and inexperienced users. Behavioral design is often referred to as usability and is the easiest to test because the product's performance can be measured when the physical features or usable parts of the product (e.g. buttons, handles, switches, etc) are changed in some way. For example, the ease of typing on a computer keyboard, the difficulty of typing on a small touchscreen device such as a smartphone, and the enjoyment of playing a computer game are all experiences at the behavioral level. Essentially, the behavioral level refers to the emotions the end-user feels as a result of accomplishing or failing to meet their goals. The experiences are usually positive when the user can use the product to complete their goals with minimum effort or difficulty. However, when the product restricts the user or requires the user to spend more time and effort to accomplish their goals due to its limitations, the user is more likely to have negative experiences.

Lastly, the reflective level (D.A. Norman, 2004) is related to the 'emotional thread of experience', which describes personal meaning derived from the use of a product (McCarthy & Wright, 2004). Its concept is based on the rationalization and intellectualization of the technology innovation to influence the behavior of the end-user (Komninos, 2019; D.A. Norman, 2004). This is the highest level of emotional design, and it involves the user weighing up the pros and cons of the product and extracting information to determine what it means to the user as an individual. An example is the user's perception of a smartwatch as a technological innovation and a luxury fashion product. As a technological innovation, the user might look for the functional and usability benefits of the smartwatch. However, as a luxury fashion product, the user might relate it to the ability to express themselves ("Does the watch look good on me?") and enhance their image ("What will my friend think when they see me wearing this watch?"). The reflective level mediates effects of the behavioral level. In this case, the user might be willing to compromise the shortcoming in the usability of the smartwatch for other non-functional benefits (e.g. reputation of the brand).

There are 4 threads of experience. The first is the sensual thread, which describes the involvement of human senses in shaping the user's experience (McCarthy & Wright, 2004). It is not only about what is perceived by the user, but also how the user reacts to what they perceive. A key factor to this sensual thread is a sense of "presence" or a sense of "being there", which can be affected by the design of the product. An illustration of presence is in virtual environments where the user is immersed in an artificially constructed space and feels the sense of presence as realism. The second thread is the emotional thread (McCarthy & Wright, 2004), which is concerned about the meanings and value judgments that users ascribe to an object (or technology product) based on their goals, values and desires. Emotions in an experience is concerned with how the user engages with a situation and the movement of events towards desirable or undesirable outcomes. The user does not exist separately from the situation nor his/her feelings toward the situation. On the other hand, the feelings experienced by an individual in a situation involving different activities at different times, or different individuals in the same situation, can be radically different. The sensual and emotional threads are intertwined – an individual's emotional response is always directed at something or someone and can form the history of experience that informs his/her sensual response the next time around. The sensual attraction to an object or technological product depends on the user's needs, desires and values at that particular time. For example, a user may be attracted by the beautiful appearance of a mobile device, but other issues such as usability and functionality may entail a higher monthly charge. These factors may outweigh the physical attractiveness of the mobile device, which will lead to a negative emotional experience for the user (e.g. feelings of disappointment or frustration).

The third is the compositional thread, which describes how the user's whole experience is affected by the relationship between the technological innovation and other products or services; or the relationship between different functions within a product (McCarthy & Wright, 2004). The experiences of users can be deliberately "framed" so that there is some structure and meaning to the user. For example, a user's experience of using Dropbox can be made up of many "frames" consisting of searching a document file from his Dropbox folder on his smartphone app, downloading the file onto his smartphone and attaching the downloaded document to a text message. The question is whether the framing of some technologies bring meaning to the experience of the user, and whether the framing of different technologies bring different meanings to the experiences in different ways for different users. If the framing of experience is meaningful through the effort of the user, he/she will be repaid by the quality of the experiences. The aesthetic quality of one's experience is dependent on whether the tasks are completed just as a detached means of getting to an end, or as personally meaningful activities that are approached creatively and enjoyed. The latter, needless to say, leads to a more enriching and better-quality experience.

Lastly, the fourth thread is spatio-temporal and it describes the user entering a state of "flow" as he becomes engrossed in his experience (McCarthy & Wright, 2004). It evokes positive feelings such as pleasure, excitement, satisfaction and happiness, but sometimes it can also lead to negative feelings such as fear and frustration, when there is a "disruption of flow". An intense emotional engagement can change one's sense of time and space. As described by McCarthy and Wright, "time may speed up or slow down, pace may increase or decrease, spaces may open up or close down" (McCarthy & Wright, 2004). For example, feelings of frustration resulting from a disruption of flow can cause the user to perceive space as being closeted and confined. In contrast, pleasure or satisfaction with a product/service can lead to a higher willingness to engage more in the product/service.

The designing of technological innovation systems require an understanding of how a person experiences the product from an interaction-centered viewpoint (Forlizzi & Battarbee, 2004). Cognitive user-product interactions require users to focus on the product at hand, thus users of the product have to learn what their actions will lead to during the interactions. To improve users' scalability of experience, stratifying the interactions combined with varied rewards will continually engage users and provide different experiences each time they interact with the products. Additional customization features to suit the user's preferences or enabling the technological innovation on a variety of platforms like smartphones and social networking sites will not only facilitate expressive interactions and co-experience, but also reinforce the users' overall experiences.

Activity-Centered Design (ACD) Approach

While the ECD approach gives designers an insight to users' experiences of the technological innovation, it does not explain how the activity of using the products affects the user. Activity Theory (AT) describes a conceptual framework for understanding how people develop purposeful, transformative interactions with the world by taking 'activity' rather than the 'person' or 'mind' as the central unit of analysis (Forlizzi & Battarbee, 2004; Kaptelinin, 1996; Kaptelinin & Nardi, 2006). While there are several interpretations of AT, the ones by Leontiev (Kaptelinin, Kuutti, & Bannon, 1995) and Engeström (Engeström, 2000) are the most common and will be discussed here. The AT concept states that the properties of the product and user truly exists only in activities, when being enacted, and not before and after the activities.

The principle on "unity of consciousness and activity" states that the human mind (consciousness) and his interaction with the environment (activity) are closely connected and mutually determine one another (Kaptelinin, 1996; Kaptelinin, et al., 1995). Activities are influenced by both the attributes of both the product (object) and its user (subject). Object-orientedness needs to be understood in this context. All human activities are directed towards objects, and therefore in order to understand the subject (user), analysis of the object (product) is necessary. A way to think about objects of activities is to think of them as objectives that provide meaning to one's actions. Activities can be evaluated on whether they help accomplish the objectives or not. As such, the activity and the subject-object relationship need to be considered in its entirely. For example, users of will know and learn how to use a technological product or its features but may not see the purpose of why they need to use the product or feature. Object-orientedness can be used to educate users on the purpose and/or importance of why the product is needed. In a broad sense, the "object" in this principle need not be related to physical objects, but can include socially/ culturally defined properties as well (Kaptelinin, et al., 1995; Kaptelinin & Nardi, 2006).

Another principle is the "hierarchical structure of activity", which states that activity in its broad sense can be analyzed through a tri-level scheme of activities, actions and operations that are dynamic and oriented towards the goals and motive of the whole activity, and thus can change with circumstances (Kaptelinin, 1996; Kaptelinin, et al., 1995; Kaptelinin & Nardi, 2006). In this context, actions are defined as conscious goal-oriented processes that are undertaken to fulfil the objectives. Different actions may be taken to meet the same goal, and goals can also have lower-level goals or sub-goals. This is like the hierarchical level of actions, which can be broken down to sub-levels of lower-level and higher-level actions too. On the other hand, operations are automatic processes that correspond to how an action is carried out and can become routinized and unconscious with practice. Operations do not have their own goals but adjust actions according to situations. The smooth transition of conscious actions to subconscious operations when using the technological product orients the user towards the objectives of learning.

However, a breakdown will disrupt the user's usage of the product and the activity and may lead to disorientation of the user or even frustration.

The third principle on "internalization-externalization" states that our mental processes are derived from external actions through the course of internalization, and is related to the socio-cultural environment (Kaptelinin, et al., 1995; Kaptelinin & Nardi, 2006). The transformation between external and internal is constantly happening and it forms the basis of activity. The process of internalization enables users to imagine a potential interaction with the product without actual interaction with the physical product, while externalization is often needed when an internalized action needs to be scaled or modified. As such, feedback mechanisms (e.g. short questions, surveys) can be incorporated with the usage of the product to identify whether users have "internalized" the knowledge that he has gained from the product through the "externalization" of his knowledge by correctly answering the questions.

The fourth principle of tool mediation is the most significant concept in AT, and it describes how a product reflects the accumulation and transmission of social knowledge, and experiences of others who have tried to solve similar problems before to make the product more efficient (Kaptelinin, 1996; Kaptelinin, et al., 1995; Kaptelinin & Nardi, 2006). The historical evidence of a product's development is reflected in the product itself, which can comprise of its structural properties, shape, material and how it should be used. This in turn influences the nature of the internalization-externalization of the user.

The last principle from Leontiev's AT states that the user's interaction with reality should also be analyzed in the context of development (Kaptelinin, et al., 1995). In AT, a system is a result of historical development under certain conditions, which will continuously re-form and develop. The system can only be understood through the analysis of its developmental transformations. Hence, "formative experiments" are conducted as part of its research methodology to monitor active participation with the developmental changes of the object of study.

Engeström's activity system model (Engeström, 2000) builds on Leontiev's framework to understand the three-way interaction between the subject, object and community based on the collective activities by groups and organizations. The scope of analysis is extended from tasks to how the subject (i.e. user) interacts with the world, including the social context. In this model, three means of mediation are added – they are the "tools" or "instruments" for subject-object interaction, "rules" for subject-community interaction and "division of labor" for community-object interaction. As an example, consider the design process for an elderly-friendly smartphone interface (Azir Rezha,

Maksom, & Naim, 2014) (Figure 3) – the tool/instrument that "connects" the subject (elderly user) to the object (smartphone interface) is the accessibility functions of the smartphone. The rules that facilitate the subject (elderly user) and community (other smartphone users) are the laws and policies that are developed for smartphone interface design, including the research disciplines that implement the technology for the elderly user. Lastly, the division of labor that enables the object (smartphone interface) to be used by the community (other smartphone users) includes the smartphone development company and its system developers and researchers. A disconnect in the accessibility functions of the smartphone will result in an interface that is not elderly-friendly. Similarly, a breakdown in communication by the smartphone company or developer to its stakeholders (elderly and other users) about the product, or a breach of the policies for interface design, will also lead to a disconnect and create problems in terms of the usage of the smartphone interface.

Figure 3. Schematic showing how Activity Theory can inform the design of an elderly-friendly smartphone interface
Adapted from Rezha et al. (Azir Rezha, et al., 2014).

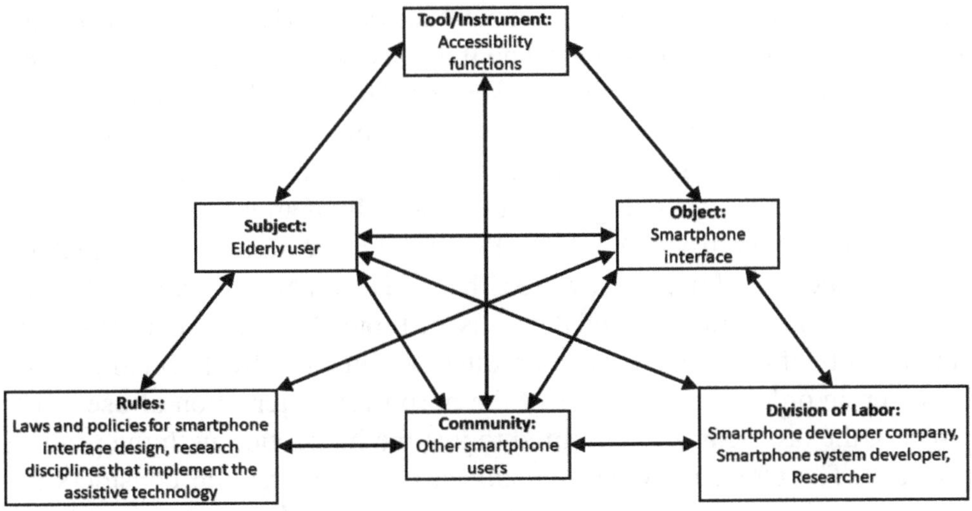

From UCD to ACD – Considerations in Technological Product Design

While the Pharmaco-cybernetic Maxims and the Ecological Systems Theory can be broadly applied to the design of digital health systems, UCD, ECD and ACD are interconnected concepts that do not usually exist alone in the design process. In UCD, the active involvement of users during the development process ensures that the product is more likely to meet users' expectations for its intended use. This improvement in satisfaction can lead to increased sales, as well as save time and costs by minimizing the need to change the product late in the design process. It also gives customers a sense of ownership in the product, thereby increasing customer loyalty through building a good brand reputation. However, designing products through UCD is expensive and certain types of data can be difficult to be translated into the design. Furthermore, developing the product will take more time, hence resulting in the product being more expensive and too complicated for general public use.

On the other hand, ECD considers a holistic perspective on users with the product or service, and their relationships with other people (e.g. designers and researchers) (Wright & McCarthy, 2010). Therefore, designers need to understand that the users' previous experiences will influence how they make sense of a new product or service, and that they will always come with their own expectations of the product or service. However, by tapping into the past experiences of users, designers can potentially uncover and challenge some of their implicit assumptions, and also stimulate their imagination and aspirations, thereby designing products that really matter to them.

Interestingly, both UCD and ACD focus on the same unit of analysis between objects and users. However, the UCD framework deals with user-product/system interaction, and the tasks are typically defined in terms of the functionality of the technological product/system (Azir Rezha, et al., 2014). However, in order to make sense of the purposeful interaction of users (i.e. subject), the tasks cannot be limited to just the interaction with the product interface. Therefore, in ACD, the subject-object interaction considers the users being in a social world, and hence, the scope of tasks is expanded to the larger context of activities that are carried out to accomplish important things regardless of the product. In AT, the study of the real-life use of the product is important as part of the subject's interaction with the world. Hence, in terms of the level of analysis, UCD often involves product-specific tasks, while in ACD, analysis tends to be on meaningful goal-directed actions. Not surprisingly, their methods of analyses are also different. UCD generally involves lab studies, while ACD gravitates towards the study of the real-life use of the product. As such, UCD studies are usually conducted over a limited time span with specific groups of users (e.g. novice or expert users), but in ACD, developmental changes in users are taken into account together with their interactions with the product, over a longer period of time. However, ACD does come with its own limitations. Because AT has a long tradition of cultural-historical psychology spanning from the 1980s, and has been used in various fields in psychology, education and ethnomethodology, among others, its scope can be ambiguous compared to other theories in the field. Furthermore, it is hard to capture and handle the time aspects in AT due to the developmental transformations that happen over time. While several checklists based on AT have been developed for human-computer interaction (HCI) practitioners (Duignan, Noble, & Biddle, 2006; Kaptelinin, Nardi, & Macaulay, 1999), those who have limited exposure or lack the basic knowledge of AT concepts may find it difficult to apply this framework in their product designs. Nonetheless, ACD can potentially help HCI practitioners by orientating their research to new directions that are overlooked or underestimated, formulating new questions in traditional or new areas that may solve HCI problems, and contribute to their self-reflection and analysis in order to better understand the values, intentions and social context of the product and its users (Kaptelinin, et al., 1995). Table 1 summarizes the key considerations of UCD, ECD and ACD in the design of technological products.

DESIGNING FOR THE iOS AND ANDROID PLATFORMS

Native applications for iOS and Android systems have different operating system-specific features. Designing for iOS is largely based on Apple's Human Interface Guidelines (Apple), while designing for Android is based on Material Design Guidelines (Google). Both guidelines by Apple and Google recommend using platform-specific navigation controls whenever possible, but in both instances, there are exceptions of apps that do not follow the standard guidelines. Native Android and iOS apps generally have different navigation patterns. Android apps tend to use a combination of tabs and a navigation drawer, which is a menu that slides in from either the left or right by pressing a "hamburger" menu icon, for users. On the other hand, there is no standard iOS control that is like the navigation drawer in iOS apps. Instead, iOS apps have a global navigation bar that contains no more than 5

Table 1. Summary of the key considerations of UCD, ECD and ACD in technological product design.

Parameter	User-centered Design (UCD)	Experience-centered Design (ECD)	Activity-centered Design (ACD)
Design focus	Focus is on the users and their needs in each phase of the design process of the technology (e.g. mHealth app).	Focus is on creating experiences beyond the product/ service (e.g. mHealth app) through creating relationships with individuals and an environment that connects on an emotional/value level to the user.	Focus is on the "activity", which is the purposeful, transformative and developing interaction between the subject (e.g. user), object (e.g. mobile device) and the world (including social context).
Design concepts	• Visibility - Affordances - Signifiers - Constraints • Mapping • Feedback • Conceptual model of the system	• Visceral level • Behavioral level • Reflective level (related to the four threads of experience): - Sensual - Emotional - Compositional - Spatio-temporal	Leontiev's Activity Theory (based on individuals acting in social contexts): • Object-orientedness • Hierarchical structure of activity • Internalization and externalization • Tool mediation • Development Engeström's activity system model (based on collective activities by groups/ organizations): • Three-way interaction between subject, object and community • Mediational means: - Tools for subject-object interaction - Rules for subject-community interaction - Division of labor for community-object interaction
Pros	• Product is more likely to meet users' expectations. • Saves time and costs by minimizing the need to change product late in the design process. • Increases user satisfaction and sense of ownership in the product.	• Considers holistic perspective on users with the product and other people. • Designers can tap on past experiences of users to uncover and challenge some of their implicit assumptions about the product.	• Considers real-life use of the product as part of the users' interaction with the world. • Analysis is on users' goal-directed actions. • Considers developmental changes in users together with their interactions with the product.
Cons	• Product can be expensive and too complicated for the general public. • Some data can be difficult to translate into the design.	• Users have their own expectations of the new product that might not have been met, based on their previous experiences.	• Scope of theory can be ambiguous. • Difficult to capture and handle time aspects. • Framework can be difficult to apply if the designer/ practitioner is not familiar with the concepts in Activity Theory.
Summary	• UCD framework focuses on how to design the technology to accommodate the needs, capabilities and behavior of the user. • Understanding the user and the needs that the technology is intended to meet requires iterative testing and observations/ feedback.	• ECD framework is about the experiences that the technology delivers, in order to fulfill the needs/values of the user, which in turn creates meaning and emotion.	• ACD framework focuses on how the real-life use of the technology is part of the user's interaction with the world.

destinations at the bottom of the screen (SteelKiwi, 2018). Another observable difference is the date picker, which appears as a reel-styled slot machine date selector in iOS, but in a calendar-styled custom control on the Android platform (Kennedy, 2020; SteelKiwi, 2018). Buttons are also different on both platforms – the primary call-to-action buttons on Android devices are usually floating action buttons, such as the compose button in email apps or the new post button in social networking apps. The analogous design of these call-to-action buttons in iOS apps are usually located on the upper-right of the screen or at the bottom-center of the tab bar (Kennedy, 2020; SteelKiwi, 2018). In addition, selection controls in Android apps typically appear in the form of an in-place dropdown menu or as a modal dialog that slides up the foreground listing the options, while the previous screen peeks through the top and recedes into the background (Kennedy, 2020; SteelKiwi, 2018). There are other differences in the two platforms, such as interaction patterns and visual styling of components. A non-exhaustive list of design element differences is provided in Table 2.

The advent of various mobile app building software (ThinkMobiles; Turner, 2019) and frameworks have enabled developers who have no coding knowledge or experience to enter into the app market. These frameworks have led to the ability to build mobile-responsive and/or cross-platform applications. The traditional mindset of designing for "iOS" or "Android" has converged to simply designing for "smartphone users". If you think of a person using a palm-sized touchscreen device, designing the user interface makes better sense if buttons are finger-sized, back buttons appear at the top-left of the screen, and navigation is at the bottom of the screen, where it is easy for the thumb to reach. If the navigation bar is at the top, it should be supplemented with swiping for better usability. Similarly, for the selection of option lists, the "switches" in iOS should look and behave like checkboxes, which are universally understood as controls for on/off states (Ou, 2019). This approach to designing for human interaction (rather than for platforms) have resulted in many responsive web-apps that do not distinguish between Android and iOS users. Many game apps, Airbnb and YouTube, have defined their own styles that do not distinguish between Android or iOS. Rather, their styles are just "wrapped in a smartphone". A major advantage of using only one design for both platforms is efficiency – there is no need to maintain two separate platform designs and a single code base can potentially be used as well, thereby eliminating the need for separate Android and iOS developers. Having one design also means that users of all devices will get a consistent experience with the app, regardless of platform. From a designer's perspective,

Table 2. Differences in the design elements of Android and iOS platforms.

Design Element	Android	iOS	Design Notes
Minimum tap target size	48 x 48 dp	44 x 44 pt	Android apps tend to have a slightly cleaner, more airy appearance than iOS.
Main app navigation	Main parts or "destinations" are shown in a variety of different places	Destination tabs are displayed as 2-5 icons across screen bottom	iOS default apps do not have profile or settings-related tabs, discourage actions in the tab bar, and make search appears last.
Secondary app navigation	Destinations are shown in a side menu that can be accessed by a "hamburger" button	Destinations that do not fit the bottom tab bar are placed in a "More" tab	Although iOS does not encourage the use of "hamburger" buttons, many third-party iOS apps do have one.
Primary call-to-action button	Usually as a floating action button on bottom-right of screen	Usually on upper-right of screen or at the center of the tab bar	Some apps have exceptions, whereby page actions on iOS will appear at the bottom and Android at the top.
Secondary actions	Top-right of screen	On-page user interface	--
Selection controls (single-choice lists)	Options are listed through an in-place dropdown menu or a modal confirmation dialogue	Options are listed as a picker control that is anchored at the bottom of screen or inline with the content	--
Selection controls (multiple-choice lists)	Checkbox list or list with switches	List with switches or checkmarks for selected items	For longer lists of options or to allow multi-selection, a dedicated picker screen (full screen) can be used.
Date picker	Custom control is used for picking dates	Appearance is like any other picker control, but with columns for day, month and year	In both platforms, inclusion of the year is optional.
"Back" pattern	Back buttons are usually on upper-left of screen. Android 9 and older phones have a permanent "Back" button on bottom-left of screen. On Android 10 and newer phones, back navigation can be done by swiping from either side of screen in	Back navigation can be done by pressing "Back" on top-left of screen, swiping left-to-right, pressing "Done" on top-right of screen, or swiping down on screen content	--
Undo pattern	Some alerts appear in the center of screen, and can appear as "snackbars" if no user input is required	Alerts appear in the center of screen or as slide up "action panels" from the screen bottom	"Snackbars" provide a way to feedback to the user that their action was a success. Actions such as "undo" can be added onto the snackbar.

there also isn't a need to be fixated on which style fits the Android or iOS conventions. On the other hand, if the intention is just to create an app for a single platform, then designing based on a native Android or iOS convention is probably the way to go. However, if limitations in budget and resources exist, one uniform design can be considered. Other factors like the technology used, app features needed, as well as expectations of the target audience should also be considered as part of the design process.

DESIGN CONSIDERATIONS IN THE DEVELOPMENT OF mHEALTH APPS FOR MEDICATION ADHERENCE

This sub-chapter further discusses the pharmaco-cybernetic frameworks through the creation of a mHealth medication adherence app. The most crucial aspect of designing an app for any health-related purpose is to ensure that end users will be able to use the product with little or no difficulty. For patients, user-friendliness is generally associated with its aesthetics and ease-of-use, rather than number and type of functionalities (Bernhard et al., 2018; Bhandari, Neben, & Chang, 2015; Mohammed, Ibrahim, & Cavus, 2018). Hence, the development of clinically-relevant and culturally-sensitive medication adherence apps requires the application of health behavior theories and UCD approaches (Bernhard, et al., 2018; Groshek, Oldenburg, Sarasohn-Kahn, & Sitler, 2015; Mao, Vredenburg, Smith, & Carey, 2005; McCurdie et al., 2012; Mohr, Schueller, Montague, Burns, & Rashidi, 2014; Whiteley, Brown, Lally, Heck, & van den Berg, 2018). The development of such an app can and should be based on the identified design requirements from the perspectives of patients, caregivers and pharmacists, as well as iterative evaluations on its usability and acceptability. The rest of this book will further illustrate the design and development of medication adherence apps through the application of the IM approach, UCD principles, quality standards and theories of technology acceptance.

THE PLACE OF HEALTH BEHAVIOR THEORIES IN THE DEVELOPMENT OF mHEALTH INTERVENTIONS

An effective intervention to promote medication adherence must address the determinants of non-adherence. This requires a clear understanding of the relationships between the patients' adherence behavior and its determinants. Health behavior models and frameworks are crucial to facilitate the identification of potentially modifiable determinants of non-adherence and the corresponding behavioral change techniques (BCTs) (Chiang, Guo, Amico, Atkins, & Lester, 2018; Direito et al., 2018; Holmes, Hughes, & Morrison, 2014; Lamort-Bouche et al., 2018; Lin, Clark, Tu, Bosworth, & Zullig, 2017; Patton et al., 2018; Presseau et al., 2016). Grounding interventions in behavioral theory makes them more effective (Glanz & Bishop, 2010; Webb, Joseph, Yardley, & Michie, 2010). It also ensures the replicability of interventions by providing clear guidance on the process of development (Chiang, et al., 2018; Direito, et al., 2018; Heath, Cooke, & Cameron, 2015; Lau et al., 2018).

The IM approach is a commonly used health behavior framework in the development of health apps, including those used for medication adherence (Athilingam, Clochesy, & Labrador, 2018; Direito, et al., 2018; Heath, et al., 2015; Oosterom-Calo, Te Velde, Stut, & Brug, 2015). The IM approach is also commonly applied in the development of interventions for cancer patients (Lamort-Bouche, et al., 2018). Essentially, the IM approach prescribes a specific set of steps in the development of interventions (Figure 4) (Bartholomew, Parcel, Kok, Gottlieb, & Fernandez, 2011). The 1st step is to establish a participatory team and conduct a needs assessment to help identify the target population, the magnitude and determinants of the health problem together with its impacts. MHealth developers are encouraged to employ a variety of research methodologies in their needs assessment process, such as systematic reviews, qualitative in-depth interviews and quantitative surveys (Peters, 2014). It is also recommended to engage in a multi-theory approach to explain the relationship between the identified variables and adherence behavior (Gerjo Kok, 2014). In the 2nd step, matrices of change objectives are developed. At this stage, the change objectives for the factors that influence the behavior and relevant sub-behaviors are articulated. The 3rd step involves selection of theory-based BCTs. The IM approach provides a detailed list of BCTs that are grounded in theory (Bartholomew, et al., 2011; G. Kok et al., 2016). Moreover, the theoretical domains framework (TDF) (Cane, O'Connor, & Michie, 2012) and the BCT taxonomy (Michie et al., 2013) are often suggested for use in mapping intervention components to behavioral determinants and BCTs. The 4th step is program production, which involves merging of the previously identified BCTs into one consistent program. At this stage, pilot testing and refinement of the program is done in order to cater for widespread adoption. The focus in the 5th step is on program adoption

Figure 4. Steps in the Intervention Mapping (IM) approach.
Adapted from Bartholomew et al. (Bartholomew, et al., 2011).

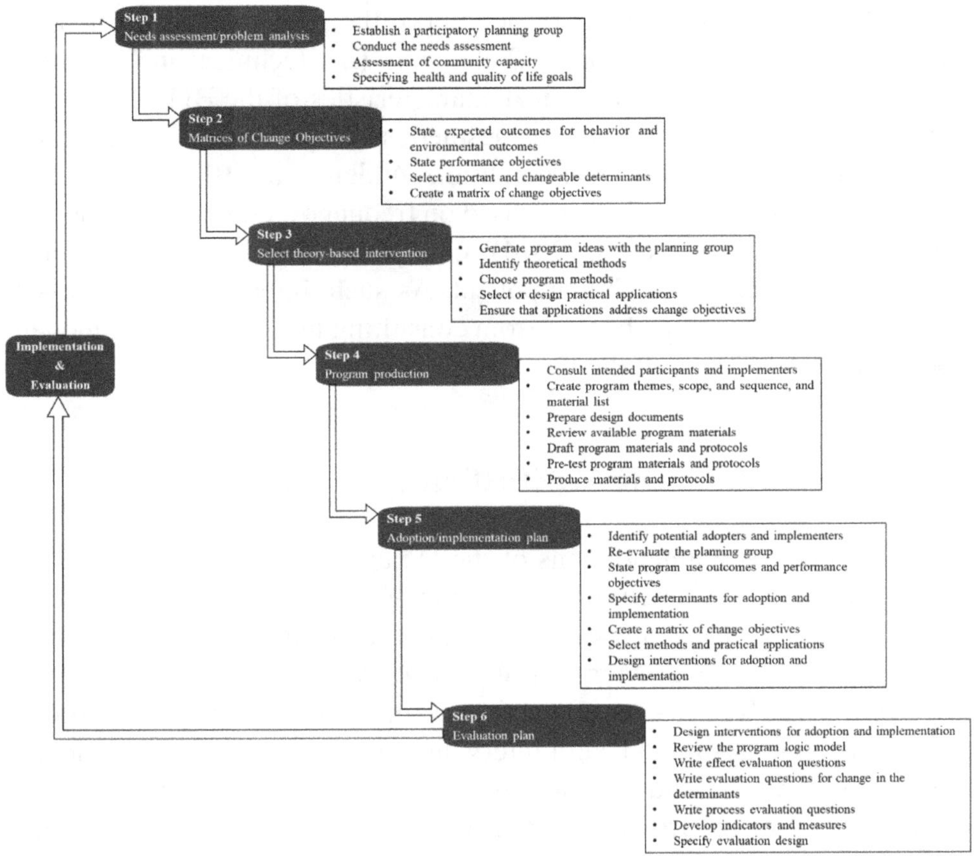

and implementation. Here, the program developers identify the determinants of adoption and implementation of the intervention, and devise strategies to promote sustainable adoption by the target population. The 6th and final step is to propose an evaluation plan for the intervention. This is done by setting indicators based on the performance and change objectives identified in the prior steps and specifying the design of the evaluation (Bartholomew, et al., 2011).

In cases where information technology (IT) interventions are involved, the IM approach can be complemented by IT-specific protocols such as the Behavioral Intervention Technology (BIT) model to provide the technological framework required to integrate the intervention methods into an IT-based program (Crutzen, 2014; Mohr, et al., 2014). The BIT model includes both theoretical and technological instantiation (BIT-Tech) components. The theoretical component describes the ways for setting the clinical and usage aims of the intervention and identification of the relevant BCTs. The BIT-Tech component describes the BIT elements (i.e. technical instantiations to be included in the BIT); technical characteristics of the BIT elements in terms of their medium, complexity, aesthetics and personalization; and the nature of the workflow (i.e., the conditions under which BIT interventions are delivered and whether they are based on frequency, condition, tunnelling or user-defined) (Mohr, et al., 2014). Compared to IM, the BIT model's strengths lie in the BIT-Tech component. As such, intervention developers using the IM approach can benefit from consulting the BIT-Tech component especially in the 4th step of the IM (Crutzen, 2014).

UCD OF MEDICATION ADHERENCE APPS

In line with the recommendations of the IM approach and the BIT model, the design and development process of medication adherence apps should involve end users through iterative cycles of prototyping and usability testing (McCurdie, et al., 2012; Mohr, et al., 2014; Whittaker, Merry, Dorey, & Maddison, 2012). The lack of end user involvement in the development process of many technology-based health interventions leads to the lack of relevant functionalities in the end product and minimal adoption (Alpert, Morris, Thomson, Matin, & Brown, 2018; Birnbaum, Lewis, Rosen, & Ranney, 2015). Hence, the development process should include patients, caregivers and healthcare professionals who are potential end users (Birnbaum, et al., 2015). For the design of medication adherence apps, the UCD approach is useful as it involves an iterative process of development that is informed by the needs and understanding of a specific end user group, so that it ensures the usefulness and ease-of-use of the app (Mao, et al., 2005; McCurdie, et al., 2012; Mohr, et al., 2014).

The first stage of the UCD process follows the first 3 steps of the IM approach. At this stage, a thorough assessment of user needs should be conducted to identify the intended use and required features of the app (Bernhard, et al., 2018; McCurdie, et al., 2012). The process employs a mixed methods study design with quantitative and qualitative components to obtain in-depth understanding of users' opinions (Darlow & Wen, 2016; McCurdie, et al., 2012; Yardley et al., 2016). An inductive approach of analysis will inform the design principles and functional requirements of the app (Birnbaum, et al.,

2015; McCurdie, et al., 2012). The next stage, which corresponds to step 4 of the IM approach, is prototype design and system development. This stage involves the generation of simple sketches and wireframes of the proposed app and continued engagement with potential users to elicit feedback that enables further refinement of the app into a working prototype. Refinement and optimization of the app is possible through formative research that allows the developers to discover new features or flaws in the original design (Wachtler et al., 2018; Whittaker, et al., 2012; Yardley, et al., 2016). The use of physical prototypes at this stage can help stimulate conversation and elicit more in-depth understanding of the users' opinions regarding design requirements (Williamson, Gorman, & Jimison, 2014). The last stage in the UCD process is the evaluation of the prototype app using walkthroughs and usability testing (McCurdie, et al., 2012). This is in line with the pilot testing recommendations in step 4 of the IM approach (Bartholomew, et al., 2011).

Methods and Considerations for Usability Testing

Usability testing in UCD is essential as it contributes to the refinement of the prototype app and provides inputs for the design of similar future interventions (Georgsson & Staggers, 2016; Jacobs & Graham, 2016; Jake-Schoffman et al., 2017; Sedlmayr, Schoffler, Prokosch, & Sedlmayr, 2019). Since usability is all about assessing how easy user interfaces are to use (Nielsen, 2012), the primary purpose of usability testing is therefore to identify issues that influence the ease-of-use and pleasantness of the app user interface. The usability testing process is recommended to employ qualitative evaluations complemented by quantitative measurements using tools such as the system usability scale (SUS) (Bangor, Kortum, & Miller, 2008; Lyles, Sarkar, & Osborn, 2014). This process generally involves identifying potential end-users of the product (typically of up to 5 participants), giving them representative tasks to do on the interface and observing them while they do the tasks (Nielsen, 2012). The end-users are usually encouraged to think aloud while doing the tasks (McCurdie, et al., 2012). This think-aloud method helps developers to identify issues in the design of the prototype system that users might find difficult or confusing. Such issues can include words used in the different features of the app and the way the different functions are integrated. It is recommended to record the think-aloud sessions to ensure that important points are noted. Here, the recording methods can range from simple note taking to more sophisticated systems that track user actions (Lewis & Rieman, 1994).

Usability issues identified in the testing process can be examined relative to established usability standards to facilitate the refinement of the user interface. In this regard, developers can use Nielsen's heuristics, which are widely accepted for computer-based user interfaces and consist of 10 usability principles (Table 3) (Nielsen, 1995). When it comes to mobile apps, Nielsen's heuristics should be tailored to the unique aspects of the mobile platform. In this regard, the Smartphone Mobile App heuRisTics (SMART) tool (Joyce, Lilley, Barker, & Jefferies, 2016), which comprises of 12 heuristics that are tailored to smartphone apps based on traditional heuristics and expert opinion, can be employed.

Table 3. General and mobile-specific heuristics for consideration in usability testing.

Nielsen's Usability Heuristics for General User Interfaces	Smartphone Mobile App Heuristics (SMART) for Mobile-specific Applications
• Visibility of system status	• Provide immediate notification of application status
• Match between system and the real world	• Use a theme and consistent terms, as well as conventions and standards familiar to the user • Use the camera, microphone and sensors when appropriate to lessen the users' workload
• User control and freedom	• Allow configuration options and shortcuts
• Consistency and standards	• Display an overlay pointing out the main features when appropriate or requested • Each interface should focus on one task
• Recognition rather than recall	• Intuitive interfaces make for easier user journeys
• Flexibility and efficiency of use	• Cater for diverse mobile environments
• Aesthetic and minimalist design	• Design a visually pleasing interface • Facilitate easier input
• Error prevention • Help users recognize, diagnose, and recover from errors	• Prevent problems where possible; assist users should a problem occur
• Help and documentation	• Design a clear navigable path to task completion

REFERENCES

Alpert, J. M., Morris, B. B., Thomson, M. D., Matin, K., & Brown, R. F. (2018). Implications of patient portal transparency in oncology: Qualitative interview study on the experiences of patients, oncologists, and medical informaticists. *JMIR Cancer*, *4*(1), e5. doi:10.2196/cancer.8993 PMID:29581090

American Society of Hospital Pharmacists. (1993). ASHP statement on pharmaceutical care. *American Journal of Hospital Pharmacy*, *50*(8), 1720–1723. doi:10.1093/ajhp/50.8.1720 PMID:8427270

Apple. (n.d.). *iOS design themes*. Retrieved 1 Mar, 2020, from https://developer.apple.com/design/human-interface-guidelines/ios/overview/themes/

Athilingam, P., Clochesy, J. M., & Labrador, M. A. (2018). Intervention mapping approach in the design of an interactive mobile health application to improve self-care in heart failure. *Computers, Informatics, Nursing*, *36*(2), 90–97. doi:10.1097/CIN.0000000000000383 PMID:28901967

Azir Rezha, N., Maksom, Z., & Naim, C. (2014). Tackling design issues on elderly smartphone interface design using activity centered design approach. *Journal of Engineering and Applied Sciences (Asian Research Publishing Network)*, *9*(8), 1190–1196.

Bangor, A., Kortum, P. T., & Miller, J. T. (2008). An empirical evaluation of the system usability scale. *International Journal of Human-Computer Interaction*, *24*(6), 574–594. doi:10.1080/10447310802205776

Bartholomew, L. K., Parcel, G. S., Kok, G., Gottlieb, N. H., & Fernandez, M. E. (2011). *Planning Health Promotion Programs: An Intervention Mapping Approach* (3rd ed.). San Francisco, CA: Jossey-Bass.

Bernhard, G., Mahler, C., Seidling, H. M., Stützle, M., Ose, D., Baudendistel, I., ... Szecsenyi, J. (2018). Developing a shared patient-centered, web-based medication platform for Type 2 diabetes patients and their health care providers: Qualitative study on user requirements. *Journal of Medical Internet Research*, *20*(3), e105. doi:10.2196/jmir.8666 PMID:29588269

Bhandari, U., Neben, T., & Chang, K. (2015). Understanding visual appeal and quality perceptions of mobile apps: An emotional perspective. In M. Kurosu (Ed.), Lecture Notes in Computer Science: Vol. 9169. *Human-Computer Interaction: Design and Evaluation. HCI2015* (pp. 451–459). Cham: Springer.

Bhavnani, S. P., Narula, J., & Sengupta, P. P. (2016). Mobile technology and the digitization of healthcare. *European Heart Journal*, *37*(18), 1428–1438. doi:10.1093/eurheartj/ehv770 PMID:26873093

Birnbaum, F., Lewis, D., Rosen, R. K., & Ranney, M. L. (2015). Patient engagement and the design of digital health. *Academic Emergency Medicine*, *22*(6), 754–756. doi:10.1111/acem.12692 PMID:25997375

Cane, J., O'Connor, D., & Michie, S. (2012). Validation of the theoretical domains framework for use in behaviour change and implementation research. *Implementation Science; IS*, *7*(1), 37. doi:10.1186/1748-5908-7-37 PMID:22530986

Chan, A., & Yap, K. Y. (2010). Detection and management of oncology drug interactions: Can we do better? *Maturitas*, *65*(3), 181–182. doi:10.1016/j.maturitas.2009.12.001 PMID:20036470

Chiang, N., Guo, M., Amico, K. R., Atkins, L., & Lester, R. T. (2018). Interactive two-way mHealth interventions for improving medication adherence: An evaluation using the behaviour change wheel framework. *JMIR mHealth and uHealth*, *6*(4), e87. doi:10.2196/mhealth.9187 PMID:29650504

Crutzen, R. (2014). The behavioral intervention technology model and intervention mapping: The best of both worlds. *Journal of Medical Internet Research*, *16*(8), e188. doi:10.2196/jmir.3620 PMID:25095730

Cut, M. (2017, Nov 16). Digital natives and digital immigrants — how are they different. *Digital Reflections.* Retrieved 28 Jul, 2019, from https://medium.com/digital-reflections/digital-natives-and-digital-immigrants-how-are-they-different-e849b0a8a1d3

Dailey, J., Kalis, B., & Sather, T. (2015). The next eHealth wave for silver surfers: Health management. *Accenture Insight Driven Health*, 1-4. Retrieved from https://www.accenture.com/_acnmedia/accenture/conversion-assets/dotcom/documents/global/pdf/dualpub_15/accenture-health-management-silver-surfers-pov.pdf

Darlow, S., & Wen, K.-Y. (2016). Development testing of mobile health interventions for cancer patient self-management: A review. *Health Informatics Journal*, *22*(3), 633–650. doi:10.1177/1460458215577994 PMID:25916831

Direito, A., Walsh, D., Hinbarji, M., Albatal, R., Tooley, M., Whittaker, R., & Maddison, R. (2018). Using the intervention mapping and behavioral intervention technology frameworks: Development of an mHealth intervention for physical activity and sedentary behavior change. *Health Education & Behavior*, *45*(3), 331–348. doi:10.1177/1090198117742438 PMID:29216765

Duignan, M., Noble, J., & Biddle, R. (2006). Activity theory for design from checklist to interview. In T. Clemmensen, P. Campos, R. Orngreen, A. M. Pejtersen, & W. Wong (Eds.), *Human Work Interaction Design: Designing for Human Work. HWID 2006. IFIP International Federation for Information Processing* (Vol. 221, pp. 1–25). Boston, MA: Springer. doi:10.1007/978-0-387-36792-7_1

Ee, R. W. X., Yap, K. Z., & Yap, K. Y. (2018). Herbopolis - A mobile serious game to educate players on herbal medicines. *Complementary Therapies in Medicine*, *39*, 68–79. doi:10.1016/j.ctim.2018.05.004 PMID:30012395

Energy Resourcing. (n.d.). *6 Things you need to know about Generation C*. Retrieved 27 Mar, 2020, from https://energyresourcing.com/blog/6-things-you-need-to-know-about-generation-c/

Engeström, Y. (2000). Activity theory as a framework for analyzing and redesigning work. *Ergonomics*, *43*(7), 960–974. doi:10.1080/001401300409143 PMID:10929830

Forlizzi, J., & Battarbee, K. (2004). Understanding experience in interactive systems. In *DIS'04: Proceedings of the 5th Conference on Designing Interactive Systems: Processes, Practices, Methods, and Techniques* (pp. 261-268). ACM.

Georgsson, M., & Staggers, N. (2016). Quantifying usability: An evaluation of a diabetes mHealth system on effectiveness, efficiency, and satisfaction metrics with associated user characteristics. *Journal of the American Medical Informatics Association*, *23*(1), 5–11. doi:10.1093/jamia/ocv099 PMID:26377990

Glanz, K., & Bishop, D. B. (2010). The role of behavioral science theory in development and implementation of public health interventions. *Annual Review of Public Health*, *31*(1), 399–418. doi:10.1146/annurev.publhealth.012809.103604 PMID:20070207

Google. (n.d.). *Material design*. Retrieved 1 Mar, 2020, from https://material.io/design/

Groshek, M. R., Oldenburg, J., Sarasohn-Kahn, J., & Sitler, B. (2015). *mHealth app essentials: Patient engagement, considerations, and implementation.* Retrieved 18 Aug, 2019, from https://www.himss.org/mhealth-app-essentials-patient-engagement-considerations-and-implementation

Heath, G., Cooke, R., & Cameron, E. (2015). A theory-based approach for developing interventions to change patient behaviours: A medication adherence example from paediatric secondary care. *Health Care*, *3*(4), 1228–1242. doi:10.3390/healthcare3041228 PMID:27417822

Holmes, E. A., Hughes, D. A., & Morrison, V. L. (2014). Predicting adherence to medications using health psychology theories: A systematic review of 20 years of empirical research. *Value in Health*, *17*(8), 863–876. doi:10.1016/j.jval.2014.08.2671 PMID:25498782

Internet Society (ISOC). (n.d.). *The Internet Engineering Task Force (IETF).* Retrieved 2 Aug, 2019, from https://www.ietf.org/

Jacobs, M. A., & Graham, A. L. (2016). Iterative development and evaluation methods of mHealth behavior change interventions. *Current Opinion in Psychology*, *9*, 33–37. doi:10.1016/j.copsyc.2015.09.001

Jake-Schoffman, D. E., Silfee, V. J., Waring, M. E., Boudreaux, E. D., Sadasivam, R. S., Mullen, S. P., ... Pagoto, S. L. (2017). Methods for evaluating the content, usability, and efficacy of commercial mobile health apps. *JMIR mHealth and uHealth*, *5*(12), e190. doi:10.2196/mhealth.8758 PMID:29254914

Jean-Guilhem. (n.d.). *World Wide Web Consortium (W3C).* Retrieved 10 Jul, 2019, from http://www.w3.org/

Joyce, G., Lilley, M., Barker, T., & Jefferies, A. (2016). *Mobile application usability: Heuristic evaluation and evaluation of heuristics. In Advances in Human Factors, Software, and Systems Engineering* (pp. 77–86). Springer International Publishing.

Kaptelinin, V. (1996). Activity theory: Implications for human-computer interaction. In B. A. Nardi (Ed.), *Context and Consciousness: Activity Theory and Human-Computer Interaction* (Vol. 1, pp. 103–116). Cambridge, MA, USA: MIT Press.

Kaptelinin, V., Kuutti, K., & Bannon, L. (1995). Activity theory: Basic concepts and applications. In B. Blumenthal, J. Gornostaev, & C. Unger (Eds.), Lecture Notes in Computer Science: Vol. 1015. *Human-Computer Interaction. EWHCI 1995* (pp. 189–201). Berlin: Springer.

Kaptelinin, V., & Nardi, B. A. (2006). *Activity theory in a nutshell. Acting with Technology: Activity Theory and Interaction Design* (pp. 29–72). Cambridge, MA: MIT Press.

Kaptelinin, V., Nardi, B. A., & Macaulay, C. (1999). Methods & tools: The activity checklist: A tool for representing the "space" of context. *Interactions, 6*(4), 27-39. doi:10.1145/306412.306431

Kennedy, E. D. (2020, Feb 22). *iOS vs. Android app UI design: The complete guide*. Retrieved 1 Mar, 2020, from https://learnui.design/blog/ios-vs-android-app-ui-design-complete-guide.html#undo

Kok, G. (2014). A practical guide to effective behavior change: How to apply theory- and evidence-based behavior change methods in an intervention. *The European Health Psychologist, 16*(5), 156–170.

Kok, G., Gottlieb, N. H., Peters, G. J., Mullen, P. D., Parcel, G. S., Ruiter, R. A., ... Bartholomew, L. K. (2016). A taxonomy of behaviour change methods: An intervention mapping approach. *Health Psychology Review, 10*(3), 297–312. doi:10.1080/17437199.2015.1077155 PMID:26262912

Komninos, A. (2019, Jul). *Norman's three levels of design*. Retrieved 1 Aug, 2019, from https://www.interaction-design.org/literature/article/norman-s-three-levels-of-design

Lamort-Bouche, M., Sarnin, P., Kok, G., Rouat, S., Peron, J., Letrilliart, L., & Fassier, J. B. (2018). Interventions developed with the Intervention Mapping protocol in the field of cancer: A systematic review. *Psycho-Oncology, 27*(4), 1138–1149. doi:10.1002/pon.4611 PMID:29247578

Lau, Y., Cheng, L. J., Chi, C., Tsai, C., Ong, K. W., Ho-Lim, S. S. T., ... Tan, K. L. (2018). Development of a healthy lifestyle mobile app for overweight pregnant women: Qualitative study. *JMIR mHealth and uHealth, 6*(4), e91. doi:10.2196/mhealth.9718 PMID:29685868

Lewis, C., & Rieman, J. (1994). *Task-centered user interface design: A practical introduction*. Retrieved 11 Jun, 2017, from http://hcibib.org/tcuid/index.html

Liaskos, J., & Diomidus, M. (2002). Multimedia technologies in education. *Studies in Health Technology and Informatics*, *65*, 359–372. PMID:15460236

Lin, C., Clark, R., Tu, P., Bosworth, H. B., & Zullig, L. L. (2017). Breast cancer oral anti-cancer medication adherence: A systematic review of psychosocial motivators and barriers. *Breast Cancer Research and Treatment*, *165*(2), 247–260. doi:10.100710549-017-4317-2 PMID:28573448

Lyles, C. R., Sarkar, U., & Osborn, C. Y. (2014). Getting a technology-based diabetes intervention ready for primetime: A review of usability testing studies. *Current Diabetes Reports*, *14*(10), 534. doi:10.100711892-014-0534-9 PMID:25173689

Manovel, I., & Sather, T. (2017). Silver surf's up: Senior citizens are riding the digital health wave. *Accenture Insight Driven Health*, 1-9. Retrieved from https://www.accenture.com/t00010101t000000__w__/au-en/_acnmedia/pdf-47/accenture-health-silver-surfers-in-australia.pdf#zoom=50

Mao, J.-Y., Vredenburg, K., Smith, P. W., & Carey, T. (2005). The state of user-centered design practice. *Communications of the ACM*, *48*(3), 105–109. doi:10.1145/1047671.1047677

McCarthy, J., & Wright, P. (2004). *The threads of experience. In Technology as Experience* (pp. 79–104). Cambridge, MA: MIT press.

McCurdie, T., Taneva, S., Casselman, M., Yeung, M., McDaniel, C., Ho, W., & Cafazzo, J. (2012). mHealth consumer apps: The case for user-centered design. *Biomedical Instrumentation & Technology*, *46*(s2), 49–56. doi:10.2345/0899-8205-46.s2.49 PMID:23039777

Michie, S., Richardson, M., Johnston, M., Abraham, C., Francis, J., Hardeman, W., ... Wood, C. E. (2013). The behavior change technique taxonomy (v1) of 93 hierarchically clustered techniques: Building an international consensus for the reporting of behavior change interventions. *Annals of Behavioral Medicine*, *46*(1), 81–95. doi:10.100712160-013-9486-6 PMID:23512568

Mohammed, H. B. M., Ibrahim, D., & Cavus, N. (2018). Mobile device based smart medication reminder for older people with disabilities. *Quality & Quantity*, *52*(S2), 1329–1342. doi:10.100711135-018-0707-8

Mohr, D. C., Schueller, S. M., Montague, E., Burns, M. N., & Rashidi, P. (2014). The behavioral intervention technology model: An integrated conceptual and technological framework for eHealth and mHealth interventions. *Journal of Medical Internet Research*, *16*(6), e146. doi:10.2196/jmir.3077 PMID:24905070

Nielsen, J. (1995). *10 Usability heuristics for user interface design*. Retrieved 12 Sep, 2017, from https://www.nngroup.com/articles/ten-usability-heuristics/

Nielsen, J. (2012). *Usability 101: Introduction to usability*. Retrieved 30 May, 2018, from https://www.nngroup.com/articles/usability-101-introduction-to-usability/

Norman, D. (2013). *The Design of Everyday Things: Revised and Expanded Edition* (1st ed.). Philadelphia: Basic Books.

Norman, D. A. (2002a). Emotion and design: Attractive things work better. *Interactions Magazine*, *9*(4), 36–42. doi:10.1145/543434.543435

Norman, D. A. (2002b). *The psychopathology of everyday things. In The Design of Everyday Things* (pp. 1–33). Basic Books. USA.

Norman, D. A. (2004). *Three levels of design: Visceral, behavioral, and reflective. In Emotional Design: Why We Love (or Hate) Everyday Things* (pp. 63–98). New York, NY: Basic Books.

Oosterom-Calo, R., Te Velde, S. J., Stut, W., & Brug, J. (2015). Development of Motivate4Change using the intervention mapping protocol: An interactive technology physical activity and medication adherence promotion program for hospitalized heart failure patients. *JMIR Research Protocols*, *4*(3), e88. doi:10.2196/resprot.4282 PMID:26195072

Ou, A. (2019). *You don't always need to follow native Android or iOS patterns when designing an app*. Retrieved 1 Mar, 2020, from https://uxplanet.org/you-dont-always-need-to-follow-native-android-or-ios-ui-patterns-when-designing-an-app-2a361a21c342

Patton, D. E., Cadogan, C. A., Ryan, C., Francis, J. J., Gormley, G. J., Passmore, P., ... Hughes, C. M. (2018). Improving adherence to multiple medications in older people in primary care: Selecting intervention components to address patient-reported barriers and facilitators. *Health Expectations*, *21*(1), 138–148. doi:10.1111/hex.12595 PMID:28766816

Peters, G.-J. Y. (2014). A practical guide to effective behavior change: How to identify what to change in the first place. *The European Health Psychologist, 16*(5), 142–155.

Pickett, P. (2019, Jan 13). *The characteristics of Generation C.* Retrieved 27 Mar, 2020, from https://www.thebalancecareers.com/who-is-generation-c-and-what-are-they-all-about-2071937

Preece, J., Sharp, H., & Rogers, Y. (2015). *Interaction Design: Beyond Human-Computer Interaction* (4th ed.). West Sussex, UK: John Wiley & Sons.

Presseau, J., Schwalm, J. D., Grimshaw, J. M., Witteman, H. O., Natarajan, M. K., Linklater, S., ... Ivers, N. M. (2016). Identifying determinants of medication adherence following myocardial infarction using the Theoretical Domains Framework and the Health Action Process Approach. *Psychology & Health, 32*(10), 1176–1194. doi:10.1080/08870446.2016.1260724 PMID:27997220

Sedlmayr, B., Schoffler, J., Prokosch, H. U., & Sedlmayr, M. (2019). User-centered design of a mobile medication management. *Informatics for Health & Social Care, 44*(2), 152–163. doi:10.1080/17538157.2018.1437042 PMID:29504838

Soegaard, M. (2019, May). *Laws of proximity, uniform connectedness, and continuation – Gestalt principles (2).* Retrieved 31 Jul, 2019, from https://www.interaction-design.org/literature/article/laws-of-proximity-uniform-connectedness-and-continuation-gestalt-principles-2

SteelKiwi. (2018, Aug 3). *Differences between designing native iOS apps and native Android apps.* Retrieved 1 Mar, 2020, from https://medium.muz.li/differences-between-designing-native-ios-apps-and-native-android-apps-e71256dfa1ca

Sullivan, T. (2019, Mar 15). *Silver Tsunami is coming to healthcare: Time to prepare.* Retrieved 28 Jul, 2019, from https://www.healthcareitnews.com/news/silver-tsunami-coming-healthcare-time-prepare

The Nielsen Company (US) LLC. (2012, Feb 23). *Introducing Generation C Americans 18-34 are the most connected.* Retrieved 28 Jul, 2019, from https://www.nielsen.com/us/en/insights/article/2012/introducing-generation-c/

The Psychology Notes HQ. (2019, May 3). *What is Bronfenbrenner's Ecological Systems Theory?* Retrieved 30 Jul, 2019, from https://www.psychologynoteshq.com/bronfenbrenner-ecological-theory/

ThinkMobiles. (n.d.). *Top-20 app development software platforms*. Retrieved 1 Mar, 2020, from https://thinkmobiles.com/blog/best-app-development-software/

Turner, B. (2019, Dec 26). *Best mobile app development software of 2020*. Retrieved 1 Mar, 2020, from https://www.techradar.com/au/best/best-mobile-app-development-software

US Food and Drug Administration. (2020, Mar 26). *Digital health*. Retrieved 31 Mar, 2020, from https://www.fda.gov/medical-devices/digital-health

Wachtler, C., Coe, A., Davidson, S., Fletcher, S., Mendoza, A., Sterling, L., & Gunn, J. (2018). Development of a mobile clinical prediction tool to estimate future depression severity and guide treatment in primary care: User-centered design. *JMIR mHealth and uHealth*, *6*(4), e95. doi:10.2196/mhealth.9502 PMID:29685864

Webb, T. L., Joseph, J., Yardley, L., & Michie, S. (2010). Using the internet to promote health behavior change: A systematic review and meta-analysis of the impact of theoretical basis, use of behavior change techniques, and mode of delivery on efficacy. *Journal of Medical Internet Research*, *12*(1), e4. doi:10.2196/jmir.1376 PMID:20164043

Whiteley, L., Brown, L., Lally, M., Heck, N., & van den Berg, J. J. (2018). A mobile gaming intervention to increase adherence to antiretroviral treatment for youth living with HIV: Development guided by the information, motivation, and behavioral skills model. *JMIR mHealth and uHealth*, *6*(4), e96. doi:10.2196/mhealth.8155 PMID:29685863

Whittaker, R., Merry, S., Dorey, E., & Maddison, R. (2012). A development and evaluation process for mHealth interventions: Examples from New Zealand. *Journal of Health Communication*, *17*(Suppl 1), 11–21. doi:10.1080/10810730.2011.649103 PMID:22548594

Wikipedia. (2019, Jul 27). *Digital health*. Retrieved 29 Jul, 2019, from https://en.wikipedia.org/wiki/Digital_health

Williamson, S. S., Gorman, P. N., & Jimison, H. B. (2014). A mobile/web app for long distance caregivers of older adults: Functional requirements and design implications from a user centered design process. *AMIA Annual Symposium Proceedings - AMIA Symposium. AMIA Symposium*, *2014*, 1960–1969. PMID:25954469

Wright, P., & McCarthy, J. (2010). *Experience-Centered Design: Designers, Users, and Communities in Dialogue*. Morgan & Claypool.

Yap, K. Y., Chan, A., & Chui, W. K. (2009). Improving pharmaceutical care in oncology by pharmacoinformatics: The evolving role of informatics and the internet for drug therapy. *Lancet Oncology*, *10*(10), 1011–1019. doi:10.1016/S1470-2045(09)70104-4 PMID:19796753

Yap, K. Y., Chuang, X., Lee, A. J. M., Lee, R. Z., Lim, L., Lim, J. J., & Ranasinghe, N. (2009). Pharmaco-cybernetics as an interactive component of pharma-culture: Empowering drug knowledge through user-, experience- and activity-centered designs. *International Journal of Computer Science Issues*, *3*, 1–13.

Yap, K. Y., & Lim, K. J. (2012). Merging the old with the new: A cybermedicine marriage for oncology interactions with traditional herbal therapies and complementary medicines. *Tang Humanitas Medicine*, *2*(2), e18. doi:10.5667/tang.2012.0004

Yardley, L., Spring, B. J., Riper, H., Morrison, L. G., Crane, D. H., Curtis, K., ... Blandford, A. (2016). Understanding and promoting effective engagement with digital behavior change interventions. *American Journal of Preventive Medicine*, *51*(5), 833–842. doi:10.1016/j.amepre.2016.06.015 PMID:27745683

Chapter 4
The Need for Quality Assessment of mHealth Interventions

ABSTRACT

With growing numbers of mHealth interventions, there is a need to evaluate the quality of existing apps based on quality assessment criteria that are grounded in published literature and health behavior research. These criteria can help identify the quality of mHealth apps from the perspectives of reliability, feature usefulness and feature convenience. This chapter will discuss the various quality criteria that are relevant for mHealth apps that target drug-related problems, as well as for medication management, through the development of two quality assessment tools. In addition to reliability, usability and privacy criteria, other feature criteria related to tele-monitoring, interaction checkers, dose calculators, medication information provision, medication records, as well as tele-support, tele-collaboration and personalization/contextualization, will be discussed. This chapter aims to provide guidance to mobile app developers, clinicians and patients on the types of quality parameters to consider in apps that are designed for pharmaceutical care and medication management.

DOI: 10.4018/978-1-7998-3832-6.ch004

INTRODUCTION

The use of mobile technologies in health care provision has paved the way for a new domain known as mobile health, or mHealth (Istepanian, Pattichis, & Laxminarayan, 2006; WHO Global Observatory for eHealth, 2011). The rapid advancement of smartphones and mHealth apps, together with advanced features such as Bluetooth, accelerometers, and 3G/4G networks, are currently supporting patient care activities in many health systems (Boulos, Brewer, Karimkhani, Buller, & Dellavalle, 2014; Istepanian, et al., 2006; WHO Global Observatory for eHealth, 2011). As of 2012, there were approximately 40,000 healthcare apps, of which 30% targeted clinicians, while the remaining 70% targeted the general consumer (BioSpace, 2012; Greenspun & Coughlin, 2012). Up to 63.5% of clinicians used apps in their clinical practices and 1 in 5 people with smartphones downloaded an app with a health-related purpose (Fox & Duggan, 2012; Franko & Tirrell, 2012).

According to the recently released U.S. Food and Drug Administration (FDA) guidelines, regulatory oversight is applied to mobile apps that satisfy the definition of a medical device. Depending on the level of risk the use of a medical app poses to patient safety, the FDA may require app developers to apply for premarket notification (510k) or premarket approval (US Food and Drug Administration, 2019). However, most health-related apps in the app stores do not fall under the FDA's regulatory oversight. Moreover, little is known about the quality of mHealth apps used by clinicians and patients in healthcare settings. Therefore, this can be a concern for the increasing number of consumers who download these apps. There is an increasing need for robust quality evaluation of mHealth apps to better inform both developers and end-users (e.g. clinicians and patients).

Several studies have described the use of apps for medication information (Aungst, 2013; Mosa, Yoo, & Sheets, 2012). In 2009, a medical apps review platform, known as iMedicalApps, was developed. iMedicalApps became a leading online mHealth resource for healthcare professionals, patients and healthcare analysts; and has since been regarded as the "go-to" resource for reviews in medical technology and healthcare apps by various reputable media outlets. This platform was also referred by the Cochrane Collaboration as an evidence-based trusted website (Husain & Misra) . However, there has been little focus on apps that addressed DRPs, particularly on medication adherence (Ali, Teo, Goh, Chew, & Yap, 2018; Loy, Ali, & Yap, 2016).

QUALITY EVALUATION OF mHEALTH INTERVENTIONS TARGETING DRUG-RELATED PROBLEMS

Loy et. al. developed a quality assessment tool for evaluating medical apps that targeted DRPs (Loy, et al., 2016). The quality assessment criteria were developed based on 70 articles from the journal literature and the iMedicalApps website. These criteria were classified into 2 major categories of quality: (i) "appropriateness of the app to serve its intended function", and (ii) "general quality". The first category was based on the features of the apps, which could be broadly categorized into 5 categories: monitoring, medication interaction checker, dose calculator, medication information, and medication records. On the other hand, the second category included sections on the reliability, usability, and privacy of apps. The quality assessment tool was developed such that mHealth apps could be rated for their general quality based on a total score of 38 points and assessed for the different features that were listed under the appropriate category. As the number of criteria for each feature varied for different apps, the scores for each section would also vary, and thus the maximum possible score in this section would be different based on the feature(s) evaluated. Table 1 shows the list of criteria for each feature, as well as the general quality criteria used in the quality assessment tool (Loy, et al., 2016).

The authors had previously screened the top 400 paid and free medical apps on the iTunes and Google Play stores to evaluate using their quality assessment tool (Loy, et al., 2016). Apps were included for assessment if they were available in English and contained 1 or more of the 5 features that the tool was designed to evaluate. From the 400 apps, only 59 (14.8%) apps fulfilled the inclusion criteria, of which 5 were available on both platforms. There were 27 apps with monitoring features, 17 apps with medication information features, 14 dose calculators, 8 apps with medication record features, and 6 medication interaction checkers. Six apps contained multiple features, but there were no apps that contained all 5 features.

Once an app was identified to contain any 1 or more of the features, the app would be evaluated under the corresponding assessment criteria under the section of "appropriateness of feature to serve its intended function". The maximum possible feature score for an app could vary between 8 (medication record feature) to 24 (monitoring feature). Combined with the overall quality of apps (maximum scores reliability, usability and privacy were 12, 22 and

Table 1. Quality assessment criteria for evaluating mHealth apps.

Part A: Quality Criteria for Evaluating App Features
Monitoring Feature (Max Score: 24)
· Monitoring of multiple physiological parameters · Setting target goals for physiological parameters · Ability to record symptoms · Syncing with external monitoring devices · Automatic transfer of readings from monitoring device to the app in real time · Ability to use monitoring feature in different environments · Ability for monitoring to be performed by patients themselves · Allows recording of medications taken by patient · Organization of patient's health parameters in chronological order · Trend display of monitored parameters · Ability to display a saved history of measurement results · Ability to classify the severity of medical conditions based on pre-set cutoff measurements · Ability to alert users on abnormal health parameter readings · Provision of a management plan for abnormal measurement · Security of access to patient's recorded health parameters · Back up/ storage of monitored data on device or the cloud
Medication Interaction Checker Feature (Max Score: 18)
· Ability to search medication by generic and brand names · Ability to display a list of possible interactions associated with a single medication · Detection of multiple drug interactions concurrently · Detection of interactions with complementary and alternative medicines · Details of interaction effects · Categorization of interactions according to severity · Comprehensiveness of the interaction database · Ability to perform interaction checks with medication lists · Presence/Absence of spelling or grammatical errors · Review of interaction content
Dose Calculator Feature (Max Score: 11)
· Dose calculations based on weight of patient · Dose calculations of antibiotics · Dose calculations based on renal/ liver function · Calculations of intravenous (IV) drip rate · Dose equivalent conversions of medications within the same pharmacologic class · Provision of a formula and/or explanation on how a calculation is derived · Drug administration instructions · Consistency of units of medications · Content review · Evidence base/citation reference of calculation formula
Medication Information Feature (Max Score: 22)
· Search function for information on specific drugs/medications · Ability to search for drug/medication information based on multiple categories · Ability to provide core and supplementary information about the drug/medication · Ability to provide information on whether the medication can be purchased over the counter or requires a prescription · Information for special populations · Black box warnings about a drug/medication, where applicable · Pill identifier feature · Comprehensiveness of the database · Evidence summary of a medication's therapeutic use with supporting reference citations · Presence/Absence of spelling or grammatical errors · Content review

continued on following page

Table 1. Continued

Medication Records Feature (Max Score: 8)
· Ability to input patient's biodata and current medications · Ability for users to edit their medication list · Adherence and reminder feature to allow users to record their medication consumption patterns · Ability to let users add basic therapeutic information regarding their medications · Ability to alert users on medication allergies and/or interactions based on their active medication list · Security of access to patient's medication records · Ability to transfer and store data to an external storage device or the cloud
Part B: General Criteria
Reliability (Max Score: 12)
· Target audience is clearly defined · Section header accurately reflects the content within the section · Provision of names and credentials of the app creators/authors · Disclaimer provided which states that the information provided by the app will not replace a healthcare professional's judgment · Declaration of sources of funding · Declaration of conflicts of interests · Presence/Absence of bias · Accreditation by a third-party certification · Provision of date of last update
Usability (Max Score: 22)
· Intuitiveness to use · Ease of navigation of app · Organization of screen layout · Readable default font size on screen · Clear and understandable language by a layperson · Presence/Absence of a help function/feature · Accessibility of the app features from any part/page of the app · Ability of app to be started/used in the absence of an internet connection · Presence/Absence of broken links · Adaptability of the user interface to portrait and/or landscape views · Customization based on user preference · Presence/Absence of bookmark feature · Availability of contact details of developer or feedback section · Robustness of app
Privacy (Max Score: 4)
· Details of privacy policy · Details of content sharing

Adapted from Loy et al. (Loy, et al., 2016).

4 respectively), the total possible scores of the apps could range from 46 for apps with medication record features to 62 for those with monitoring features.

From their analysis, they found that apps with medication interaction checkers and apps with monitoring features had the highest and lowest overall qualities (66.9% versus 54.8%). Paid Apple (58.1%) and Android apps (59.4%) also had higher overall quality than their free app counterparts (Apple, 55.8%; Android, 59.1%). In general, reliability of free and paid apps across both platforms were poor (25% each). However, the usability of paid apps was better than free apps (79.6% versus 68.2%), but worse in terms of privacy (25.0% versus 50.0%).

The Cancer.Net mobile app ranked the highest (79.0%) among the monitoring apps, followed by apps that monitored blood pressure and heart rate (66.1%-67.7%) (Table 2). At the other end of the scale, apps that monitored visual, hearing and temperature changes had the lowest quality scores (30.6%-38.7%) (Loy, et al., 2016). Most monitoring apps did not allow users to set target goals for physiological parameters (e.g. body temperature, blood glucose and heart rate) or provide a management plan when an abnormal reading was measured, and only a few apps allowed syncing of data from blood pressure devices via Bluetooth.

On the other hand, Medscape ranked the highest (76.8%) among all the medication interaction checkers. Most of the apps that were evaluated were unable to provide users with a list of all possible interactions associated with a single medication, while half could not detect interactions with herbal medicines. Free dose calculator apps scored higher for overall quality compared to paid ones. The highest-scoring apps with dose calculator features were Medscape (75.5%), MedCalc (67.3%) and Epocrates (61.2%). Majority of the dose calculator apps could not calculate dose requirement for antibiotics, nor provide administration instructions after calculation of doses.

Among the medication information apps, free apps (Apple 63.3%, Android 60.0%) generally had higher overall quality scores than paid apps (Apple 58.3%, Android 51.7%) (Loy, et al., 2016). Medscape and Epocrates were the top-ranking apps (71.7% each) in this category. However, most apps could not identify medications based on their physical parameters (e.g. shape, color, imprint), nor provide supporting references for the medication information provided. In contrast, paid apps with medication record features ranked higher than free apps in terms of overall quality (64.1% versus 42.4%). The top-ranked medication record apps were Pillboxie and Med Helper Pro Pill Reminder (67.4% each). However, more than half of the evaluated apps were unable to provide medication reminders, track medication schedules, and alert users to potentially allergy-causing medications based on users' active medication lists.

QUALITY EVALUATION OF mHEALTH INTERVENTIONS TARGETING MEDICATION ADHERENCE

In recent years, many mHealth apps have also been developed for medication adherence. As such, having a comprehensive set of quality criteria that is grounded in health behavior research can help identify the required features needed for adherence apps (Morrissey, Corbett, Walsh, & Molloy, 2016).

Table 2. Top-ranking mHealth apps evaluated based on the quality evaluation tool developed by Loy et al. (Loy, et al., 2016).

Feature	Rank	Score	Application Name
Monitoring feature	1	79.0%	Cancer.Net Mobile
	2	67.7%	Blood Pressure Diary Pro HeartWise Blood Pressure Tracker iBP Blood Pressure (Apple)
	3	66.1%	Blood Pressure Monitor – Family Lite BP Blood Pressure (Android)
	4	64.5%	Manage My Pain Pro
	5	62.9%	Blood Pressure Diary
	6	61.3%	Blood Pressure Companion iHeart - Pulse Reader
	7	59.7%	Blood Pressure (My Heart) Headache Diary Pro
	8	56.5%	Blood Pressure Companion Free
	9	54.8%	BP Tracker - Blood Pressure Tracker
	10	53.2%	Blood Pressure Blood Pressure - Smart Blood Pressure (SmartBP) BP Tracker
Medication interaction checker	1	76.8%	Medscape (Apple and Android)
	2	69.6%	Skyscape Medical Resources (RxDrugs)
	3	64.3%	Epocrates (Apple)
	4	58.9%	Epocrates (Android)
	5	57.1%	Drugs.com Medication Guide
Dose Calculator	1	75.5%	Medscape (Apple and Android)
	2	67.3%	MedCalc
	3	61.2%	Epocrates (Apple)
	4	59.2%	Mediquation Medical Calculator Calculate by QxMD (Android)
	5	57.1%	Calculate by QxMD (Apple) Epocrates (Android)
	6	55.1%	Lippincott Nursing Drug Handbooks Pedi STAT
	7	51%	MedCalc 3000 Complete
	8	44.9%	IV Drips Medical Calculator Paramedic Meds
Medication information	1	71.7%	Medscape Epocrates (Apple)
	2	66.7%	Epocrates (Android)
	3	63.3%	Lippincott Nursing Drug Handbooks MIMS (Apple)
	4	61.7%	MIMS (Android) Skyscape Medical Resources (RxDrugs)
	5	60%	Micromedex Drug Information
	6	58.3%	Drugs.com Medication Guide
	7	53.3%	Drugs & Medications
	8	51.7%	Johns Hopkins ABX Guide MIMS Singapore
	9	40%	iPharmacy
	10	36.7%	Antibiotics pocket
Medication record	1	67.4%	Med Helper Pro Pill Reminder Pillboxie
	2	65.2%	My Medical Info
	3	63.0%	My Medical
	4	56.5%	Family Medical Info
	5	45.7%	Pill Monitor Free–Medication Reminders and Logs
	6	43.5%	Drugs.com Medication Guide
	7	39.1%	iPharmacy

Table 3. Quality appraisal criteria for medication adherence apps used in published studies.

General Information and Category of Quality Criteria Used in Published Studies	Number of Criteria in Each Category				
	Dayer et al. 2013 (L. Dayer, et al., 2013) n (%)	Gal et al. 2015 (Gal, et al., 2015) n (%)	Heldenbrand et al. 2016 (Heldenbrand, et al., 2016); Dayer et al. 2017 (L. E. Dayer, et al., 2017) n (%)	Santo et al. 2016 (Santo, et al., 2016) n (%)	Haase et al. 2017 (Haase, et al., 2017) n (%)
· Targeted disease/ medication	General	Contraceptives	General	General	General
· How quality criteria were developed	Author consensus	Author consensus	Author consensus	Literature review and author consensus	Not specified
· Privacy policy and disclaimers (compliance with Health Insurance Portability and Accountability Act, availability of disclaimers, privacy policy)	1 (7.7)		2 (5.0)	1 (5.0)	1 (7.7)
· Capacity to schedule complex dosing regimens	1 (7.7)		1 (2.5)	1 (5.0)	
· Medication list (name of medications and medication pictures)		2 (16.7)	2 (5.0)	1 (5.0)	1 (7.7)
· Monitoring medication adherence (monitor missed and taken doses)	1 (7.7)		2 (5.0)	3 (15.0)	3 (23.1)
· Medication information (provision of up-to-date and well-cited medication information)					1 (7.7)
· Health information			12 (30.0)		
· Reminders/alerts (options for reminders including sound, vibration, and displayed alerts)	1 (7.7)	9 (75.0)	5 (12.5)	4 (20.0)	2 (15.4)
· Backup for data (cloud or device-based backup mechanism for user-input data)	1 (7.7)		1 (2.5)		
· Sharing and collaboration (sharing of data with caregivers or healthcare professionals and support mechanisms for patients)	2 (15.4)		3 (7.5)	3 (15.0)	3 (23.1)
· Personalization (keep personal medical records, check interactions, enable password protected account and facilitate refill orders)			4 (10.0)	1 (5.0)	2 (15.4)
· Accessibility (language, cost, updates, multiple platforms)	3 (23.1)		4 (10.0)	4 (20.0)	
· Feature convenience (easy entry of medication list and reminders, ability to snooze and postpone reminders)	3 (23.1)	1 (8.3)	4 (10.0)	2 (10.0)	
Total	13 (100)	12 (100)	40 (100)	20 (100)	13 (100)

Furthermore, it is generally recommended that tools should be developed for the systematic appraisal of apps so as to identify apps that can be useful for patients (Academy of Medical Sciences and the Royal Academy of Engineering, 2015). This is particularly important because the plethora of adherence apps are often criticised for their lack of features that are needed to improve adherence (L. Dayer, Heldenbrand, Anderson, Gubbins, & Martin, 2013; Morrissey, et al., 2016).

The medical apps rating scale developed by Stoyanov et al. and mHealth apps usability evaluation guidelines introduced by the Health Care Information and Management Systems Society are examples of quality assessment tools that have been developed for general mHealth apps (Healthcare Information and Management Systems Society (HIMSS), 2012; Stoyanov et al., 2015). However, these tools lack specificity to medication adherence apps. There have been attempts by various researchers to come up with quality criteria for medication adherence apps (Table 3). However, the quality criteria in these tools were developed based on consensus among the researchers rather than a systematic review of the literature (L. Dayer, et al., 2013; L. E. Dayer et al., 2017; Gal, Zite, & Wallace, 2015; Haase, Farris, & Dorsch, 2017; Heldenbrand et al., 2016; Santo et al., 2016). Moreover, the evaluation criteria heavily focused on medication reminders, the ability to keep and share medication lists and the availability of the app on multiple smartphone operating systems (OSs). Despite the importance of including credible medication information and side-effect management tools in adherence apps, the available quality criteria lacked focus on these issues (Morrissey, et al., 2016).

A comprehensive quality appraisal tool, which addresses essential behavioral change techniques (BCTs) suggested by adherence theories can work as a checklist for quality control in the design and development of adherence apps. The *Med*ication *Ad*herence *App Q*uality assessment tool (MedAd-AppQ) is one such tool that was developed based on BCT (Ali, Chan, Leow, Chew, & Yap, 2019; Ali et al., 2019; Ali, Leow, Chew, & Yap, 2018; Ali, Teo, et al., 2018). The original version of MedAd-AppQ comprised of 24 items in its quality criteria (Table 4) (Ali, Teo, et al., 2018). These 24 items were classified into different sections and sub-sections based on the quality construct that was measured by each item. Three major sections of content reliability (7 criteria), feature usefulness (15 criteria), and feature convenience (2 criteria) were developed. The content reliability criteria were categorized into 2 subsections related to the details of the app developer and the presence of disclaimers and privacy policy. The feature usefulness section evaluated app features that were related to the scheduling of varied dosing regimens,

Table 4. Quality assessment criteria in the MedAd-AppQ tool for medication management apps.

Category	Quality Criteria in MedAd-AppQ
	Content Reliability [Score: 11]
· Details of Developer and Target Audience	· Brief description of the app purpose and intended audience · Availability of contact details of the developer · Availability of names and credentials of the developers · Declaration of conflicts of interests
· Privacy Policy and Disclaimers	· Information on privacy policy · Presence of disclaimer declaring that app is not meant to replace the advice of a health professional · Declaration on sources of funding
	Feature Usefulness [Score: 31]
· Data Backup Capability	· Ability to backup medical data (e.g. on the phone, on the cloud, or synced with an online account)
	Tele-support Features
· Capacity to Schedule Varied Dosing Regimens	· Scheduling of medication tapers · Custom scheduling of medication regimen frequencies · Custom scheduling medications with varied dosing times
· Reminder and Alerts	· Ability to set reminders for medication time* · Medication refill reminder feature · Medical appointment reminder feature · Ability to generate medication reminders without Internet connectivity
· Drug/Disease Information	· Provision of medication information · Provision of disease-related information · Other features for identification of medications (e.g. images or photos of medications)
	Tele-monitoring Features
· Capacity to Monitor Issues with Medication Management	· Ability to track signs and symptoms of medication side-effects/ adverse drug reactions · Ability to track medication adherence by recording taken and missed doses
	Tele-collaboration Features
· Capacity to Facilitate Collaboration in Medication Management	· Ability for users to share their medication list and medication use patterns with other relevant parties · Ability to provide medication reminders for other third-party users · Alert feature for family/ caregivers if patient misses a dose
	Feature Convenience [Score: 3]
· Feature Convenience	· Autocomplete and/or text recognition/2D barcode scanning feature for convenient entry of user's medication list · Snooze/postpone function
	Personalization/ Contextualization Capability [Score: 18]
· Personalization/ Contextualization Capability*	· Security access to patient's medication records · Feature to input patient's biodata · Ability for users to choose who they share their content and/or monitoring data · Ability to save and edit medication list · Ability to let users add personalized notes on therapeutic information about their medications · Tailored medication information based on user's medication list · Ability to detect medication interactions and allergies based on user's medication list · Management support for medication management problems · Ability to provide pharmacy locations to facilitate filling and re-filling of prescriptions

Adapted from Ali et al. (Ali, Teo, et al., 2018).

* Additional criteria added to the final version of MedAd-AppQ

tracking and backup capabilities, provision of disease/drug information and presence of reminders/alerts. The last section was on feature convenience and this was not split into sub-sections.

In general, a reasonable level of inter-rater reliability was observed for MedAd-AppQ. The correlation coefficient values of >0.60 for most of its subsections showed strong correlations between the ratings of the evaluators. The results of the inter-rater reliability test were used to modify MedAd-AppQ and the modified tool was used to evaluate the quality of apps identified in the updated search. Based on an evaluation of 52 medication adherence apps on the iOS and Android platforms (Ali, Teo, et al., 2018), Ali et. al. had identified more than half of the apps (20 iOS, 74.1%; 17 Android, 68.0%) to score less than 50% in terms of quality. There were only 3 apps from each platform that scored 27/43 (62.8%) or more, but there was none that scored more than 28/43 (65.1%). The first 2 of the top 3 apps (GenieMD, Medisafe) had the same scores of 28/43 (65.1%) and the third app (CareZone) scored 27/43 (62.8%). There were no statistically significant differences between the median scores of apps on the Android and iOS platforms. Furthermore, the differences in the median scores of the free and paid apps were not statistically significant for all quality criteria sub-sections except the drug/disease information quality criteria where paid apps had significantly higher scores compared to free apps (14.3% versus 0%, $p = 0.032$).

Some unique features were identified among the top-ranked apps. For example, one of the apps used a text recognition system for convenient entry of medication names. The app enabled patients to take a picture of the medication labels using the smartphone camera, then used a text recognition algorithm to update the patient's medication list. As a result, this app had the highest score on the feature convenience section of MedAd-AppQ. Another unique feature found in 4 apps was a system that could alert a caregiver in the case of a patient's missed dose. This was particularly relevant, as the involvement of caregivers in medication management could potentially improve the patients' perceived social support and help in enhancing medication adherence (Nieuwlaat et al., 2014).

On the other hand, most of the evaluated apps were also lacking some features. None of the apps had the ability to conveniently schedule medication dose tapers. Only one app from each platform provided disease-related information (Android 1/25, 4.0%; iOS 1/27, 3.7%) and two apps from each platform had medication information (Android 2/25, 8.0%; iOS 2/27, 7.4%). Only four apps from each platform had an alert feature for missed doses (Android 4/25, 16.0%; iOS 4/27, 14.8%). Despite the presence of recording features for patients' symptoms related to medication side-effects in 9 apps on each platform (Android 9/25, 36.0%; iOS 9/27, 33.3%), none of them provided recommendations for self-management or real-time clinician management of such symptoms.

In order to maximize patient benefits from the interventions, provisions of personalized and contextualized adherence services are also advocated (Car, Tan, Huang, Sloot, & Franklin, 2017; Finitsis, Pellowski, & Johnson, 2014; Free et al., 2013; Hugtenburg, Timmers, Elders, Vervloet, & van Dijk, 2013; Liu et al., 2015). To respond to these requirements, MedAd-AppQ was modified by adding criteria from the quality assessment tool developed by Loy et. al. (Loy, et al., 2016), due to its robust development process from a systematic review of the literature and the fact that it also consisted of quality criteria for the evaluation of adherence app contextualization and personalization (Loy, et al., 2016). As such, a total of nine criteria were added to MedAd-AppQ so as to enhance its ability to measure the quality attributes of contextualization and personalization. Additionally, more options were included to the existing quality criteria in MedAd-AppQ, and the original criteria under feature usefulness were also categorized into domains related to tele-support, tele-monitoring and tele-collaboration. As such, the final version of MedAd-AppQ comprised of 34 quality criteria categorized into 4 sections – content reliability (11 points), feature usefulness (31 points), feature convenience (3 points) and personalization/contextualization (18 points) (Table 4). The final criteria in the tool was based on the literature on assessing the credibility and reliability of health apps (Ali, Teo, et al., 2018; Huckvale, Car, Morrison, & Car, 2012; Lewis, 2013; Loy, et al., 2016).

QUALITY CONSIDERATIONS FOR DESIGNING mHEALTH APPS

In the absence of clear recommendations on which app to use for medication management and adherence from regulatory authorities, clinicians can potentially use the tools described in this chapter to help them in their recommendation of appropriate mHealth apps to patients. Based on the quality tools described by Loy et al. (Loy, et al., 2016) and Ali et al. (Ali, Teo, et al., 2018), the quality assessment criteria for mHealth apps can be categorized into the general criteria of reliability, usability and privacy, as well as specific usefulness criteria of the different features in the apps (Appendix). As the number of quality criteria for each feature is different, it is expected that the overall quality scores for each feature will be also be different. In accordance to the methodology for app comparison by Loy et al. (Loy, et al., 2016), the weightages of each section of the quality assessment tool can be calculated as percentages of the raw scores. Similarly, the general criteria can also be calculated as a percentage based on the composite scores (39 points) for reliability (13 points, 33%), usability (22 points, 56%) and privacy (4 points, 10%). For ease of understanding, let's assume that each mHealth app has only one medication management feature. The quality weightage scores for feature usefulness (as a percentage of the total app score) are highest for medication adherence (52/91 points, 57%), monitoring (24/63 points, 38%), medication information (22/61 points, 36%) and medication interaction checker apps (18/57 points, 32%). (Table 5). This is in part due to the fact that there are more criteria to consider for these features. The feature usefulness score for medication adherence apps is double that of the other features as it also contains some overlapping criteria in the other features.

Table 5. Quality assessment scores for various medication management features based on feature usefulness and general quality.

	Quality Scores (%)					
App Feature	**Monitoring**	**Medication Information**	**Medication Interaction Checker**	**Medication Records**	**Dose Calculator**	**Medication Adherence**
Quality Criteria						
Feature Usefulness	24 (38)	22 (36)	18 (32)	8 (17)	11 (22)	52 (57)
General Quality · Reliability (13 points) · Usability (22 points) · Privacy (4 points)	39 (62)	39 (64)	39 (68)	39 (83)	39 (78)	39 (43)
Total score of app	63 (100)	61 (100)	57 (100)	47 (100)	50 (100)	91 (100)

Adapted from Loy et al. and Ali et al. (Loy, et al., 2016) and (Ali, Teo, et al., 2018).

Another major quality consideration for mHealth apps is security. While privacy has been addressed from the user's perspective in the quality tools, security is dependent on the technological, physical or administrative safeguards present in the mHealth system to protect any identifiable health data from unauthorized access (Martínez-Pérez, de la Torre-Díez, & López-Coronado, 2015). Studies have shown that the usage of mobile devices by clinicians and patients are much faster than the speed (Martínez-Pérez, et al., 2015) at which security and privacy protection features are implemented on the devices. Furthermore, the laws regulating privacy and security in mHealth are general and broad and are not able to catch up with the rapid advancements in digital health technologies (Martínez-Pérez, et al., 2015). As such, the threats in relation to unauthorized access to patients' health information, misuse of patient identities and unauthorized disclosure of personal information is very real (Avancha, Baxi, & Kotz, 2012), especially for mHealth apps that provide linked access to electronic or patient health records. These threats can be intentional or unintentional, and can be due to human missteps, fraud or malice, or technological gaps such information technology (IT) vulnerabilities and malware. The recent cybersecurity attacks on the electronic health records in Australia (Braue, 2019) and Singapore (Kwang, 2018) indicate the need to step up security in the healthcare sector. There are various frameworks and standards in security and privacy (Council of the European Union & European Parliament, 2016; FTC Staff Report, 2013; US Department of Health & Human Services) that may differ in different countries. Similarly, there are many technologies that have targeted this issue, for example, biometric/radio-frequency identification (RFID) authentications, attribute-based encryption/decryption, smart-emergency access control, and more recently, blockchain (Ichikawa, Kashiyama, & Ueno, 2017; Lu & Sinnott, 2020; Saha, Amin, Kunal, Vollala, & Dwivedi, 2019). These frameworks, standards and technologies are beyond the scope of this book. However, Martínez-Pérez and colleagues have put forward a list of security and privacy recommendations that should be considered for mHealth apps (Table 6). Developers are encouraged to refer to their publication for more details (Martínez-Pérez, et al., 2015).

Nonetheless, mHealth app developers are encouraged to consult the quality assessment criteria (Appendix) listed in this chapter to develop better medication management apps or upgrade existing ones. For example, developers of medication adherence apps should consider including more functionalities than just simple medication reminders. The functionalities of medication adherence apps can be enhanced in the areas of side-effect management, provision of medication-related and disease-related information, and ability to program complex medication schedules to cater to patients

Table 6. Security and privacy considerations for designing mHealth apps.

Factor for Consideration	Recommendation
Access control	Access control should be patient centered. Users should be able to control who accesses their information.
Authentication	Unique ID and password needed. Password should be complex with at least 7 characters, combination of numbers and letters, including one capital letter and one special character. Multifactor authentication can also be used.
Security and confidentiality	Advanced Encryption Standard (AES) should be used to encrypt the personal health information. The cryptographic key must have at least 128 bits.
Integrity	A symmetric key-based authentication code must be used, but a public key-based digital signature is preferred.
Privacy policy	Privacy policy should include purpose of collection, who will use the data, privacy methods used, user rights and contact method. Should also include a section for minors, requiring consent of a parent/guardian.
Data transfer	A Transport Layer Security (TLS) with at least 128-bit encryption should be used. Virtual Private Networks (VPNs) can also be used.
Data retention	Data retention policy should be included. Data should be kept only for as long as the initial purpose requires.
Body Area Network (BAN) communication	Cryptographic methods must be used for authentication and key distribution. Mobile device can be identified and authenticated by its International Mobile Equipment Identity (IMEI) or Subscriber Identity Module (SIM) card number. User's biometric patterns can be used for encryption and decryption.
Breach Notification	Relevant authorities and affected users must be notified within 1-3 days in the case of a data breach. Affected users should be compensated for the possible damage caused by the breach.

Adapted from Martínez-Pérez, et al. (Martínez-Pérez, et al., 2015).

with chronic diseases who are often on polypharmacy. A practical approach to developing more advanced adherence apps would be to tap into the electronic health record systems in hospitals, but it would require additional quality considerations in regard to the security features of the app. This will enable clinicians to monitor their patients easily and make tailored clinical and educational interventions in real time. Involvement of electronic health information systems will also help in the scheduling of complex medication regimens (L. Dayer, et al., 2013).

REFERENCES

Academy of Medical Sciences and the Royal Academy of Engineering. (2015). *Health apps: Regulation and quality control.* Retrieved 20 Feb, 2016, from https://acmedsci.ac.uk/policy/policy-projects/health-apps-regulation-and-quality-control

Ali, E. E., Chan, S. S. L., Leow, J. L., Chew, L., & Yap, K. Y. (2019). User acceptance of an app-based adherence intervention: Perspectives from patients taking oral anticancer medications. *Journal of Oncology Pharmacy Practice*, *25*(2), 390–397. doi:10.1177/1078155218778106 PMID:29792123

Ali, E. E., Chan, S. S. L., Poh, H. Y., Susanto, Y. A., Suganya, T., Leow, J. L., ... Yap, K. Y. (2019). Design considerations in the development of app-based oral anticancer medication management systems: A qualitative evaluation of pharmacists' and patients' perspectives. *Journal of Medical Systems*, *43*(3), 63. doi:10.100710916-019-1168-x PMID:30726518

Ali, E. E., Leow, J. L., Chew, L., & Yap, K. Y. (2018). Patients' perception of app-based educational and behavioural interventions for enhancing oral anticancer medication adherence. *Journal of Cancer Education*, *33*(6), 1306–1313. doi:10.100713187-017-1248-x PMID:28707206

Ali, E. E., Teo, A. K. S., Goh, S. X. L., Chew, L., & Yap, K. Y. (2018). MedAd-AppQ: A quality assessment tool for medication adherence apps on iOS and android platforms. *Research in Social & Administrative Pharmacy*, *14*(12), 1125–1133. doi:10.1016/j.sapharm.2018.01.006 PMID:29402755

Aungst, T. D. (2013). Medical applications for pharmacists using mobile devices. *The Annals of Pharmacotherapy*, *47*(7-8), 1088–1095. doi:10.1345/aph.1S035 PMID:23821609

Avancha, S., Baxi, A., & Kotz, D. (2012). Privacy in mobile technology for personal healthcare. *Association for Computing Machinery Computing Surveys*, *45*(1), 3. doi:10.1145/2379776.2379779

BioSpace. (2012, Aug 6). *GlobalData release: mHealth: Healthcare goes mobile*. Retrieved 7 Aug, 2019, from https://www.biospace.com/article/releases/-b-globaldata-b-release-mhealth-healthcare-goes-mobile-/

Boulos, M. N., Brewer, A. C., Karimkhani, C., Buller, D. B., & Dellavalle, R. P. (2014). Mobile medical and health apps: State of the art, concerns, regulatory control and certification. *Online Journal of Public Health Informatics*, *5*(3), 229. doi:10.5210/ojphi.v5i3.4814 PMID:24683442

Braue, D. (2019, Oct 2). Ransomware strike cripples regional Victorian hospitals. *CSO Online*. Retrieved from https://www.csoonline.com/article/3501694/ransomware-strike-cripples-regional-victorian-hospitals.html

Car, J., Tan, W. S., Huang, Z., Sloot, P., & Franklin, B. D. (2017). eHealth in the future of medications management: Personalisation, monitoring and adherence. *BMC Medicine*, *15*(1), 73. doi:10.118612916-017-0838-0 PMID:28376771

Council of the European Union & European Parliament. (2016). *Regulation (EU) 2016/679 of the European Parliament and of the Council of 27 April 2016 on the protection of natural persons with regard to the processing of personal data and on the free movement of such data, and repealing Directive 95/46/EC (General Data Protection Regulation)*. Retrieved 20 Feb, 2020, from https://op.europa.eu/en/publication-detail/-/publication/3e485e15-11bd-11e6-ba9a-01aa75ed71a1/language-en

Dayer, L., Heldenbrand, S., Anderson, P., Gubbins, P., & Martin, B. (2013). Smartphone medication adherence apps: Potential benefits to patients and providers. *Journal of the American Pharmacists Association*, *53*(2), 172–181. doi:10.1331/JAPhA.2013.12202 PMID:23571625

Dayer, L. E., Shilling, R., Van Valkenburg, M., Martin, B. C., Gubbins, P. O., Hadden, K., & Heldenbrand, S. (2017). Assessing the medication adherence app marketplace from the health professional and consumer vantage points. *JMIR mHealth and uHealth*, *5*(4), e45. doi:10.2196/mhealth.6582 PMID:28428169

Finitsis, D. J., Pellowski, J. A., & Johnson, B. T. (2014). Text message intervention designs to promote adherence to antiretroviral therapy (ART): A meta-analysis of randomized controlled trials. *PLoS One*, *9*(2), e88166. doi:10.1371/journal.pone.0088166 PMID:24505411

Fox, S., & Duggan, M. (2012, Nov 8). *Mobile health 2012*. Retrieved 8 Aug, 2019, from https://www.pewinternet.org/2012/11/08/mobile-health-2012/

Franko, O. I., & Tirrell, T. F. (2012). Smartphone app use among medical providers in ACGME training programs. *Journal of Medical Systems, 36*(5), 3135–3139. doi:10.100710916-011-9798-7 PMID:22052129

Free, C., Phillips, G., Watson, L., Galli, L., Felix, L., Edwards, P., ... Haines, A. (2013). The effectiveness of mobile-health technologies to improve health care service delivery processes: A systematic review and meta-analysis. *PLoS Medicine, 10*(1), e1001363. doi:10.1371/journal.pmed.1001363 PMID:23458994

Gal, N., Zite, N. B., & Wallace, L. S. (2015). Evaluation of smartphone oral contraceptive reminder applications. *Research in Social & Administrative Pharmacy, 11*(4), 584–587. doi:10.1016/j.sapharm.2014.11.001 PMID:25640888

Greenspun, H., & Coughlin, S. (2012). *mHealth in an mWorld: How mobile technology is transforming health care.* Retrieved 11 Aug, 2019, from https://www2.deloitte.com/content/dam/Deloitte/us/Documents/life-sciences-health-care/us-lhsc-mhealth-in-an-mworld-103014.pdf

Haase, J., Farris, K. B., & Dorsch, M. P. (2017). Mobile applications to improve medication adherence. *Telemedicine Journal and e-Health, 23*(2), 75–79. doi:10.1089/tmj.2015.0227 PMID:27248315

Healthcare Information and Management Systems Society (HIMSS). (2012, Jul 1). *Selecting a mobile app: Evaluating the usability of medical applications.* Retrieved 11 Aug, 2019, from https://www.himss.org/selecting-mobile-app-evaluating-usability-medical-applications-0?ItemNumber=28900

Heldenbrand, S., Martin, B. C., Gubbins, P. O., Hadden, K., Renna, C., Shilling, R., & Dayer, L. (2016). Assessment of medication adherence app features, functionality, and health literacy level and the creation of a searchable web-based adherence app resource for health care professionals and patients. *Journal of the American Pharmacists Association, 56*(3), 293–302. doi:10.1016/j.japh.2015.12.014 PMID:27067551

Huckvale, K., Car, M., Morrison, C., & Car, J. (2012). Apps for asthma self-management: A systematic assessment of content and tools. *BMC Medicine, 10*(1), 144. doi:10.1186/1741-7015-10-144 PMID:23171675

Hugtenburg, J. G., Timmers, L., Elders, P. J., Vervloet, M., & van Dijk, L. (2013). Definitions, variants, and causes of nonadherence with medication: A challenge for tailored interventions. *Patient Preference and Adherence*, *7*, 675–682. doi:10.2147/PPA.S29549 PMID:23874088

Husain, I., & Misra, S. (n.d.). *About iMedicalApps*. Retrieved 30 Jul, 2019, from https://www.imedicalapps.com/about/

Ichikawa, D., Kashiyama, M., & Ueno, T. (2017). Tamper-resistant mobile health using blockchain technology. *JMIR mHealth and uHealth*, *5*(7), e111. doi:10.2196/mhealth.7938 PMID:28747296

Istepanian, R. S. H., Pattichis, C. S., & Laxminarayan, S. (2006). Ubiquitous m-health systems and the convergence towards 4G mobile technologies. In R. S. H. Istepanian, S. Laxminarayan, & C. S. Pattichis (Eds.), *M-Health. Topics in Biomedical Engineering* (pp. 3–14). Boston, MA: Springer. doi:10.1007/0-387-26559-7_1

Kwang, K. (2018, Sep 21). COI for SingHealth cyberattack: IT gaps, staff missteps contributed to incident, says Solicitor-General, *Channel News Asia*. Retrieved from https://www.channelnewsasia.com/news/singapore/singhealth-cyberattack-committee-inquiry-staff-hack-10744182?cid=h3_referral_inarticlelinks_24082018_cna

Lewis, T. L. (2013). A systematic self-certification model for mobile medical apps. *Journal of Medical Internet Research*, *15*(4), e89. doi:10.2196/jmir.2446 PMID:23615332

Liu, X., Lewis, J. J., Zhang, H., Lu, W., Zhang, S., Zheng, G., ... Fielding, K. L. (2015). Effectiveness of electronic reminders to improve medication adherence in tuberculosis patients: A cluster-randomised trial. *PLoS Medicine*, *12*(9), e1001876. doi:10.1371/journal.pmed.1001876 PMID:26372470

Loy, J. S., Ali, E. E., & Yap, K. Y. (2016). Quality assessment of medical apps that target medication-related problems. *Journal of Managed Care & Specialty Pharmacy*, *22*(10), 1124–1140. doi:10.18553/jmcp.2016.22.10.1124 PMID:27668561

Lu, Y., & Sinnott, R. O. (2020). *Security and privacy solutions for smart healthcare systems. In Innovation in Health Informatics* (pp. 189–216). Elsevier.

Martínez-Pérez, B., de la Torre-Díez, I., & López-Coronado, M. (2015). Privacy and security in mobile health apps: A review and recommendations. *Journal of Medical Systems*, *39*(1), 181. doi:10.100710916-014-0181-3 PMID:25486895

Morrissey, E. C., Corbett, T. K., Walsh, J. C., & Molloy, G. J. (2016). Behavior change techniques in apps for medication adherence: A content analysis. *American Journal of Preventive Medicine*, *50*(5), e143–e146. doi:10.1016/j.amepre.2015.09.034 PMID:26597504

Mosa, A. S. M., Yoo, I., & Sheets, L. (2012). A systematic review of healthcare applications for smartphones. *BMC Medical Informatics and Decision Making*, *12*(1), 67. doi:10.1186/1472-6947-12-67 PMID:22781312

Nieuwlaat, R., Wilczynski, N., Navarro, T., Hobson, N., Jeffery, R., Keepanasseril, A., ... Haynes, R. B. (2014). Interventions for enhancing medication adherence. *Cochrane Database of Systematic Reviews*, *11*, CD000011. doi:10.1002/14651858.CD000011.pub4 PMID:25412402

Saha, A., Amin, R., Kunal, S., Vollala, S., & Dwivedi, S. K. (2019). Review on "Blockchain technology based medical healthcare system with privacy issues". *Security and Privacy*, *2*(5), e83. doi:10.1002py2.83

Santo, K., Richtering, S. S., Chalmers, J., Thiagalingam, A., Chow, C. K., & Redfern, J. (2016). Mobile phone apps to improve medication adherence: A systematic stepwise process to identify high-quality apps. *JMIR mHealth and uHealth*, *4*(4), e132. doi:10.2196/mhealth.6742 PMID:27913373

FTC Staff Report (2013). *Mobile privacy disclosures: Building trust through transparency*. Retrieved 20 Feb, 2020, from https://www.ftc.gov/reports/mobile-privacy-disclosures-building-trust-through-transparency-federal-trade-commission

Stoyanov, S. R., Hides, L., Kavanagh, D. J., Zelenko, O., Tjondronegoro, D., & Mani, M. (2015). Mobile app rating scale: A new tool for assessing the quality of health mobile apps. *JMIR mHealth and uHealth*, *3*(1), e27. doi:10.2196/mhealth.3422 PMID:25760773

US Department of Health & Human Services. (n.d.). *Summary of the HIPAA Privacy Rule*. Retrieved 20 Feb, 2020, from https://www.hhs.gov/hipaa/for-professionals/privacy/laws-regulations/index.html

US Food and Drug Administration. (2019, Nov 5). *Device software functions including mobile medical applications.* Retrieved 27 Mar, 2020, from https://www.fda.gov/medical-devices/digital-health/device-software-functions-including-mobile-medical-applications

WHO Global Observatory for eHealth. (2011). *mHealth: New horizons for health through mobile technologies: Second global survey on eHealth.* Retrieved from https://apps.who.int/iris/handle/10665/44607

APPENDIX

Table 7. Overall quality assessment criteria for evaluating mHealth apps.

Part A: Quality Assessment Criteria for Specific Mobile App Features	
Monitoring feature* [Max score: 24]	**Medication information feature* [Max score: 22]**
Monitoring of multiple physiological parameters **[0]** No **[1]** Yes	Search function for information on specific drugs/medications **[0]** No **[1]** Yes
Allows the setting of target goals for physiological parameters **[0]** No **[1]** Yes	Ability to search for drug/medication information based on multiple categories (e.g. generic name, brand name, disease/medical condition) **[0]** No **[1]** Yes
Ability to record symptoms **[0]** No **[1]** Yes, only subjective symptoms **[2]** Yes, objective symptoms	Ability to provide core information (medication name, indication, dosing instruction, contraindication, and side effects) and supplementary information (precaution, drug interaction) about the drug/medication **[0]** No, not all core information provided **[1]** Yes, only core information provided **[2]** Yes, both core and supplementary information provided
Syncing with external monitoring devices (e.g. blood pressure monitor, glucometer) **[0]** Yes **[1]** No (skip next question)	Ability to provide information on whether the medication can be purchased over the counter or requires a prescription **[0]** No **[1]** Yes
Automatic transfer of readings from monitoring device to the app in real time **[0]** No, manual entry needed **[1]** Yes, manual syncing by user **[2]** Yes, automatic syncing in real time	Information for special populations (e.g. pediatrics, pregnancy, renal/liver dysfunction) **[0]** No **[1]** Yes
Ability to use monitoring feature in different environments **[0]** No **[1]** Yes	Black box warnings about a drug/medication, where applicable Correctly classified as a black box warning **[0]** No **[1]** Yes Comprehensiveness of information provided regarding black box warning **[0]** No information provided **[1]** Some information provided **[2]** All information provided Provision of relevant resources regarding black box warning **[0]** No **[1]** Yes
Ability for monitoring to be performed by patients themselves **[0]** No **[1]** Yes	Pill identifier feature **[0]** None **[1]** Yes, but does not include pictures of medications **[2]** Yes, also includes pictures of medications
Allows recording of medication(s) taken by patient (e.g. medication name, dose, frequency) **[0]** No **[1]** Yes, only medication name **[2]** Yes, medication name + dose/timing/frequency **[3]** Yes, medication name + dose + timing/frequency	Comprehensiveness of the database (e.g. number of medications in the database) **[0]** No details provided **[1]** Standalone app with no information on comprehensiveness of database **[2]** Standalone app with information on comprehensiveness of database provided **[3]** App follows a parent database, but has no information on comprehensiveness of database **[4]** App follows a parent database and information on comprehensiveness of database provided
Organization of patient's health parameters (e.g. vitals) in chronological order **[0]** No **[1]** Yes	Evidence summary of a medication's therapeutic use with supporting reference citations **[0]** None provided **[1]** Either evidence summary or supporting references provided **[2]** Both evidence summary and supporting references provided
Trend display of monitored parameter(s) (e.g. graph) **[0]** No **[1]** Yes	Presence/Absence of spelling or grammatical errors **[0]** Major errors that compromise level of understanding **[1]** Minor errors that do not compromise level of understanding **[2]** No errors present
Ability to display a saved history of measurement results **[0]** No **[1]** Yes, display is based on limited number of records **[2]** Yes, display can be based on selected time frames (weeks, months, years)	Content review (e.g. internally or externally) **[0]** Not reviewed/not stated **[1]** Reviewed internally **[2]** Reviewed externally
Ability to classify the severity of medical condition(s) based on pre-set cutoff measurements **[0]** No **[1]** Yes, but classification is not evidence-based **[2]** Yes, classification is evidence-based	
Ability to alert users on abnormal health parameter readings **[0]** No alerts **[1]** Yes, alerts are qualitative (e.g. color-coded) **[2]** Yes, alerts are quantitative (high/low or normal ranges provided)	
Provision of a management plan for an abnormal measurement **[0]** None provided **[1]** Yes, general management plan provided **[2]** Yes, patient-specific management plan provided	
Security of access to patient's recorded health parameters (e.g. password/pin) **[0]** No **[1]** Yes	
Back up/ storage of monitored data on device or the cloud **[0]** No data storage feature **[1]** Data are non-transferable (stored on device itself) **[2]** Data are transferable (to external storage device/cloud)	

continued on following page

Table 7. Continued

<table>
<tr><th>Medication interaction checker feature* [Max score: 18]</th><th>Medication records feature* [Max score: 8]</th></tr>
<tr><td rowspan="3">Ability to search medication by generic and brand names
[0] No search function
[1] Yes, search by either generic or brand name
[2] Yes, search by both generic and brand name

Ability to display a list of possible interactions associated with a single medication
[0] No **[1]** Yes

Detection of multiple drug interactions concurrently
[0] No **[1]** Yes

Detection of interactions with complementary and alternative medicines
[0] No **[1]** Yes

Details of interaction effects (e.g. severity, mechanism, management plan)
[0] Only one parameter provided
[1] Two parameters provided
[2] All three parameters provided

Categorization of interactions according to severity
[0] None provided
[1] Classification rubric provided without supporting evidence
[2] Classification rubric provided with supporting evidence

Comprehensiveness of the interaction database (e.g. number of medications/ interactions detected by the database)
[0] No details provided
[1] Standalone app with no information on comprehensiveness of database
[2] Standalone app with information on comprehensiveness of database provided
[3] App follows a parent database, but has no information on comprehensiveness of database
[4] App follows a parent database and information on comprehensiveness of database provided

Ability to perform interaction checks against previously saved medication lists
[0] No **[1]** Yes

Presence/Absence of spelling or grammatical errors in the interaction content
[0] Major errors that compromise level of understanding
[1] Minor errors that do not compromise level of understanding
[2] No errors present

Review of interaction content (e.g. internally or externally)
[0] Not reviewed/not stated
[1] Reviewed internally
[2] Reviewed externally</td>
<td>Ability to input patient's biodata (age, weight, allergy, medical history, medical condition) and current medications
[0] Not all data can be input
[1] Both biodata and current medications can be input

Ability for users to edit their medication list
[0] No **[1]** Yes

Adherence and reminder feature to allow users to record their medication consumption patterns
[0] No such feature
[1] Recording function available but no medication reminder
[2] Both recording function and medication reminder available

Ability to let users add basic therapeutic information regarding their medications
[0] No **[1]** Yes

Ability to alert users on medication allergies and/or interactions based on their active medication list
[0] No **[1]** Yes

Security of access to patient's medication records (e.g. password/pin)
[0] No **[1]** Yes

Ability to transfer and store data on an external storage device or the cloud
[0] Data are non-transferable (stored on device itself)
[1] Data are transferable (to external storage device/cloud)</td></tr>
<tr><th>Dose calculator feature* [Max score: 11]</th></tr>
<tr><td>Dose calculations based on weight of patient
[0] No **[1]** Yes

Dose calculations of antibiotics
[0] No **[1]** Yes

Dose calculations based on renal/ liver function
[0] No **[1]** Yes

Calculations of intravenous (IV) drip rate
[0] No **[1]** Yes

Dose equivalent conversions of medications within the same pharmacologic class
[0] No **[1]** Yes

Provision of a formula and/or explanation on how a calculation is derived
[0] No **[1]** Yes

Provision of drug administration instructions
[0] No **[1]** Yes

Consistency of units of medications throughout the calculation
[0] No **[1]** Yes

Content review (e.g. internally or externally)
[0] Not reviewed/not stated
[1] Reviewed internally
[2] Reviewed externally

Evidence base/citation reference of calculation formula
[0] No **[1]** Yes</td></tr>
</table>

continued on following page

Table 7. Continued

Medication adherence feature [Max score: 52]**

Ability to backup medical data, including medication list, adherence patterns, biodata
[0] No backup functionality
[1] Backup is done locally on the phone
[2] Backup is done manually on the cloud
[3] Backup is synced automatically with an online account

Tele-support features:
Scheduling of medication tapers
[0] No **[1]** Yes

Custom scheduling of medication regimen frequencies
[0] Not customizable at all
[1] Customizable to a limited extent
[2] Mostly customizable

Custom scheduling of medications with varied dosing times
[0] Not customizable at all
[1] Customizable to a limited extent
[2] Mostly customizable

Ability to set medication reminders
[0] No **[1]** Yes

Medication refill reminder feature
[0] No **[1]** Yes

Medical appointment reminder feature
[0] No **[1]** Yes

Ability to generate medication reminders without Internet connectivity
[0] Internet connectivity required
[1] Internet connectivity not required

Provision of medication information
[0] None provided
[1] Yes, but no proper citations or date of last update
[2] Yes, with either proper citations or date of last update
[3] Yes, with both proper citations and date of last update

Provision of disease-related information
[0] None provided
[1] Yes, but no proper citations or date of last update
[2] Yes, with either proper citations or date of last update
[3] Yes, with both proper citations and date of last update

Features for identification of medications other than generic names
[0] No other features available
[1] Yes, shapes and colors of medication provided
[2] Yes, photos from a medication image database provided
[3] Yes, users can take a picture of their own medications

Tele-monitoring features:
Ability to track signs and symptoms of medication side-effects/ adverse drug reactions
[0] No feature available
[1] Symptom tracking feature available
[2] Symptom tracking feature available with self-management recommendations
[3] Symptom tracking feature available with real-time management by healthcare professionals

Ability to track medication adherence by recording taken and missed doses
[0] No feature available
[1] Manual recording of either taken or missed doses
[2] Manual recording of both taken and missed doses
[3] Automatic recording of taken and missed doses (e.g. by a medication event monitoring system)

Tele-collaboration features:
Ability for users to share their medication list and medication use patterns with other relevant parties (e.g. health professionals, family or caregivers)
[0] No feature available
[1] Feature only allows sharing of either medication list or medication use pattern
[2] Feature allows both sharing of medication list and medication use pattern

Ability to provide medication reminders for other third-party users (e.g. family members)
[0] No **[1]** Yes

Alert feature for family/ caregivers if patient misses a dose
[0] No **[1]** Yes

Medication list entry is by autocomplete and/or text recognition/2D barcode scanning
[0] No feature available
[1] Either autocomplete or text recognition/barcode scanning feature available
[2] Both autocomplete and text recognition/barcode scanning features available

Availability of snooze/postpone function
[0] No **[1]** Yes

Security access to patient's medication records (e.g. password/pin)
[0] No **[1]** Yes

Feature to input patient's biodata (age, weight, allergy, medical history, medical condition)
[0] No biodata can be input
[1] Some biodata can be input
[2] All biodata can be input

Ability for users to choose who they share their content and/or monitoring data
[0] No **[1]** Yes

Ability to save and edit medication list
[0] None
[1] Allows saving of medication list only
[2] Allows both saving and editing of medication list

Ability to let users add personalized notes on therapeutic information about their medications
[0] No **[1]** Yes

Provision of tailored medication information based on user's medication list
[0] No **[1]** Yes

Ability to detect medication interactions and allergies based on the user's medication list
[0] None
[1] Manual detection of either medication interactions or allergies by user (no auto-detection feature)
[2] Manual detection of both medication interactions and allergies by user (no auto-detection feature)
[3] Auto-detects either medication interactions or allergies, with manual detection of the other by user
[4] Auto-detects both medication interactions and allergies based on user's medication list

Management support for medication management problems (e.g. medication non-adherence)
[0] None provided
[1] General management support provided
[2] Specific management support provided tailored to the patient

Ability to provide pharmacy locations to facilitate filling and re-filling of prescriptions
[0] None
[1] Generic list of pharmacies within a single organization provided without regard to user's location
[2] Generic list of pharmacies from multiple organizations provided without regard to user's location
[3] GPS/other location mechanism available to identify a list of pharmacies within a single organization
[4] GPS/other location mechanism available to identify a list of pharmacies from multiple organizations

continued on following page

Table 7. Continued

Part B: General Quality Assessment Criteria for Reliability, Usability and Privacy		
Reliability* [Max score: 13]	**Usability* [Max score: 22]**	**Privacy* [Max score: 4]**
Target audience is clearly defined **[0]** No **[1]** Yes Purpose of app is clearly defined** **[0]** No **[1]** Yes Section header accurately reflects the content within the section **[0]** No **[1]** Yes Provision of names and credentials of the app creators/authors **[0]** None stated **[1]** Either names or credentials stated **[2]** Both names and credentials stated Disclaimer which states that the information provided by the app will not replace a healthcare professional's judgment is provided **[0]** No **[1]** Yes Declaration of sources of funding **[0]** Not clearly stated **[1]** Clearly stated Declaration of conflicts of interests **[0]** Not stated **[1]** Conflict of interest stated clearly **[2]** Stated clearly that no conflicts of interest exist Presence/Absence of bias (e.g. advertisements) **[0]** Presence **[1]** Absence Accreditation by a third-party certification (e.g. medical/ government organization) **[0]** No **[1]** Yes Provision of date of last update **[0]** Not stated **[1]** Frequency of update provided without actual date of last update **[2]** Actual date of last updated provided	Intuitive to use **[0]** No **[1]** Yes Ease of navigation of app **[0]** Major user interface problems that compromise ease of navigation **[1]** Minor user interface problems that do not compromise ease of navigation **[2]** No user interface problems present Organization of screen layout (e.g. well-organized / cluttered) **[0]** Cluttered / Not well-organized **[1]** Not cluttered / Well-organized Readable default font size on screen **[0]** Non-readable by default, can only be viewed on a larger screen **[1]** Non-readable by default, but user can zoom in and pan the screen **[2]** Readable by default Clear and understandable language by a layperson **[0]** Not at all **[1]** Sometimes **[2]** Most of the time **[3]** All the time Presence/Absence of a help function/feature **[0]** Absence **[1]** Presence Accessibility of the app features from any part/page of the app **[0]** No **[1]** Yes Ability of app to be started/used in the absence of an internet connection **[0]** Can only be used with an internet connection **[1]** Can be used without an internet connection Presence/Absence of broken links **[0]** Many broken links **[1]** Few broken links **[2]** No broken links Adaptability of the user interface to portrait and landscape views when phone is rotated **[0]** No **[1]** Yes Customizable based on user preference **[0]** Not customizable at all **[1]** Customizable to a limited extent **[2]** Mostly customizable Presence/Absence of bookmark feature for quick access **[0]** Absence **[1]** Presence Availability of contact details of developer or feedback section **[0]** No **[1]** Yes Robustness of app (How often does it crash unexpectedly) **[0]** Frequently **[1]** Occasionally **[2]** Rarely **[3]** Never	Details of privacy policy **[0]** None present **[1]** Only mentions collection of user data **[2]** Mentions both collection of user data and how it is being used Content sharing (e.g. does user control what to share and who to share with) Users can control what content to share **[0]** No **[1]** Yes Users can control who to share content with **[0]** No **[1]** Yes
* Quality criteria from the quality assessment tool by Loy et al. (Loy, et al., 2016) ** Quality criteria from the MedAd-AppQ tool by Ali et al. (Ali, Teo, et al., 2018)		

(Adapted from the quality assessment tools by Loy et al. and Ali et al. (Ali, Teo, et al., 2018; Loy, et al., 2016))

Chapter 5
Acceptability and Adoption of mHealth Interventions for Medication Adherence

ABSTRACT

The success of medication adherence apps depends on user acceptance and usage of the apps in their daily lives. It is essential for app developers to gain an in-depth understanding of the factors that can influence the acceptance of mHealth apps for adherence. It has been suggested that end users' acceptance of a technology-based health intervention can be studied through evaluation of their behavioral intention to use the intervention. Hence, it is important to continuously engage the target audience (e.g. clinicians, patients, caregivers) for their perceptions, experiences and feedback about the technological intervention, in this case, medication adherence apps. Factors such as socio-demographics and prior use of mobile technologies can influence user acceptance and adoption of mHealth apps. This chapter introduces the evolution of the Technology Acceptance Model (TAM) and the Unified Theory of Acceptance and Use of Technology (UTAUT). In addition, the application of the UTAUT2 model is described through a case study in Singapore that determined the factors which influenced the acceptability of mHealth-based adherence interventions among healthcare institutions in Singapore.

DOI: 10.4018/978-1-7998-3832-6.ch005

INTRODUCTION

As previously described in Chapter 3, the IM approach is a health behavior framework that prescribes a specific set of steps in the development of interventions, such as mHealth apps. The success of an app ultimately depends on the acceptance and usage by its target audience (Alkhaldi et al., 2016; Car, Tan, Huang, Sloot, & Franklin, 2017; Venkatesh, Thong, & Xu, 2016), such as patients for medication adherence apps. Therefore, in line with Step 5 of the IM approach (Chapter 3, Figure 4), developers should seek to gain an in-depth understanding of the factors that can influence patient acceptance of their mHealth app for adherence (Bartholomew, Parcel, Kok, Gottlieb, & Fernandez, 2011; Car, et al., 2017). It has been suggested that end users' acceptance of a technology-based health intervention can be studied through evaluation of their behavioral intention to use the intervention, which is a reliable predictor of actual use (Holden & Karsh, 2010). Although there is a paucity of information on the acceptability of medication adherence apps for chronic conditions, studies for other aspects of healthcare in various disease conditions suggest that apps generally have favorable acceptance among patients and healthcare professionals (Azevedo, Bernardes, Fonseca, & Lima, 2015; Berkowitz, Zullig, Koontz, & Smith, 2017; de Vries et al., 2018; K. A. Kessel, Vogel, Schmidt-Graf, & Combs, 2016; Kerstin Anne Kessel et al., 2017). These studies show that different socio-demographic characteristics, such as younger age and male gender (Azevedo, et al., 2015; Crilly et al., 2019; Kerstin Anne Kessel, et al., 2017), and prior use of mobile technologies (e.g. SMS or apps) (Azevedo, et al., 2015; de Vries, et al., 2018) can significantly influence patients' and healthcare professionals' interests in using or recommending the use of mHealth apps.

MODELS TO FACILITATE ADOPTION OF mHEALTH TECHNOLOGIES

The Technology Acceptance Model (TAM)

Apart from socio-demographics, a more in-depth analysis of the determinants of patients' acceptance of adherence apps is necessary to facilitate widespread adoption (Car, et al., 2017). This can be done by utilizing structured models such as Fred Davis' Technology Acceptance Model (TAM) (Becker, 2016; Car, et al., 2017; Davis, 1989; Lee & Han, 2015). Originated from the psychological theory of reasoned action (TRA) and theory of planned behavior (TPB), the TAM has been a model that has been used by various researchers to understand the predictors of human behavior towards an individual's acceptance (or rejection) of technology (Madden, Ellen, & Ajzen, 1992; Marangunić & Granić, 2014). Originally developed as a generic model for information systems, the TAM has since gained much attention in the health information technology acceptance literature (Davis, 1989; Holden & Karsh, 2010). In essence, the TRA suggested that behavioral intention was a predictor of one's actual behavior, and the intention mediated the influence of attitude on the behavior (Marangunić & Granić, 2014). In this theory, "attitude" was defined as a person's positive or negative evaluation of an object, was affective and based on a set of beliefs about the object of behavior (e.g. having a credit card is convenient) (Lai, 2017). Another factor that determined behavioral intention was the person's subjective norms (i.e. social pressures put on him/her) about engaging in the behavior (e.g. my peers use a credit card and it is a status symbol to have one) (Figure 1) (Lai, 2017; Marangunić & Granić, 2014). However, a major limitation of the TRA was the model's inability to deal with individuals who had little (or felt that they had little) control over their behaviors and attitudes (Ajzen; Marangunić & Granić, 2014). Thus, a third element of perceived behavioral control was added, resulting in a newer theory known as the TPB (Ajzen; Lai, 2017; Marangunić & Granić, 2014). The perceived behavior control element was the control that users perceived which might limit their behavior and would be informed by the individual's beliefs about the opportunities and resources needed to engage in the behavior (e.g. what are the requirements for applying for a credit card and am I eligible to apply?) (Ajzen; Lai, 2017; Marangunić & Granić, 2014).

When applied to users' acceptance of a technological system, these theories did not manage to explain the system acceptance or rejection. Hence, Fred Davis proposed the TAM through adaptation of the TRA and TPB, whereby he considered the actual use of the system as a behavior (Davis, 1985; Marangunić & Granić, 2014). The TAM had two main differences from the TRA and TPB. The first difference was the omission of subjective norm in predicting the actual behavior and only considered the person's attitude towards the behavior. The rationale for its omission was because no relevant perceived social norms would exist for the users of newly developed systems, since they would be encountering the system for the first time and thus would not be able to receive any cues from referents to draw any normative inferences

Figure 1. Schematic of the theory of reasoned action (TRA) showing the additional element (grey box) that resulted in the newer theory of planned behavior (TPB).
Adapted from Madden et al. (Madden, et al., 1992).

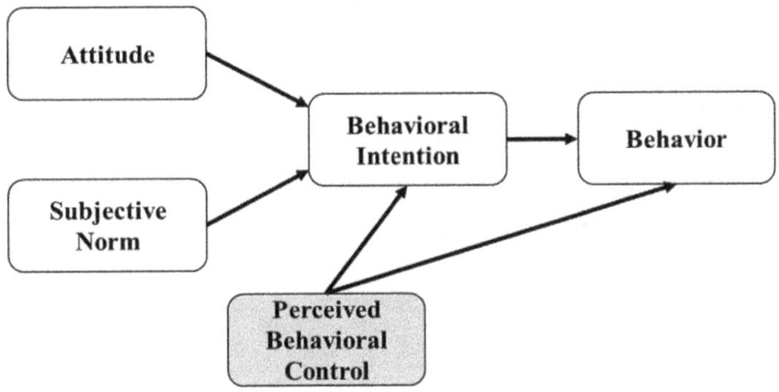

(Davis, 1985). Davis also proposed the omission of behavioral intention since the measurements of a person's motivation to use a new technological system would only take place after the system was demonstrated to the user. A behavioral intention would not have been formed prior to its measurement (i.e. absence of intention or when an individual had not decided either way) – a phenomenon he called "intention instability". He suggested that the users' attitude would predict the behavior better than their intention (Davis, 1985).

The second difference was the inclusion of two distinct beliefs that could predict the attitude of users towards their use of a system – perceived usefulness and perceived ease of use (Davis, 1985, 1989; Lai, 2017; Marangunić & Granić, 2014; Venkatesh & Bala, 2008). Perceived usefulness was the degree to which a user believed that the use of a particular system would improve his/her action or job performance. Perceived ease of use, on the other hand, referred to the degree to which the user believed that using the particular system would be free of effort. Davis hypothesized that perceived ease of use would directly influence the perceived usefulness, and both these beliefs would be directly influenced by the system design characteristics (Figure 2). However, it was found that attitude did not fully mediate perceived usefulness and perceived ease of use, but both these beliefs had a direct influence on behavioral intention. Therefore, a parsimonious TAM was suggested, whereby the attitude construct was removed from the model. The final TAM model added behavioral intention as a new variable, which was directly influenced by both perceived usefulness and perceived ease of use.

Another change that was brought to the original TAM was the addition of five external variables, which might influence the perceived usefulness

Figure 2. Technology Acceptance Model (TAM), showing the original TAM proposed by Davis (1985) and the final TAM version in which the attitude construct was removed, and behavioral intention was added as a new variable.
Adapted from Marangunić et al. (Marangunić & Granić, 2014) and (Lai, 2017).

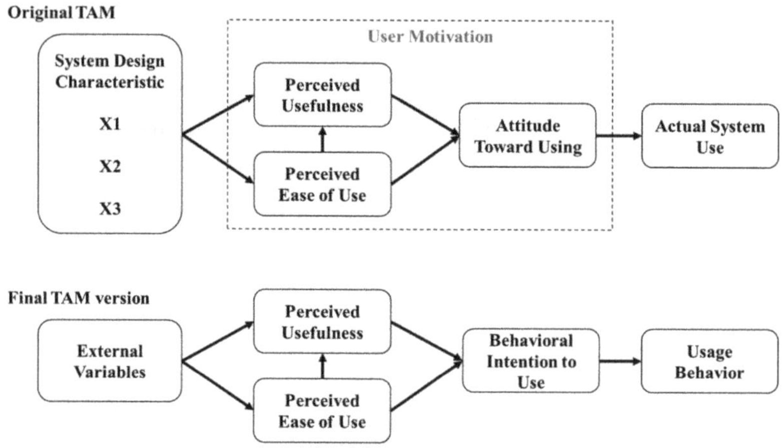

of the user of the technological system. This extended model was known as the TAM2 (Figure 3), which proposed that the user's perceived usefulness of the technology could be influenced by his/her mental assessment of the match between important work goals and the consequences of performing the job tasks using the technology (Lai, 2017). These variables included: (i) the others' influence on the user's decision on whether to use the technology (subjective norm); (ii) the user's desire to maintain a favorable standing among others (image); (iii) the degree to which the technology was applicable to the user's job (job relevance); (iv) the extent to which the technology adequately performed its intended purpose/ required tasks (output quality); and (v) the tangibility of the results produced by the technology (result demonstrability). Additionally, two moderating factors for subjective norm were also included – experience and voluntariness. Studies showed that TAM2 worked well in both voluntary and mandatory environments (Lai, 2017).

A more integrated model, known as the TAM3, was further proposed by Venkatesh and Bala by combining the TAM2 with the model of determinants of perceived ease of use (Lai, 2017; Venkatesh & Bala, 2008) (Figure 4 and Table 1). The latter model proposed that there were two main categories of determinants of perceived ease of use – anchors and adjustments. Anchor determinants would drive the initial judgments of perceived ease of use toward the new system based on the user's general beliefs regarding computers and

Figure 3. Technology Acceptance Model 2 (TAM2), showing the external variables and moderating factors influencing perceived usefulness and subjective norm.
Adapted from Marangunić et al. and Lai (Marangunić & Granić, 2014) and (Lai, 2017).

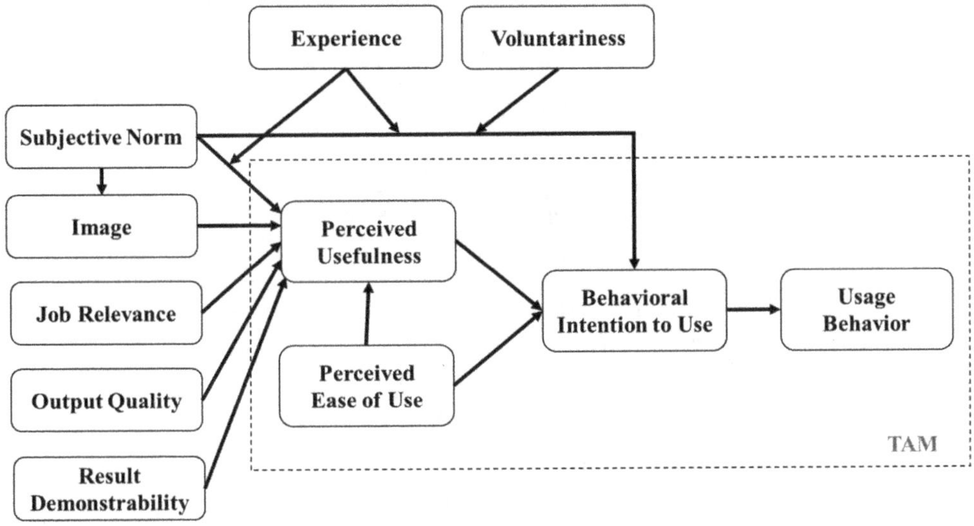

computer usage, while adjustment determinants would influence perceived ease of use after the user gains direct hands-on experience with the new system. The four anchors proposed were: (i) computer self-efficacy (i.e. user's control beliefs regarding his/her personal ability to use the system to perform specific tasks/job); (ii) computer anxiety (i.e. degree of user's apprehension and/or fear in using computers); (iii) computer playfulness (i.e. user's intrinsic motivation to use the system); and (iv) perceptions of external control (i.e. user's control beliefs on the organizational and technical resource availability to support the usage of the system). On the other hand, the two adjustments were: (i) perceived enjoyment (i.e. extent to which the user perceived the system to be enjoyable other than the performance consequences resulting from the usage of the system), and (ii) objective usability (i.e. the actual level of effort required to complete specific tasks with the system, rather than the user's perception). With increasing experience of the user with the new system, the roles of computer self-efficacy and perceptions of external control would continue to be strong, but the effects of computer anxiety and computer playfulness would diminish over time. Furthermore, the effects of adjustments on the user's perceived ease of use would be stronger with more hands-on experience with the new system.

Figure 4. Technology Acceptance Model 3 (TAM3), showing the combination of TAM2 (dotted lines) with the model of determinants of perceived ease of use.
Adapted from Venkatesh et al. and Lai (Venkatesh & Bala, 2008) and (Lai, 2017).

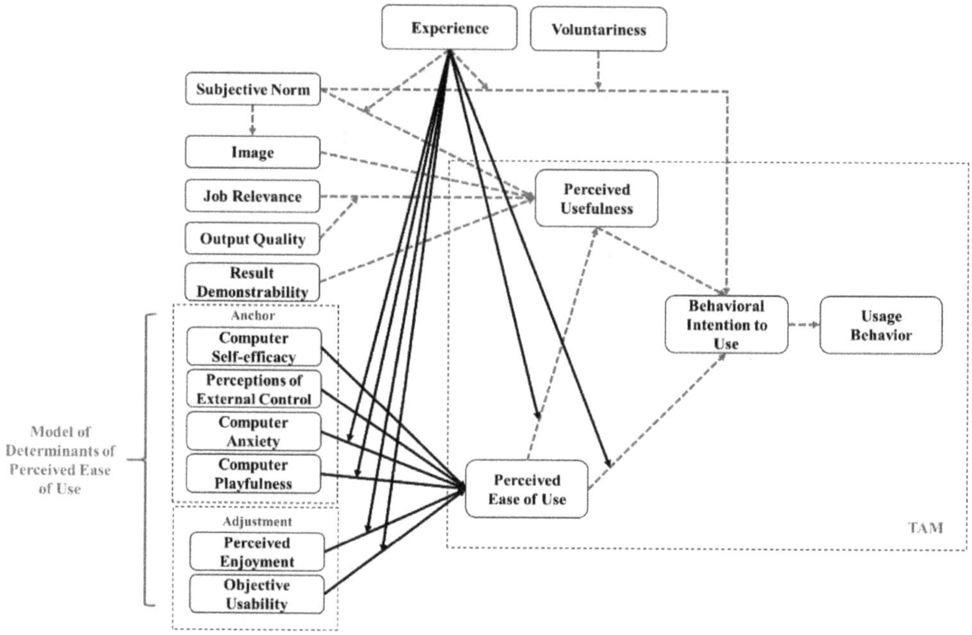

Arguably, the TAM has become one of the most influential theories for researchers studying the adoption of various technologies. Therefore, it is not surprising that this model has been extended through the introduction of new factors and variables from a vast number of studies (Marangunić & Granić, 2014). These include external predictors, factors from other theories of technology acceptance to increase the predictive validity of TAM, contextual factors that may have a moderating effect on TAM, and usage measures for operationalizing actual system usage (Figure 5). As technology advances in the era of digital health, there will no doubt be more studies that will explore the potential of the TAM in previously unexplored domains, in order to contribute to its predictive accuracy and applicability.

The Unified Theory Of Acceptance And Use Of Technology (Utaut) Model

The Unified Theory of Acceptance and Use of Technology (UTAUT) model is an extension of the TAM2 and is based on a review and synthesis of 8

Table 1. Definitions and measurement items of the various constructs of the Technology Acceptance Model 3 (TAM3).

Constructs	Definitions	Measurement Items*
Behavioral Intention	Individual's intention to perform a specific behavior	• Assuming I had access to the system, I intend to use it. • Given that I had access to the system, I predict that I would use it. • I plan to use the system in the next <n> months.
Use (Usage behavior)	Self-reported usage behavior	• On average, how much time do you spend on the system each day?
Perceived Usefulness	Degree to which a user believes that the use of a particular system will improve his/her action or job performance	• Using the system improves my performance in my job. • Using the system in my job increases my productivity. • Using the system enhances my effectiveness in my job. • I find the system to be useful in my job.
Determinants of Perceived Usefulness		
Perceived Ease of Use	Degree to which the user believes that using the system will be free of effort	• My interaction with the system is clear and understandable. • Interacting with the system does not require a lot of my mental effort. • I find the system to be easy to use. • I find it easy to get the system to do what I want it to do.
Subjective Norm	Others' influence on the user's decision on whether to use the system	• People who influence my behavior think that I should use the system. • People who are important to me think that I should use the system. • The senior management of this business has been helpful in the use of the system. • In general, the organization has supported the use of the system.
Image	User's desire to maintain a favorable social status standing among others	• People in my organization who use the system have more prestige than those who do not. • People in my organization who use the system have a high profile. • Having the system is a status symbol in my organization.
Job Relevance	Degree to which the user believes that the system is applicable to his/her job	• In my job, usage of the system is important. • In my job, usage of the system is relevant. • The use of the system is pertinent to my various job-related tasks.
Output Quality	Degree to which the system adequately performs its intended purpose/ required tasks	• The quality of the output I get from the system is high. • I have no problem with the quality of the system's output. • I rate the results from the system to be excellent.
Result Demonstrability	Tangibility of the results produced by the system	• I have no difficulty telling others about the results of using the system. • I believe I could communicate to others the consequences of using the system. • The results of using the system are apparent to me. • I would have difficulty explaining why using the system may or may not be beneficial.
Moderators of Perceived Usefulness		
Experience **	Hands-on experience with the specific system	-
Voluntariness	Degree of user's willingness to use the system	• My use of the system is voluntary. • My supervisor does not require me to use the system. • Although it might be helpful, using the system is certainly not compulsory in my job.
Determinants of Perceived Ease of Use		
Computer Self-Efficacy ⁺	Degree to which the user believes regarding his/her ability to use the system to perform a specific task/job	• I could complete the job using a software package if: o there was no one around to tell me what to do as I go. o I had just the built-in help facility for assistance. o someone showed me how to do it first. o I had used similar packages before this one to do the same job.
Perceptions of External Control	Degree to which the user believes that organizational and technical resources are available to support the usage of the system	• I have control over using the system. • I have the resources necessary to use the system. • Given the resources, opportunities and knowledge it takes to use the system, it would be easy for me to use the system. • The system is not compatible with other systems I use.

continued on following page

Table 1. Continued

Constructs	Definitions	Measurement Items*
Computer Anxiety	Degree of the user's apprehension and/or fear in using computers	• Computers do not scare me at all. • Working with a computer makes me nervous. • Computers make me feel uncomfortable. • Computers make me feel uneasy.
Computer Playfulness	Degree of the user's intrinsic motivation (or cognitive spontaneity) to use the system	• The following questions ask you how you would characterize yourself when you use computers: o spontaneous o creative o playful o unoriginal
Perceived Enjoyment	Degree to which the user perceives the system to be enjoyable other than the performance consequences resulting from the usage of the system	• I find using the system to be enjoyable. • The actual process of using the system is pleasant. • I have fun using the system.
Objective Usability ++	Comparison of systems based on the actual level of effort required to complete specific tasks with the system, rather than the user's perception	-

Adapted from Venkatesh et al. and Lai (Venkatesh & Bala, 2008) and (Lai, 2017).

* Generally, measurement items were based on a 7-point Likert scale (1: strongly disagree – 7: strongly agree).

** Experience was coded as an ordinal variable.

+Computer self-efficacy was based on a 10-point Guttman scale

++No specific items were used to measure objective usability. It was measured as a ratio of time spent by the user to the time spent by an expert on the same set of tasks.

theories/models of technology use (Venkatesh, Thong, & Xu, 2012). Originally conceived to predict the behavioral intention of technology use primarily in organizational contexts, the UTAUT model comprises of 4 key constructs that influence a user's behavioral intention to use a technology (Figure 6 and Table 2) (Lai, 2017; Venkatesh, et al., 2012). The first – performance expectancy – is the extent to which the usage of a technology will benefit the user in performing certain activities. Secondly, effort expectancy is the extent of ease associated with the user's technology use. Third is social influence, which is the extent to which the user's social circle (e.g. family and friends) influences their use of the technology. Lastly, facilitating conditions are the user's perceptions regarding the available support and resources to perform the use behavior. The first 3 constructs (i.e. performance expectancy, effort expectancy and social influence) influence the user's behavioral intention to use the technology, while the last construct (i.e. facilitating conditions) and behavioral intention determine the user's technology use behavior. In addition, there are 4 key moderators of age, gender, experience and voluntariness (Lai, 2017; Venkatesh, et al., 2012).

On the other hand, the UTAUT2 is developed as an extension to the original UTAUT so that the model can be tailored to a consumer use context (Venkatesh,

Figure 5. Four categories of modifications to the Technology Acceptance Model (TAM) from various studies.
Adapted from Marangunić et al. (Marangunić & Granić, 2014).

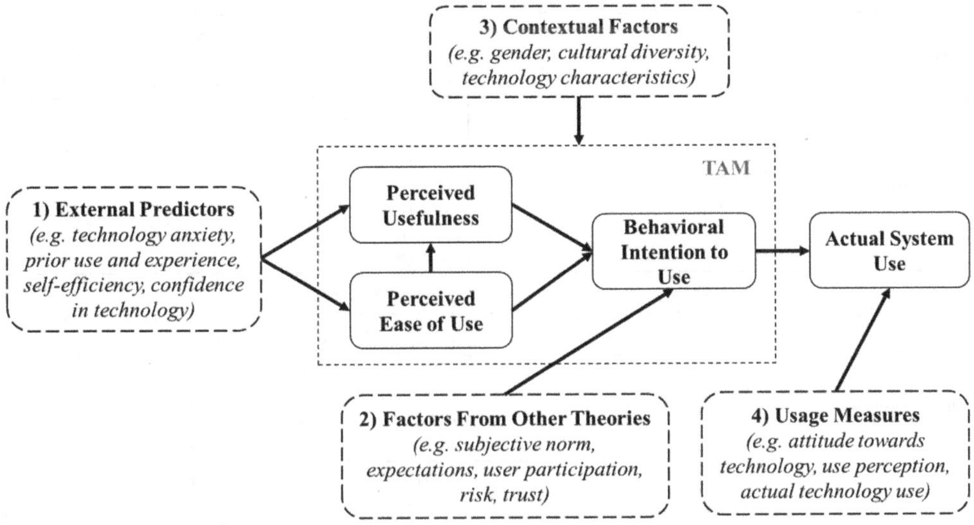

Figure 6. The Unified Theory of Acceptance and Use of Technology 2 (UTAUT2) model, encompassing the original version of UTAUT (shown as dotted lines).
Adapted from Venkatesh et al. (Venkatesh, Morris, Davis, & Davis, 2003) and (Venkatesh, et al., 2012).

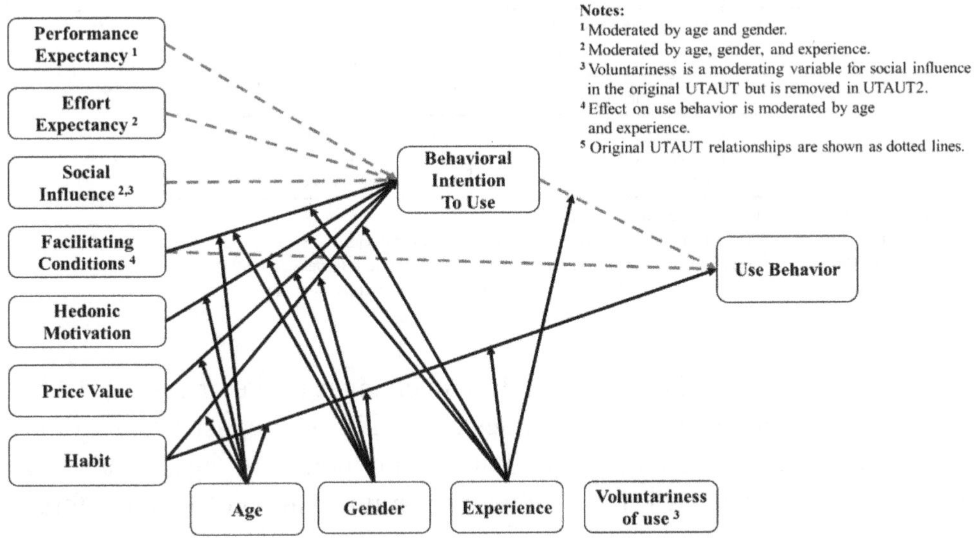

Table 2. Definitions and items used to estimate the Unified Theory of Acceptance and Use of Technology 2 (UTAUT2) on users of mobile Internet technology.

Constructs	Definitions	Items Used to Estimate UTAUT2 *
Behavioral Intention	Individual's intention to use a technology	• I intend to continue using mobile Internet in the future. • I will always try to use mobile Internet in my daily life. • I plan to continue to use mobile Internet frequently.
Use Behavior **	Self-reported usage behavior	• Please choose your usage frequency for each of the following: o SMS o MMS o Ringtone and logo download o Java games o Browse websites o Mobile e-mail
Performance Expectancy	Degree to which the usage of a technology will benefit the user in performing certain activities	• I find mobile Internet useful in my daily life. • Using mobile Internet helps me accomplish things more quickly. • Using mobile Internet increases my productivity.
Effort Expectancy	Degree of ease associated with the user's technology use	• Learning how to use mobile Internet is easy for me. • My interaction with mobile Internet is clear and understandable. • I find mobile Internet easy to use. • It is easy for me to become skilful at using mobile Internet.
Social Influence	Degree to which the user's social circle influences their use of the technology	• People who are important to me think that I should use mobile Internet. • People who influence my behavior think that I should use mobile Internet. • People whose opinions that I value prefer that I use mobile Internet.
Facilitating Conditions	User's perceptions regarding the available support and resources to perform the use behavior	• I have the resources necessary to use mobile Internet. • I have the knowledge necessary to use mobile Internet. • Mobile Internet is compatible with other technologies I use. • I can get help from others when I have difficulties using mobile Internet.
Hedonic Motivation	The fun or pleasure derived from using a technology	• Using mobile Internet is: o fun. o enjoyable. o very entertaining.
Price Value	The cognitive trade-off between the user's perceived benefits of the technology and the monetary value of using it	• Mobile Internet is reasonably priced. • Mobile Internet is a good value for the money. • At the current price, mobile Internet provides a good value.
Habit	Degree to which the user performs a behavior automatically due to learning	• The use of mobile Internet has become a habit for me. • I am addicted to using mobile Internet. • I must use mobile Internet.

Adapted from Venkatesh et al. (Venkatesh, et al., 2012).
* Generally, items were measured based on a 7-point Likert scale (strongly disagree – strongly agree).
** Use was measured as a composite index of variety and frequency of mobile Internet use.
Frequency was based on a 7-point Likert scale ranging from "never" to "many times per day".

et al., 2012). In particular, there are 3 main changes to the original UTAUT model. Firstly, the UTAUT2 comprises of 3 additional constructs (hedonic motivation, price value and habit) that are moderated by age, gender and experience (Figure 6 and Table 2). Hedonic (or intrinsic) motivation refers to the fun or pleasure derived from using a technology (i.e. perceived enjoyment) and has been found to influence the acceptance and use of technology in the consumer context. Price value refers to the cognitive trade-off between the user's perceived benefits of the technology and the monetary value of using it. The price value construct has a significant impact on consumers' technology use because unlike in the organizational context whereby employees do not have to bear the monetary cost of using the technology, consumers generally have to bear this cost themselves. Habit refers to the degree to which the user performs a behavior automatically due to learning. Secondly, voluntariness has been removed as a moderating variable because it was theorized that most consumer behaviors are completely voluntary, thus there is no variance in the voluntariness construct. Lastly, another direct relationship has been added from facilitating conditions to behavioral intention on top of the existing relationship between facilitating conditions and technology use behavior.

Models Used By Studies To Evaluate Acceptance Of mHealth Technologies

Studies that used TAM-based models to evaluate acceptance of mHealth have confirmed their predictive powers (Holden & Karsh, 2010; Lim et al., 2011; Rai, Chen, Pye, & Baird, 2013; Sun, Wang, Guo, & Peng, 2013; Xue et al., 2012). In some cases, the studies included constructs from health behavior-related models such as the health belief model, theory of planned behavior and protection motivation theory in addition to the known constructs in the TAM and its variants (Rai, et al., 2013; Sun, et al., 2013). The studies varied in terms of the constructs that were identified as predictors of intention to use mHealth. However, the most commonly reported constructs were performance expectancy (perceived usefulness), effort expectancy (perceived ease of use), subjective norm, self-efficacy, personal innovativeness towards mobile services, perceived healthiness and perceived vulnerability to chronic disease (Lim, et al., 2011; Rai, et al., 2013; Sun, et al., 2013; Xue, et al., 2012).

ACCEPTABILITY OF mHEALTH ADHERENCE INTERVENTIONS AMONG HEALTHCARE PROFESSIONALS: CASE STUDY OF PHARMACISTS IN SINGAPORE

In the context of app-based adherence interventions, it is crucial to secure the support of pharmacy managers, informatics pharmacists and other senior pharmacists for the successful deployment of the app. While there are studies showing the acceptance of mHealth interventions by healthcare professionals, there is a paucity of information about their acceptance of adherence apps (Berkowitz, et al., 2017; de Vries, et al., 2018; K. A. Kessel, et al., 2016). Furthermore, there is a dearth of information regarding pharmacy managers' and pharmacists' opinions about adherence apps and the factors that influence their deployment in the context of healthcare institutions in Singapore.

A cross-sectional survey aimed to identify healthcare professional's acceptance of mobile app-based adherence interventions was conducted among pharmacy managers, senior pharmacists and informatics pharmacists working in different healthcare facilities in Singapore. The questionnaire was designed to include sections on socio-demographic characteristics; services provided to improve medication adherence and level of technology usage; acceptance of app-based interventions for medication adherence and the barriers to adoption/continued use of adherence apps. The section on acceptance of adherence apps contained questions adapted from the UTAUT2 (Venkatesh, et al., 2012). The respondents' acceptance of adherence apps was measured using one item asking their intentions to recommend the implementation/ continued usage of such apps at their institutions. The use of only one of the three items in the behavioral intention construct in UTAUT2 was helpful in improving the clarity of the questions. This was in line with studies, which reported that the use of three items as part of the construct could be confusing to respondents (Ortega Egea & Román González, 2011).

In order to adapt to the nature of the study population, the UTAUT2 constructs that were focused on individuals and difficult to translate to organization-level decision making, such as hedonic motivation (e.g. using app is fun, enjoyable, very entertaining) and habit (e.g. use of app has become a habit for me, I am addicted to using apps; I must use app) were excluded. In contrast, additional constructs on respondents' attitudes towards the use of adherence apps and their perceived organizational intentions to implement or continue the use of adherence apps were added. This was done in order to better understand the respondents' reasons for their acceptance of adherence apps in patient care. For all items, participants were required to rate their degree of agreement on a scale of 1 (strongly disagree) to 5 (strongly agree). The last section of the questionnaire focused on the barriers to adoption of adherence apps.

The response rate of the study was 88.2% (97 out of 110 surveys). The proportion of senior pharmacists, pharmacy managers and informatics

Table 3. Adherence programmes provided by respondents' institutions. (N=97)

Components of the Intervention	n	(%)
Patient education and counselling		
Face-to-face education by a pharmacist	65	(67.0)
Printed educational materials	49	(50.5)
Behavioural counselling by a pharmacist	26	(26.8)
Motivational interviewing by a pharmacist	21	(21.6)
Web-based educational interventions	4	(4.1)
Number of institutions using one or more interventions in this category	**67**	**(69.1)**
Dose organisers and tailoring to daily routines		
Tailoring medication regimen to patients' lifestyle	30	(30.9)
Pillboxes	24	(24.7)
Daily dose blister packaging	22	(22.7)
Number of institutions using one or more interventions in this category	**46**	**(47.4)**
Support mechanisms for patients		
Involving patients' family in managing adherence	42	(43.3)
Support groups directed at adherence	1	(1.0)
Number of institutions using one or more interventions in this category	**42**	**(43.3)**
Telepharmacy-based		
Phone call-based monitoring and support	18	(18.6)
Phone call-based education by a pharmacist	16	(16.5)
Smartphone app	10	(10.3)
Reminder phone calls	6	(6.2)
SMS reminders	3	(3.1)
Video call	1	(1.0)
Number of institutions using one or more interventions in this category	**35**	**(36.1)**

pharmacists were 56.7%, 25.8% and 17.5% respectively. Majority were from

Table 4. Currently available health apps and future priorities in the respondents' health facilities.

Purpose of the App	Respondents With Health Apps at Their Institution (n = 41)		Priorities for Future Apps (n = 42) *					
			1st		2nd		3rd	
	n	(%)	n	(%)	n	(%)	n	(%)
Provide information *(Medication, disease, healthy living)*	26	(63.4)	5	(11.9)	10	(23.8)	11	(26.2)
Filling prescription *(Finding pharmacy, price comparisons, processing refill)*	16	(39.0)	28	(66.7)	5	(11.9)	1	(2.4)
Finding healthcare facility/ clinician and managing appointment	16	(39.0)	-		-		1	(2.4)
Medication adherence	10	(24.4)	5	(11.9)	14	(33.3)	9	(21.4)
Healthy living *(Monitoring diet; exercise, sleep)*	9	(22.0)	-		2	(4.8)	3	(7.1)
Symptom checking and self-diagnosis	4	(9.8)	1	(2.4)	-		-	
Management of medication side-effects	3	(7.3)	-		2	(4.8)	4	(9.5)
Monitoring of treatment outcomes	1	(2.4)	1	(2.4)	-		-	
Smoking cessation	-		2	(4.8)	-		-	

* Percentages were calculated based on 42 of the 53 respondents who indicated the priority areas for future apps at their institutions.

the public sector (87.6%), while the rest were from private and other non-governmental sectors (12.4%). A total of 70 respondents (72.2%) reported having one or more programs for promoting patient medication adherence. Most of the respondents (69.1%) mentioned the use of programs involving educational and counselling-based interventions. Interestingly, majority of the programs were non-digital. Digital interventions were only reported by 4.1% of the respondents (Table 3).

Telepharmacy-based programs (those involving telephone/ mobile/ smartphone-based interventions) were reported by 35 (36.1%) of the respondents. Only 10 (10.3%) mentioned the use of smartphone apps for adherence. The main features of the adherence apps were medication information (8/10, 80.0%), reminders (7/10, 70.0%) and medication list (7/10, 70.0%). Less than half (41, 42.3%) of the respondents indicated that their institutions offered one or more types of health apps for patients (Table 4). The highly mentioned purposes of these apps were the provision of medication, disease and/or health information (26, 63.4%), support for prescription filling (16, 39.0%) and finding health facilities (16, 39.0%). Over half (53, 54.6%) indicated plans to develop a health app in the next two years. The top three priority areas were helping patients fill their prescriptions (28/42, 66.7%), followed by medication adherence and provision of health-related and medication-related information (5/42, 11.9% each). Other priority areas included support for smoking cessation (2/42, 4.8%), symptom checking and self-diagnosis, and monitoring of treatment outcomes (1/42, 2.4% each).

It has been suggested that app-based interventions for improving adherence should include multiple features that address the various factors associated with medication non-adherence (Ali, Teo, Goh, Chew, & Yap, 2018; Dayer et al., 2017). Similar to the current trends in the global app market, the features of adherence apps employed at the respondents' institutions were generally limited to reminders, keeping medication list and provision of medication information (Ali, Teo, et al., 2018). This was in contrast to patient demands for features that enabled the monitoring and self-management of side-effects and adherence behavior (Ali, Leow, Chew, & Yap, 2018).

Acceptance of adherence apps was measured based on respondents' intentions to recommend the implementation of such apps at their health facilities. Accordingly, the median level of intention to recommend implementation or continued utilization of adherence apps was 4.0 (interquartile range, IQR: 3.0 – 4.0) on a scale of 1 (strongly disagree) to 5 (strongly agree). Respondents' intention (median: 4.0, IQR: 3.0 – 4.0) was significantly correlated with their performance expectancy (median: 3.7, IQR: 3.3 – 4.0, $r=0.41$; $p<0.001$), social influence (median: 3.3, IQR: 3.0 – 3.7, $r=0.55$; $p<0.001$), attitude (median: 4.0, IQR: 3.3 – 4.0, $r=0.49$; $p<0.001$), and perceived organizational intention to implement or continue using adherence apps (median: 3.0, IQR: 2.0 – 4.0, $r=0.57$; $p<0.001$). These findings were consistent with the predictions of the UTAUT2 and studies in healthcare and other settings (Hernández, Jiménez, & Martín, 2008; Holden & Karsh, 2010; Venkatesh, et al., 2012). This showed the need to ensure that pharmacists appreciated the usefulness of new adherence interventions for patients (Holden & Karsh, 2010). Respondents' perceived effort expectancy (median: 3.0, IQR: 3.0 – 4.0, $r=0.24$; $p=0.020$) and the existence of facilitating factors (median: 3.3, IQR: 2.8 – 3.5, $r=0.30$; $p=0.004$) were also weakly correlated with their intentions to recommend the use of adherence apps.

Respondents' also had statistically significant differences in their scores for intention to recommend the implementation or continued use of an adherence app based on their practice setting (mean ranks 50.3 [public] versus 26.5 [private], p=0.003) and type of facility (mean ranks 52.6 [general hospital] versus 34.3 [speciality centre], p=0.048). This study also showed that the most frequently mentioned barriers to the implementation of adherence apps in their institutions were the difficulty of integrating adherence apps with current dispensing systems (76, 78.4%), lack of funding (68, 70.1%), low technology literacy levels of patients (64, 66.0%), and the high costs of implementing adherence apps (62, 63.9%). These findings reiterate the importance of addressing the needs of end users' in the design and implementation of adherence apps.

In conclusion, this study showed that adherence apps were not commonly used in health facilities in Singapore. Moreover, the available apps mainly focused on the provision of medication information and reminders. However, there was a positive acceptance of adherence apps as measured by the pharmacists' expressed intentions to recommend their use in their institutions. Future developments in medication management apps should consider including tele-monitoring and tele-support components in addition to the current focus on the facilitation of prescription filling.

REFERENCES

Ajzen, I. (n.d.). From intentions to actions: A theory of planned behavior. In J. Kuhl & J. Beckmann (Eds.), *Action Control. SSSP Springer Series in Social Psychology* (pp. 11–39). Berlin: Springer. doi:10.1007/978-3-642-69746-3_2

Ali, E. E., Leow, J. L., Chew, L., & Yap, K. Y. (2018). Patients' perception of app-based educational and behavioural interventions for enhancing oral anticancer medication adherence. *Journal of Cancer Education*, *33*(6), 1306–1313. doi:10.100713187-017-1248-x PMID:28707206

Ali, E. E., Teo, A. K. S., Goh, S. X. L., Chew, L., & Yap, K. Y. (2018). MedAd-AppQ: A quality assessment tool for medication adherence apps on iOS and android platforms. *Research in Social & Administrative Pharmacy*, *14*(12), 1125–1133. doi:10.1016/j.sapharm.2018.01.006 PMID:29402755

Alkhaldi, G., Hamilton, F. L., Lau, R., Webster, R., Michie, S., & Murray, E. (2016). The effectiveness of prompts to promote engagement with digital interventions: A systematic seview. *Journal of Medical Internet Research*, *18*(1), e6. doi:10.2196/jmir.4790 PMID:26747176

Azevedo, R., Bernardes, M., Fonseca, J., & Lima, A. (2015). Smartphone application for rheumatoid arthritis self-management: Cross-sectional study revealed the usefulness, willingness to use and patients' needs. *Rheumatology International*, *35*(10), 1675–1685. doi:10.100700296-015-3270-9 PMID:25903352

Bartholomew, L. K., Parcel, G. S., Kok, G., Gottlieb, N. H., & Fernandez, M. E. (2011). *Planning Health Promotion Programs: An Intervention Mapping Approach* (3rd ed.). San Francisco, CA: Jossey-Bass.

Becker, D. (2016). Acceptance of mobile mental health treatment applications. *Procedia Computer Science*, *98*, 220–227. doi:10.1016/j.procs.2016.09.036

Berkowitz, C. M., Zullig, L. L., Koontz, B. F., & Smith, S. K. (2017). Prescribing an app? Oncology providers' views on mobile health apps for cancer care. *JCO Clinical Cancer Informatics*, *1*(1), 1–7. doi:10.1200/CCI.17.00107 PMID:30657404

Car, J., Tan, W. S., Huang, Z., Sloot, P., & Franklin, B. D. (2017). eHealth in the future of medications management: Personalisation, monitoring and adherence. *BMC Medicine*, *15*(1), 73. doi:10.118612916-017-0838-0 PMID:28376771

Crilly, P., Hassanali, W., Khanna, G., Matharu, K., Patel, D., Patel, D., ... Kayyali, R. (2019). Community pharmacist perceptions of their role and the use of social media and mobile health applications as tools in public health. *Research in Social & Administrative Pharmacy*, *15*(1), 23–30. doi:10.1016/j.sapharm.2018.02.005 PMID:29501431

Davis, F. D. (1985). *A technology acceptance model for empirically testing new end-user information systems: Theory and results* (PhD Thesis). Massachusetts Institute of Technology. Retrieved from https://dspace.mit.edu/bitstream/handle/1721.1/15192/14927137-MIT.pdf

Davis, F. D. (1989). Perceived usefulness, perceived ease of use, and user acceptance of information technology. *Management Information Systems Quarterly*, *13*(3), 319–339. doi:10.2307/249008

Dayer, L. E., Shilling, R., Van Valkenburg, M., Martin, B. C., Gubbins, P. O., Hadden, K., & Heldenbrand, S. (2017). Assessing the medication adherence app marketplace from the health professional and consumer vantage points. *JMIR mHealth and uHealth*, *5*(4), e45. doi:10.2196/mhealth.6582 PMID:28428169

de Vries, S. T., Denig, P., Lasheras Ruiz, C., Houyez, F., Wong, L., Sutcliffe, A., & Mol, P. G. M. (2018). Interest in a mobile app for two-way risk communication: A survey study among European healthcare professionals and patients. *Drug Safety*, *41*(7), 697–712. doi:10.100740264-018-0648-0 PMID:29500800

Hernández, B., Jiménez, J., & Martín, M. J. (2008). Extending the technology acceptance model to include the IT decision-maker: A study of business management software. *Technovation*, *28*(3), 112–121. doi:10.1016/j.technovation.2007.11.002

Holden, R. J., & Karsh, B. T. (2010). The technology acceptance model: Its past and its future in health care. *Journal of Biomedical Informatics*, *43*(1), 159–172. doi:10.1016/j.jbi.2009.07.002 PMID:19615467

Kessel, K. A., Vogel, M. M., Schmidt-Graf, F., & Combs, S. E. (2016). Mobile apps in oncology: A survey on health care professionals' attitude toward telemedicine, mHealth, and oncological apps. *Journal of Medical Internet Research*, *18*(11), e312. doi:10.2196/jmir.6399 PMID:27884810

Kessel, K. A., Vogel, M. M. E., Kessel, C., Bier, H., Biedermann, T., Friess, H., ... Combs, S. E. (2017). Mobile health in oncology: A patient survey about app-assisted cancer care. *JMIR mHealth and uHealth*, *5*(6), e81. doi:10.2196/mhealth.7689 PMID:28615159

Lai, P. C. (2017). The literature review of technology adoption models and theories for the novelty technology. *Journal of Information Systems and Technology Management*, *14*(1), 21–38. doi:10.4301/S1807-17752017000100002

Lee, E., & Han, S. (2015). Determinants of adoption of mobile health services. *Online Information Review*, *39*(4), 556–573. doi:10.1108/OIR-01-2015-0007

Lim, S., Xue, L., Yen, C. C., Chang, L., Chan, H. C., Tai, B. C., ... Choolani, M. (2011). A study on Singaporean women's acceptance of using mobile phones to seek health information. *International Journal of Medical Informatics*, *80*(12), e189–e202. doi:10.1016/j.ijmedinf.2011.08.007 PMID:21956003

Madden, T. J., Ellen, P. S., & Ajzen, I. (1992). A comparison of the theory of planned behavior and the theory of reasoned action. *Personality and Social Psychology Bulletin, 18*(1), 3–9. doi:10.1177/0146167292181001

Marangunić, N., & Granić, A. (2014). Technology acceptance model: A literature review from 1986 to 2013. *Universal Access in the Information Society, 14*(1), 81–95. doi:10.100710209-014-0348-1

Ortega Egea, J. M., & Román González, M. V. (2011). Explaining physicians' acceptance of EHCR systems: An extension of TAM with trust and risk factors. *Computers in Human Behavior, 27*(1), 319–332. doi:10.1016/j.chb.2010.08.010

Rai, A., Chen, L., Pye, J., & Baird, A. (2013). Understanding determinants of consumer mobile health usage intentions, assimilation, and channel preferences. *Journal of Medical Internet Research, 15*(8), e149. doi:10.2196/jmir.2635 PMID:23912839

Sun, Y., Wang, N., Guo, X., & Peng, Z. (2013). Understanding the acceptance of mobile health services: A comparison and integration of alternative models. *Journal of Electronic Commerce Research, 14*(2), 183–199.

Venkatesh, V., & Bala, H. (2008). Technology Acceptance Model 3 and a research agenda on interventions. *Decision Sciences, 39*(2), 273–315. doi:10.1111/j.1540-5915.2008.00192.x

Venkatesh, V., Morris, M. G., Davis, G. B., & Davis, F. D. (2003). User acceptance of information technology: Toward a unified view. *Management Information Systems Quarterly, 27*(3), 425–478. doi:10.2307/30036540

Venkatesh, V., Thong, J. Y. L., & Xu, X. (2012). Consumer acceptance and use of information technology: Extending the unified theory of acceptance and use of technology. *Management Information Systems Quarterly, 36*(1), 157–178. doi:10.2307/41410412

Venkatesh, V., Thong, J. Y. L., & Xu, X. (2016). Unified theory of acceptance and use of technology: A synthesis and the road ahead. *Journal of the Association for Information Systems, 17*(5), 328–376. doi:10.17705/1jais.00428

Xue, L., Yen, C. C., Chang, L., Chan, H. C., Tai, B. C., Tan, S. B., ... Choolani, M. (2012). An exploratory study of ageing women's perception on access to health informatics via a mobile phone-based intervention. *International Journal of Medical Informatics*, *81*(9), 637–648. doi:10.1016/j.ijmedinf.2012.04.008 PMID:22658778

Chapter 6
Application of Health Behavior Frameworks in the Design of an Oral Anticancer Medication Adherence App

ABSTRACT

This chapter describes the application of the Intervention Mapping (IM) framework through a case study of the development of an in-house medication adherence mHealth app for oral anticancer medications (called MedFC). Using the behavioral intervention frameworks described previously, this chapter discusses how patients' medication adherence needs, mobile app usage, perceptions and experiences with the prototype helped inform the development of MedFC. Through iterative evaluations, this chapter will illustrate how a mHealth intervention can be developed in a holistic manner, involving its target audience in the design process.

INTRODUCTION

The advancement of smartphone technologies and its ubiquitous distribution in various parts of the world have presented a great opportunity for effective interventions that can be used to address patients' needs (E. E. Ali, Leow, Chew, & Yap, 2018; Car, Tan, Huang, Sloot, & Franklin, 2017; Deloitte, 2015; Haase, Farris, & Dorsch, 2017; Pew Research Center, 2016; Spoelstra

DOI: 10.4018/978-1-7998-3832-6.ch006

& Sansoucie, 2015). This has resulted in a plethora of apps that have targeted medication adherence, but majority of these apps have deficiencies that limit their usefulness for patients with medication adherence issues (E. E. Ali, Teo, Goh, Chew, & Yap, 2018; L. E. Dayer et al., 2017; Santo et al., 2016). One of the reasons for the suboptimal quality of these apps is because of the lack of involvement from potential end-users in the development process (Ahmed et al., 2018). There are limited studies in the literature on what makes an ideal adherence app. Research work done in this domain have either focused on specific aspects of interventions (e.g. side-effect management, education) (Hsu et al., 2017), or only provided a listing of potentially relevant app features (E. E. Ali, Leow, et al., 2018; Fishbein et al., 2017). Although studies have suggested that the usability and relevance of an mHealth app is greatly impacted by the way the health or drug information is presented to patients (Fraccaro et al., 2018; Groshek, Oldenburg, Sarasohn-Kahn, & Sitler, 2015), there is little work being done to identify the details of the app interface design. This chapter discusses how health behavior frameworks can be applied through a case example of the design requirements of a medication adherence app prototype for oral anticancer medications (OAMs), known as MedFC (E. E. Ali et al., 2019; E. E. Ali, Leow, et al., 2018). This app was developed for use by clinicians to monitor patients with cancer and on multiple medications. The system utilized near-field communication (NFC) technologies for medication labeling, and was designed to have different features with separate interfaces for clinicians, patients and caregivers (E.E. Ali et al., 2016).

MedFC was developed in accordance to IM framework, BIT-Tech, and UCD theory (E. E. Ali, Chan, Leow, Chew, & Yap, 2019; E. E. Ali, Chan, Poh, et al., 2019). The IM approach advocated an iterative process that involved six essential steps in the development of theory-based and evidence-based behavioral interventions (Please refer to Chapter 3, Figure 4) (Bartholomew, Parcel, Kok, Gottlieb, & Fernandez, 2011; Kok, 2014). Components of the BIT model that complemented the IM approach, particularly with respect to the technical instantiation of theory-based interventions, were consulted. More specifically, the development process described in this section matched with the first four steps of the IM approach and the BIT-Tech components of the BIT model.

USER INVOLVEMENT IN MEDFC DEVELOPMENT

In order to improve the quality and usability of MedFC, the UCD theory was adopted, which involved target end users at every stage of the development. Starting from the needs assessment phase, reasons for non-adherence and preferred strategies to help improve adherence were sought from patients with cancer on OAMs. The feedback from users were used to inform the design of MedFC through the adaptation of the relevant behavioral intervention strategies. Moreover, target end users were involved in the iterative testing phase of MedFC to determine the usability of the its user interface and features, and its acceptability among patients and caregivers.

STEPS IN THE DEVELOPMENT AND EVALUATION OF MEDFC

Step 1: Needs Assessment

As part of the needs assessment phase of MedFC, the target population and target behavior for the intervention was defined. The target population were patients who were taking OAMs. The process of needs assessment was informed by existing systematic reviews from the literature, which identified major determinants of OAM adherence (Greer et al., 2016; Verbrugghe, Verhaeghe, Lauwaert, Beeckman, & Van Hecke, 2013). In order to obtain context-specific information on the beliefs of patients in the context of Singapore, a series of surveys were conducted through semi-structured interviews with patients taking oral adjuvant endocrine therapies (OAETs) (Eskinder Eshetu Ali et al., 2017), capecitabine (Foo, Ali, Sia, Yap, & Chew, 2016) and epidermal growth factor receptor (EGFR) tyrosine kinase inhibitors (TKIs) (Shen, Ali, & Chew, 2017) at a local multidisciplinary cancer care facility in Singapore, which treated ~70% of the public sector cancer cases (Tan, 2017). The questionnaires were designed to obtain participants': (a) demographics, (b) therapy-related information, (c) medication adherence levels, (d) reasons for non-adherence, and (e) preferred strategies to help improve medication adherence. In these studies, patients with a total score of 4 were deemed to have high adherence levels, while scores of 3 points and 2 or less points indicated moderate and low levels of adherence respectively, based on the four-item Morisky medication adherence scale (MMAS-4) (Lavsa, Holzworth, & Ansani, 2011; Morisky &

DiMatteo, 2011). Through multivariate analyses, the authors identified that the odds of OAET adherence were almost three times higher in patients who reported having one or more comorbidities (adjusted odds ratio (OR) = 2.797, 95% confidence interval (CI) = 1.266 – 6.179) compared to those who did not have chronic conditions other than cancer. Capecitabine adherence was lower by 53% among participants who had known their cancer diagnosis for two years or more (adjusted OR = 0.470, 95% CI = 0.234 – 0.945) compared to those with lesser duration since diagnosis. Moreover, participants' living arrangement and the number of years of taking EGFR TKIs were found to significantly predict adherence – patients who lived with family or someone else were almost 13 times more likely to be adherent (adjusted OR = 12.770, 95% CI = 2.005 – 81.345) than those who lived alone. In contrast, patients who had been taking their EGFR TKIs for more than two years had almost 70% lesser odds of being adherent (adjusted OR = 0.288, 95% CI = 0.10 – 0.834).

From the studies, patients' reasons for non-adherence were also identified (Table 1). Forgetfulness was the top cited reason in all the three studies (67.7% of patients taking OAET (Eskinder Eshetu Ali, et al., 2017); 75.7% of patients taking capecitabine (Foo, et al., 2016) and 57.1% of patients on EGFR TKIs (Shen, et al., 2017)). The authors postulated that forgetfulness as a reason for non-adherence could indicate an underlying problem in the patients' behavioral skills in maintaining optimal adherence and their perception of the benefits of the medications (Irwin & Johnson, 2015; Lacey, Cate, & Broadway, 2009; Moon, Moss-Morris, Hunter, & Hughes, 2017). It was probable that patients might find it easier and more convenient to report "forgetting" to take their medicines, since it was a more socially desirable answer than reporting an intentional action not to take their medications (Atkins & Fallowfield, 2006).

The second most common reason was related to patients wanting to prevent medication side-effects (Table 1), which was similar to other adherence studies in cancer patients (Irwin & Johnson, 2015; Timmers et al., 2014; Yagasaki, Komatsu, & Takahashi, 2015). The long duration of therapy was cited as an equally important reason for non-adherence by patients taking OAET. Other reasons for non-adherence included patients' perceptions that the medications did not work, and the consumption of multiple medications (i.e. polypharmacy), among others. Interestingly, patients on capecitabine found it difficult to integrate their medication-taking behavior with their daily routines. On the other hand, patients on OAETs were non-adherent as they felt less empowered in their medication-taking behavior because they were excluded from the decision-making process.

Table 1. Patients' reasons for not taking their medications as prescribed.

Reasons for Non-adherence	OAET (n = 93)		Capecitabine (n = 74)		EGFR TKI (n = 21)	
	n	(%)*	n	(%)*	n	(%)*
Forget to take medications	63	(67.7)	56	(75.7)	12	(57.1)
Feeling worse when taking medication or wanting to prevent side-effects	18	(19.4)	20	(27.0)	4	(19.0)
Too long duration of therapy	18	(19.4)	2	(2.7)		--
Perception that the medications do not work	8	(8.6)	2	(2.7)	1	(4.8)
Taking too many medications	7	(7.5)	2	(2.7)		--
Do not need to take medication	3	(3.2)	3	(4.1)		--
Nobody checking on me	4	(4.3)	1	(1.4)		--
Do not understand verbal/written instructions	4	(4.3)	2	(2.7)	3	(14.3)
Difficulty in integrating with daily routines		--	5	(6.8)		--
Do not know how the medication works	4	(4.3)		--	1	(4.8)
Did not take part in making the decision to use the medication	3	(3.2)		--		--
Medications are too expensive	2	(2.2)		--		--
Fail to refill in time					2	(9.5)

*Percentages do not add up to 100% because a respondent could give more than one reason for non-adherence.

The reasons for non-adherence behavior in the 3 patient groups could be mapped onto the information, motivation, behavioral skills (IMB) theory, which was categorized into 3 constructs – information, motivation and behavioral skills (Figure 1). In this model, the information construct comprised of both behavior-related information and heuristics that could affect behavior-related decision making (e.g. patient's lack of knowledge on how the medication works and lack of understanding regarding the medication instructions) (S. J. Chang, Choi, Kim, & Song, 2014). On the other hand, the motivation construct comprised of personal motivation (such as attitudes toward particular health behaviors and beliefs about the intervention outcomes) and social motivation factors (including perceived social norms or support to engage in particular behaviors). For example, the patient's perception that the medications do not work, and the perceived lack of social support would de-motivate him to be adherent to his OAMs. Lastly, the behavioral skills construct represented various skills needed to perform particular health behaviors, such as difficulty of integrating medication-taking behavior with daily routines, failing to refill medications on time, patient's confusion with too many medications, and difficulties managing side-effects. All these factors

Figure 1. Integrating participants' reasons for non-adherence to the IMB model.
Adapted from the model by Fisher et al. (Fisher, Fisher, & Harman, 2003).

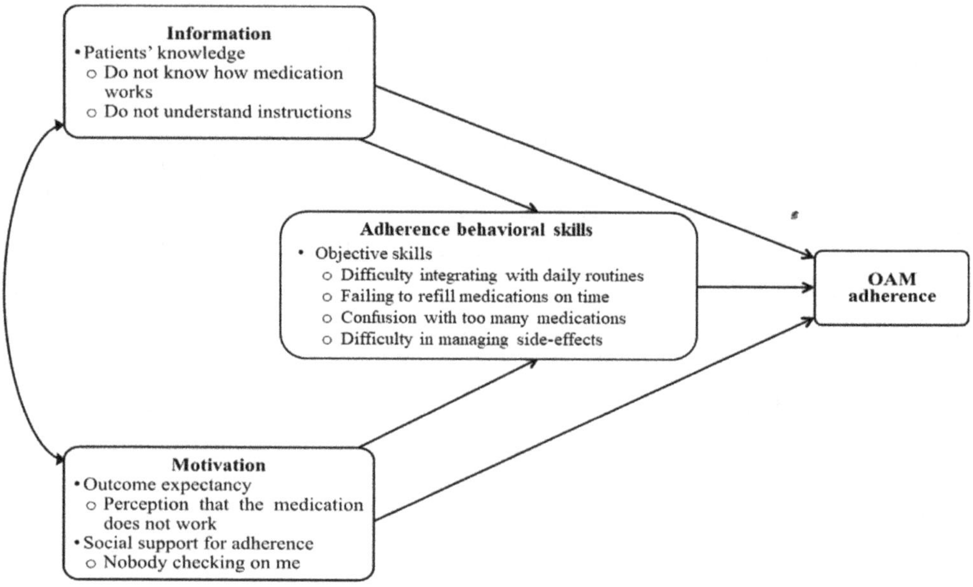

provided the theoretical basis for understanding non-adherence in the study populations and the development of potential intervention strategies (Greer, et al., 2016; Verbrugghe, et al., 2013). The factors identified in the information and motivation constructs would have direct effects on the behavioral skills construct, which in turn would directly impact health behavior (in this case, OAM adherence).

The 3 studies also identified strategies to help patients in their medication adherence. The most popular intervention strategy was education on the disease condition, benefits of medications, and management of side-effects by healthcare professionals (Table 2). The use of pillboxes and mHealth/telehealth were also popular strategies. From the capecitabine and EGFR TKI studies, integration of medication taking into daily routine and the involvement of family and other support groups were other popular strategies.

A cross-sectional study was also conducted to seek patients' demographics on smartphone ownership and health app usage, as well as their interests and perceptions of an adherence app for their OAMs (E. E. Ali, Leow, et al., 2018). The self-administered questionnaire included a list of adherence-enhancing strategies as potential features for the adherence app, which were based on

Table 2. Potential solutions suggested by respondents to facilitate adherence to OAMs.

Suggested Strategies	OAET (n = 136)		Capecitabine (n = 59)		EGFR-TKI (n = 85)	
	n	(%)*	n	(%)*	n	(%)*
Educational interventions by health professionals on disease condition, benefits of medication, management of side-effects	89	(65.4)	17	(28.8)	51	(60.0)
Use of pillbox	83	(61.0)	11	(18.6)	28	(32.9)
mHealth and other telehealth-based strategies (mobile apps, SMS, phone calls)	83	(61.0)	10	(16.9)	27	(31.8)
Involvement of family and other support groups	31	(22.8)	5	(8.5)	43	(50.6)
Monitoring of adherence by health professionals at each patient visit	61	(44.9)	6	(10.2)	6	(7.1)
More patient involvement in decision making by health professionals	41	(30.1)	3	(5.1)	11	(12.9)
Integrate medication into daily routine, alarms, change in regimen	8	(5.9)	13	(22.0)		--

*Percentages do not add up to 100% because a respondent could give more than one reason for non-adherence.

the recommended interventions for enhancing adherence – these included questions on areas of disease-related and drug-related information, tool for self-management of side-effects, monitoring adherence and medication reminders (L. Dayer, Heldenbrand, Anderson, Gubbins, & Martin, 2013; Demonceau et al., 2013; Schneider, Hess, & Gosselin, 2011). Among the 409 respondents, 211 (51.6%), 115 (28.1%), and 6 (1.5%) owned Android smartphones, iPhones and both iPhones and Android smartphones, respectively (Figure 2A). This translated to a smartphone penetration level of 81.2% (332/409) among study participants. Over a quarter (92/332, 27.7%) of smartphone owners reported using health-related apps on their smartphones. Monitoring healthy living activities (e.g. diet, exercise, sleep) was the main purpose for using health apps by majority of the respondents (61/92, 66.3%) (Figure 2B).

Among the 332 respondents who owned smartphones, 219 (66.0%) were interested in using an app for OAM adherence. Among the 69 respondents (20.8%) who were not interested in using an adherence app, the main reasons were related to perceptions that apps were either not useful to manage medications (31, 44.9%) or too difficult to use (18, 26.1%). App features that were rated on a higher importance level (i.e. "very important") included access to medication information (65.0%), access to disease-related information (60.2%) and a tool for self-management of side-effects (60.2%) (Table 3). Reminders to take medications (47.4%) and tracking missed doses (44.8%) were

Figure 2. (A) Mobile device ownership and (B) use of health apps by patients
** Percentages do not add up to 100% because participants could select multiple responses.*
*** Other types of apps included hospital-specific apps, an electronic health record app in Singapore and an app for the tracking of menstrual cycle.*

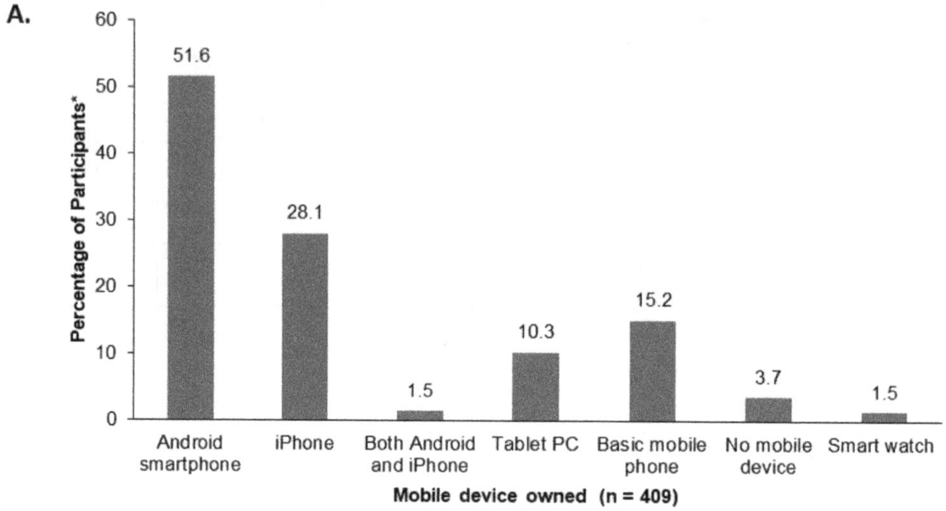

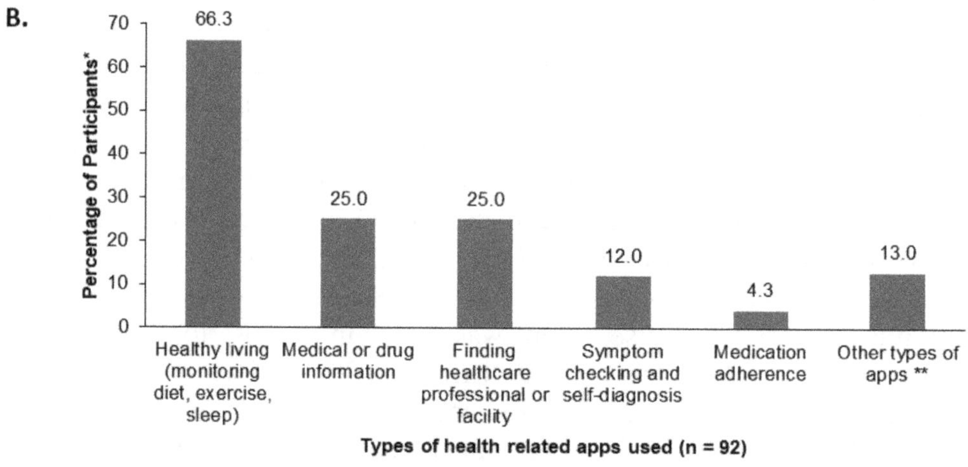

rated as "very important" by nearly half of the respondents, while the features that were rated the least important included the transmission of medication-taking patterns to health professionals (36.3%) and offline accessibility of app contents (35.0%). Being able to download the app free-of-charge was rated as "very important" by more than half of the respondents (67.7%).

Table 3. Level of importance of smartphone app features for medication adherence.

Potential Features	No. of Responses	Very Important	Moderately Important	Slightly Important	Unimportant
Access to information about your medications	360	234 (65.0)	93 (25.8)	20 (5.6)	13 (3.6)
Access to information on your disease condition	364	219 (60.2)	105 (28.8)	25 (6.9)	15 (4.1)
Tool for self-management of side-effects	364	219 (60.2)	112 (30.8)	19 (5.2)	14 (3.8)
Reminders to take your medications	361	171 (47.4)	105 (29.1)	49 (13.6)	36 (10.0)
Tracking missed and taken doses	359	161 (44.8)	108 (30.1)	51 (14.2)	39 (10.9)
Transmitting your medication usage patterns for review by your healthcare professional	358	130 (36.3)	142 (39.7)	54 (15.1)	32 (8.9)
Offline access to contents of the app	351	123 (35.0)	138 (39.3)	57 (16.2)	33 (9.4)
Can be downloaded free of charge	362	245 (67.7)	81 (22.4)	15 (4.1)	21 (5.8)

Step 2: Matrices of Change Objectives

The matrix of change objectives was created based on the results identified in the previous step. The behavioral change objective was to increase the proportion of patients who were adherent to OAMs. The IMB model explained most of the OAM adherence-related factors identified from the literature (Greer, et al., 2016; Verbrugghe, et al., 2013). However, a few factors, such as forgetfulness to take medicine and forgetfulness to refill prescription, were mapped onto part of the Theoretical Domains Framework (TDF) model (Cane, O'Connor, & Michie, 2012). Hence, the combination of the IMB and TDF models were used to develop the matrix of change objectives. The change objectives were based on the targeted determinants of a given behavior (Bartholomew, et al., 2011; Peters, 2014). Thus, the reasons for non-adherence that were identified in the previous step were re-worded to reflect the objectives of change. In contrast, the performance objectives covered the different 'preparatory behaviors' for adherence to OAMs (Peters, 2014). In the context of this study, 3 important preparatory behaviors, which were selected based on prior research and consensus among the authors, were targeted by the performance objectives (Table 4).

Table 4. Matrix of change objectives for the development of MedFC.

Performance Objectives (PO)	Targeted Determinants and Change Objectives (CO)				
	IMB-Information	IMB-Motivation		IMB-Behavioral Skills	TDF
	1. Knowledge	2. Outcome Expectancy	3. Social Support	4. Skills	5. Memory
PO1. Apply proper techniques to ensure accurate medication taking at the right time/ frequency	CO1.1.1. Explain the proper administration instructions for the medication CO1.1.2. Explain how medication works	CO1.2.1. Avoid missing doses for fear of facing side-effects	CO1.3.1. Obtain help from significant others for appropriate timing		CO1.5.1. Avoid missing doses due to forgetfulness CO1.5.2. Refill medications on time
PO2. Monitor adherence behavior and medication side-effects			CO2.3.1. Obtain support from significant others	CO2.4.1. Monitor side-effects to help in their management CO2.4.2. Monitor medication adherence behavior	
PO3. Increased ability to manage medication side-effects and other symptoms	CO3.1.1. Explain ways of side-effect management and methods to minimize missing doses			CO3.4.1. Manage side-effects and other symptoms related to medications	

Step 3: Selection of Theory-Based Intervention Methods and Practical Applications

Program ideas for MedFC were reviewed to facilitate the selection of theory-based methods (Chapter 3). Ideas for the different features of the system were drawn from the quality appraisals of the available adherence apps, patient preferences identified in the surveys and qualitative evaluations (Eskinder Eshetu Ali, et al., 2017; E. E. Ali, Leow, et al., 2018; E. E. Ali, Teo, et al., 2018) . Theoretical methods in the form of behavioral change techniques (BCTs) were identified (Bartholomew, et al., 2011; S. J. Chang, et al., 2014; Michie et al., 2013), and adapted to design the MedFC app.

Iterative qualitative interviews with potential users were used in the development of the app features of MedFC. A total of 16 pharmacists, 15 patients and 3 caregivers took part in the study. The in-house developed prototype app-based system was used to give participants an idea about the potential functions of medication management systems. This was done to gain a deeper understanding of the participants' responses. The prototype system included medication reminder, medication information, symptom reporting and adherence tracking functions in a smartphone app for patients.

At the beginning of each interview, participants were observed while they performed various medication management tasks. They were encouraged to talk about their thoughts and what they were trying to do while performing the tasks. The interviews lasted between 35 minutes to 1.5 hours and included questions on participants' overall impressions of the system and its usability, their favourite features, features that they deemed unnecessary, and suggestions for improvement. Low fidelity paper mock-ups were discussed to ensure understanding of the participants' suggestions for improvements or additions to the system. Analysis of the interview data followed inductive thematic analysis methods (Braun & Clarke, 2006). The inductive approach was employed in order to ensure in-depth understanding of participants' perceptions and opinions. Thematic analysis identified 4 main themes in the areas of monitoring medication-related problems, medication information, integration with current systems and accessibility of app content on devices other than smartphones. A summary of the list of themes, subthemes and suggested design considerations is provided in Table 5.

Consistent with the principles of UCD, the study involved potential end-users of such systems (Darlow & Wen, 2016; Groshek, et al., 2015; McCurdie et al., 2012; Mirkovic, Kaufman, & Ruland, 2014; Whittaker, Merry, Dorey, & Maddison, 2012). The use of a robust qualitative research methodology that involved important stakeholders (i.e. patients, caregivers and oncology pharmacists) in medication adherence enabled the study to address the on-going calls for the development of solutions that target the adherence needs of patients taking OAMs (Verbrugghe, et al., 2013). Based on the design suggestion and outcome expectation of MedFC users, an intervention map linking the determinants of OAM adherence to BCT methods and the app components of MedFC was created (Figure 3). This process serves as a guide to identify, target, and execute user input based on the existing BIT theory.

Table 5. Key themes, sub-themes and corresponding design suggestions identified in thematic analysis of MedFC.

Theme/Sub-theme	Design Suggestions
Theme 1. Monitoring Medication-related Problems	
Data input methods	Designated button to report taken doses Report symptoms using checklist of common symptoms with a potential for personalization, free text entries, audio-records, pictures
Displaying monitored reports/ information	Graphical visualization of trends in patients' medication consumption patterns and reported side-effects [by pharmacists] A list of symptoms and display of medication consumption records on a daily basis [by patients]
Expected mode of intervention	Near real-time management recommendation via phone calls and in app notifications Chat-based real-time support Involvement of nearby pharmacies in management of medication-related problems
Reminder options	Options to customize the number of reminders and snooze
Theme 2. Medication Information	
	Focused information on the most important aspects of medication Avoid essay type narrations Enable personalization of medication information
Theme 3. Replace or Integrate With the Current System	
Minimize the need for typing	Auto-fill features and ability to fetch medication data from patients' electronic medical records (EMRs)
Alerts/notifications in dispensing system (Tell me when something is wrong)	Enable effortless identification of abnormal medication adherence and symptom reports by the pharmacist at the point of patient care
Theme 4. Accessibility of App Content on Devices Other Than Smartphones	
	Optional provision of app contents on the web to make them accessible from PCs.

Step 4: Program Production

The MedFC system consisted of a smartphone app for patients/caregivers and a web app with different levels of access for patients/caregivers, pharmacists and other healthcare professionals (Figure 4). A clinician NFC app was also created for encoding NFC stickers, which were to be attached on the patient's medication packaging as part of the label. The mobile app for patients was developed in both NFC-enabled and non-NFC-enabled versions, and its main functionalities were medication reminders, provision of medication information (a record of the patient's medication list together with detailed information), symptom monitoring and adherence tracking. Multiple programming languages and frameworks were used to develop MedFC,

Figure 3. Intervention map linking the determinants of OAM adherence to behavioral change technique (BCT) methods and app components. (A-C) Determinants targeted based on the information, motivation, behavioral skills (IMB) construct; (D) Determinants targeted based on the theoretical domain framework (TDF) construct.

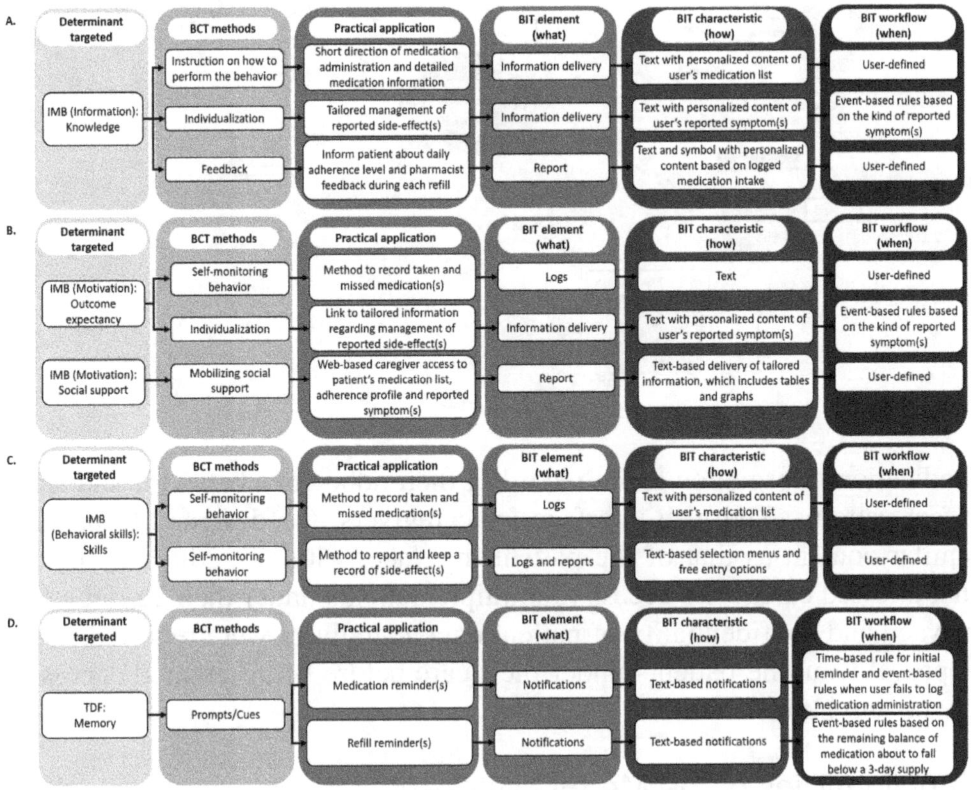

such as hypertext markup language (HTML), JavaScript and cascading style sheets for its web interface, and hypertext pre-processor (PHP) scripting for server-side scripts. The web server was configured to support secure socket layer (SSL) to ensure communications privacy over the Internet. Android Studio was used to develop the MedFC patient app and clinician NFC app.

The web app for pharmacists and other healthcare professionals allowed them to maintain a complete record of the patients' medication list, as well as track medication adherence and side-effect patterns through symptom reports (Figure 5). Moreover, the clinician could use the web interface to manage the medication database and grant access to patients/caregivers and other clinicians. On the other hand, the web interface for patients was able to provide patient-level access to their medication lists, together with detailed

Figure 4. Flowchart showing the components of the MedFC system.

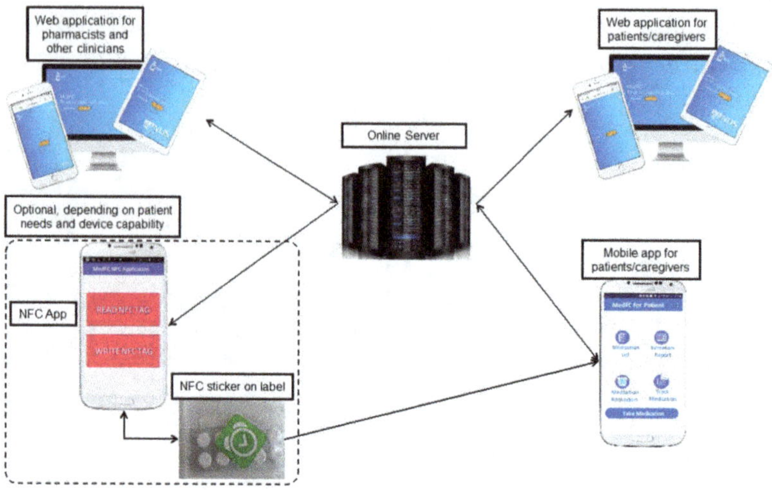

medication information and a record of their adherence behavior and side-effect patterns. The web interface for caregivers was designed to provide similar content as that of the patient interface, with an additional feature that allowed caregivers access to multiple patients under their care. Due to privacy and confidentiality of patient data, caregivers were required to get approval from the patients under their care before being granted access to the patient information.

Functionalities of the MedFC Web App

Users would have to log into the MedFC web app in order to access the medication-related information of the patient. There were 2 levels of access – one for pharmacists/healthcare professionals and another for patients/caregivers. The patient-level/caregiver-level access is discussed as part of the patient app in the later part of this chapter. Pharmacists with general-level access could create the patient's list of medications and electronically push that information to the patients' account, which would be accessible on the MedFC mobile app.

The web app also allowed pharmacists to monitor patient medication adherence trends through tabular and graphical representations of patients' medication-taking patterns. This information could be used to monitor patients between appointment periods and intervene in case of abnormal trends. The

Figure 5. Screenshots of the MedFC web app for pharmacists and healthcare professionals.

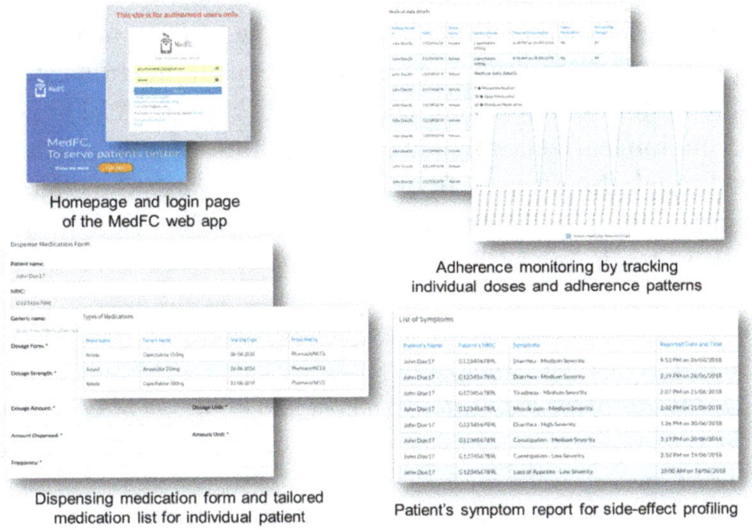

pharmacist could also use the information to counsel patients during their next visit.

Similarly, the side-effect profile of patients could also be monitored through a symptom report in the web app, so that the pharmacists could manage the patients' concerns in between appointments and/or during the patients' visits to the hospital. The prototype did not have any functionality to enable sending of notification alerts directly to the app. However, pharmacists could call the patient or caregiver to intervene in case of abnormal reports.

Functionalities of the MedFC Patient App

The MedFC patient app was an Android app designed to help patients manage their medications and side-effects. The app enabled patients to set reminders, access medication information, track daily medication consumption, and report and track their symptoms and medication side-effects. The main functionalities of the patient app are described below.

Medication List

One of the main features in MedFC was the patient medication list – a feature that aimed to address the lack of knowledge on medication information, which was cited by patients as one of the factors contributing to their non-adherence behavior. The medication list would be created by the pharmacist on the clinician web application and electronically pushed to the patient app. Its functionality was designed such that the name of each medication in the list would be linked to concise information about its indications, how to take, common side-effects and special precautions (Figure 6). A PDF copy of the patient information leaflet developed by the institution could also be accessed by patients through this feature. In order to cater towards the majority of the Singaporean population, the patient information leaflets were available both in English and Mandarin.

Figure 6. Screenshots of the medication list components of the MedFC patient app.

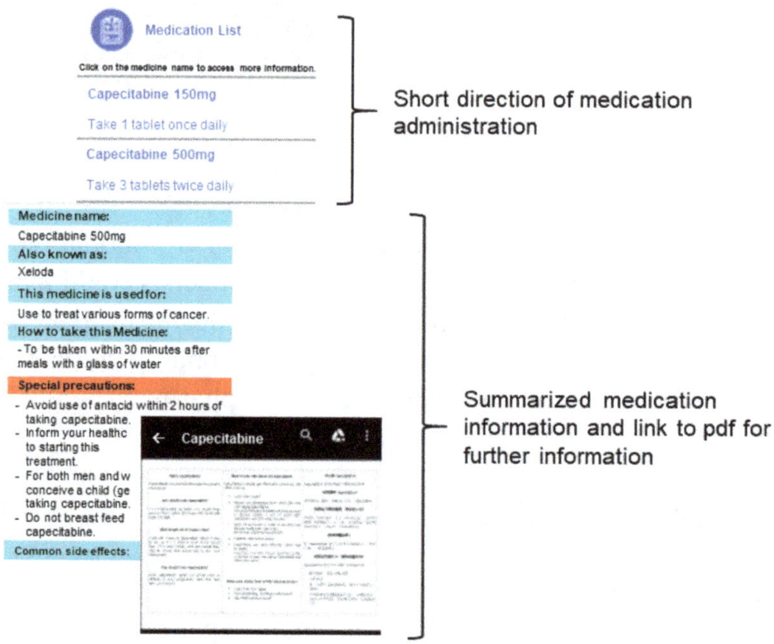

Medication Adherence Tracking

This feature was developed in response to the BCT theory of providing feedback and self-monitoring of adherence (Figure 3), so that patients could track doses that were due, taken or missed on each day. Patients could log their medication consumption patterns through one of 2 ways – (i) by tapping the medication packaging with their NFC-enabled smartphones, which would automatically register a dose of the medication and a record of the timing, or (ii) directly selecting from their list of medications and recording their administration times manually (for non-NFC-enabled phones) (Figure 7).

Figure 7. Screenshots of medication adherence tracking components of the MedFC patient app.

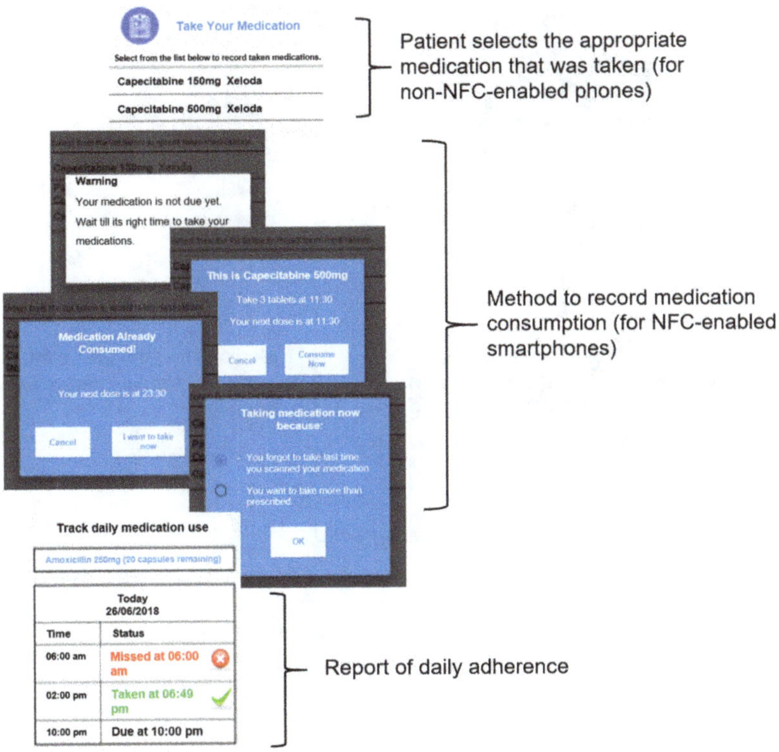

Medication Reminder

As previously reported, one of the most common reasons for medication non-adherence behavior was forgetfulness (Table 1). Therefore, developing a medication reminder feature was one of the BCT strategies aimed to enhance adherence behavior of patients. The medication reminder could be set up during consultation, when the pharmacist first created the patient's medication list on the web app. Patients could then change the timings of the medication reminders according to their needs. Patients would also have an option to select the types of alerts, for example, in the form of sound, vibration or both. In addition, the app provided an option to anonymize the reminder alerts for patients who wanted privacy and did not want the names of their medications to be displayed (Figure 8).

Figure 8. Screenshots of the medication reminder components of the MedFC patient app.

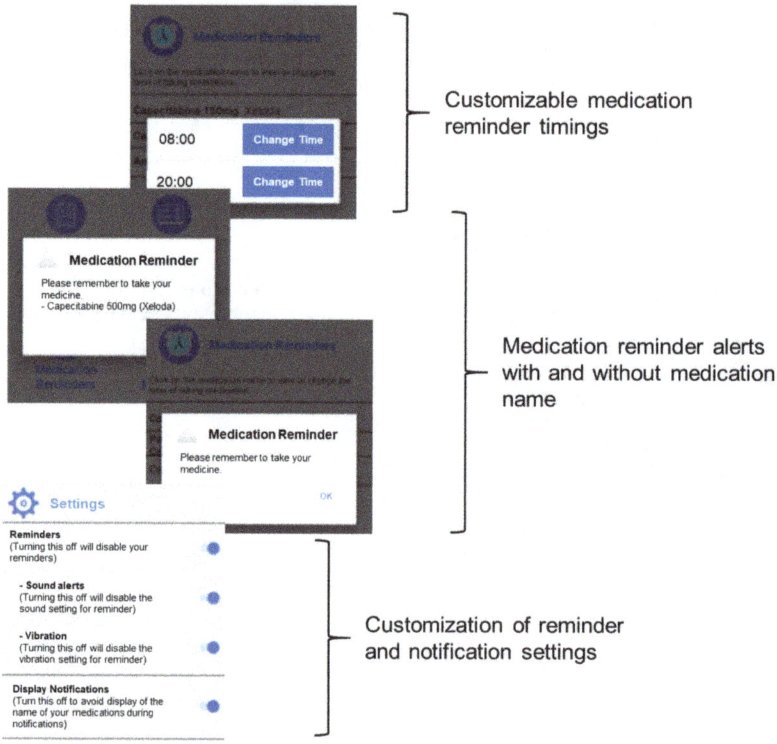

Symptom Report

The symptom report feature was also developed to address another common reason for medication non-adherence – to prevent and/or manage side-effects (Table 1). This feature allowed users to report their symptoms by either selecting from a list of symptoms or recording their symptoms in free text format (Figure 9). The app also kept a record of all reported symptoms with date and time stamps. Furthermore, whenever the patient reported

Figure 9. Screenshots of the symptom reporting feature of the MedFC patient app.

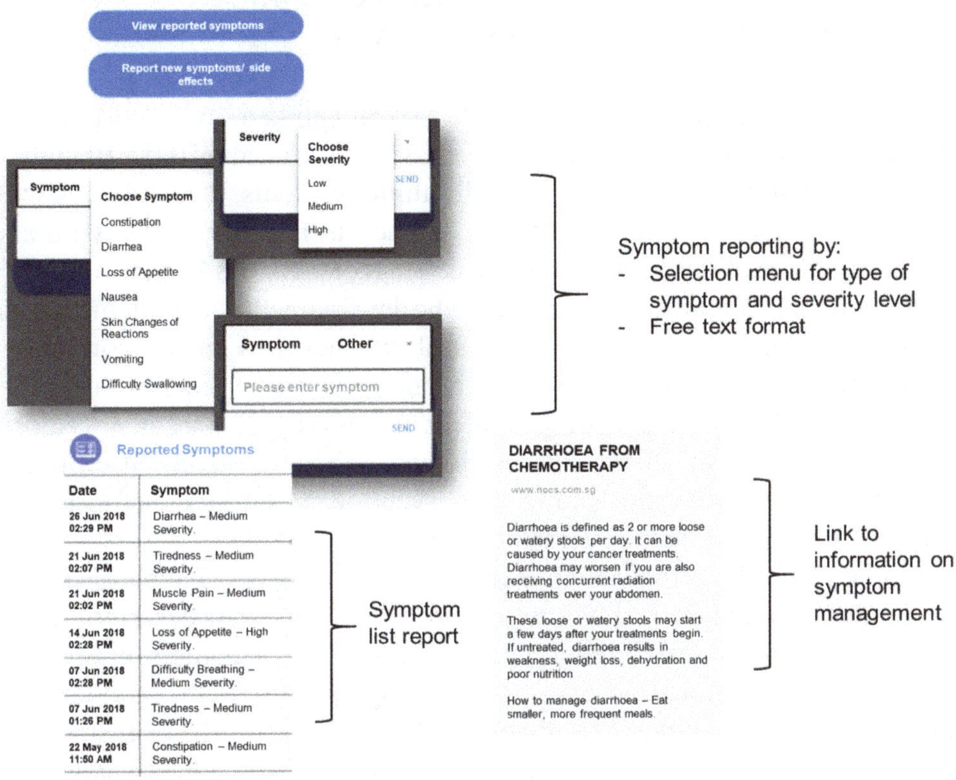

a symptom through the selection menu, a link to tailored information on possible management options for the reported symptom would be provided.

Issues of Data Security and Privacy

Access to MedFC was restricted to patients who had a valid username and password. Users had to register for an account with a valid email and they could only access the system after approval by the app administrator. In contrast to patient users who could only view their own information, users with clinician-level access could also prepare their patients' medication lists, save information under specific patients and view their patients' reported symptoms and adherence patterns. Security algorithms and protocols were employed to ensure password security and privacy of communications over the Internet.

Steps 5 and 6: Implementation and Evaluation of MedFC Usability for Enhancing Adherence to Oral Anticancer Medications (OAMs)

From patients' perspectives, the usability of an app is more important than the number and type of functionalities (Bernhard et al., 2018; Bhandari, Neben, & Chang, 2015; Mohammed, Ibrahim, & Cavus, 2018). Issues with the usability of an app can potentially impact users' interactions with and their acceptance of the app (Georgsson & Staggers, 2016). As such, usability evaluation should be an integral aspect of the development and implementation of mHealth apps. Iterative testing of usability helps to ensure continuous quality improvement of the app by enabling developers to identify usability issues early in the design and development process (Lyles, Sarkar, & Osborn, 2014; McCurdie, et al., 2012). It is also in line with Step 4 of the IM approach, which recommends the pilot testing of intervention programmes before rolling them out for widespread use (Bartholomew, et al., 2011).

Studies describing the design and development of OAM adherence apps are limited in number. Fishbein et al. provided a detailed description of a chemotherapy assistant (CORA) app, which consisted of features that enabled management of medication plans, monitoring of side-effects, and keeping notes and access to support healthy living (Fishbein, et al., 2017). In addition, Hsu et al. described a tablet app that utilized animation for educating patients on OAM adherence (Hsu, et al., 2017). However, none of these studies presented robust usability evaluations of their apps. This represented a gap in the accurate assessment of the potential level of user engagement with the apps and their future adoption by patients. There is also limited information on the usability issues that developers of similar apps should anticipate and address in their products.

The main aim of this section is to describe the usability evaluation of MedFC from the perspectives of patients and caregivers. The study described also aimed to evaluate user acceptance and feasibility of the app. In this context, feasibility referred to the degree to which MedFC could be conveniently implemented in the monitoring of patients' adherence and symptom reports.

MedFC Acceptability Evaluation

A qualitative study design using the Grounded Theory approach described by Charmaz was followed in this study (Charmaz, 2006). A total of 18 interviews were conducted with patients and caregivers. In the context of this study, participants' stated intention to use an app for the management of medication adherence determined their acceptance of the app. The factors that influenced participants' acceptance of an adherence app were classified into facilitating and hindering factors. The facilitating factors were facing difficulty in maintaining adherence and getting superior features over current methods. In contrast, the hindering factors were lower perceived competence in using apps, having to pay and the lack of options for different languages (Figure 10).

Figure 10. Consideration factors of patients and caregivers on their intention to use an adherence app.

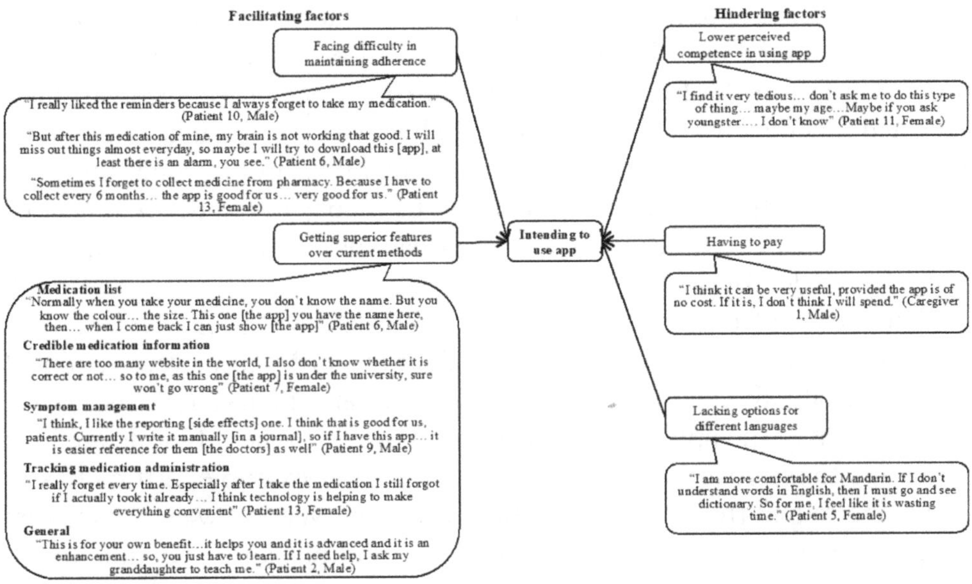

MedFC Usability Evaluation

The study involved an iterative usability evaluation of 3 different prototypes of the MedFC app and a pilot feasibility evaluation of the latest version. The second and third versions were concurrently developed based on user inputs on the first version. The first two versions utilized NFC capabilities for medication identification and confirmation of intake by patients. In contrast, the third version was the non-NFC equivalent of the second version in order to cater to non-NFC-enabled phones. Through a comprehensive usability evaluation process that comprised of participants being observed while they performed a set of medication management tasks, a self-administered questionnaire based on the System Usability Scale (SUS) and Technology Acceptance Model (TAM) for acceptance of mHealth apps (Bangor, Kortum, & Miller, 2008; Brooke, 2013; Krebs & Duncan, 2015; Loy, Ali, & Yap, 2016), and qualitative interviews, a total of 36 participants (patients and caregivers) took part in the usability evaluation study. Different participants were recruited for the usability evaluation of the first (N=15), second (N=10) and third (N=11) versions of MedFC.

The last version (Version 3) of MedFC had a SUS score of 90 (interquartile range IQR: 80–95). This score was significantly higher than the scores for Version 2 (p=0.020) and Version 1 (p=0.001) of the app (Table 6). According to the SUS, a score of above 70 indicated acceptable usability. Better apps would score in the high 70s to upper 80s, and the genuinely superior ones would score above 90 (Bangor, et al., 2008). The SUS score of 90 in this study indicated excellent usability of MedFC. In line with the findings of previous research on app-based adherence interventions for chronic conditions, the excellent usability score was a product of the theory-based development of the app with user-centered iterative modifications (Whiteley, Brown, Lally, Heck, & van den Berg, 2018).

Consistent with the recommendations for successful usability evaluation of health apps, the quantitative usability evaluations of MedFC were validated through a qualitative analysis that provided additional inputs for the successful improvement of the app. Modifications were made to the different versions of the app to improve its usability (Figure 11). For example, difficulties in navigating to and from the main menu of the first version were reduced by designing a graphical user interface with four buttons corresponding to the primary functions of the app. Furthermore, the cluttered format of medication information was reduced to only the amount and frequency of dosing. Another modification, which was critical to the excellent usability score of the last MedFC version, was the removal of the NFC scanning function, which seemed to hinder the Smartphone Mobile App heuRisTics (SMART) to "facilitate easier input". These findings were consistent to the literature, which suggested that problems in the data input requirements of health apps were known to influence their acceptance and continued usage by end users (Krebs & Duncan, 2015; Laing et al., 2014).

Table 6. Usability scores of the different versions of MedFC based on the System Usability Scale (SUS).

Usability Scale	Evaluated Version of MedFC					
	Version 1		Version 2		Version 3	
	Median*	(IQR)	Median*	(IQR)	Median*	(IQR)
I would like to use this system frequently.	3	(3; 4)	3	(2; 3)	4	(3; 4)
I found the system unnecessarily complex.	3	(2; 3)	3	(3; 3)	4	(4; 4)
I thought the system was easy to use.	3	(2; 3)	3	(3; 3)	4	(3; 4)
I would need the support of a technical person.	3	(1; 4)	3	(2; 3)	4	(2; 4)
The various functions were well integrated.	3	(2; 3)	3	(3; 3)	3	(3; 4)
I thought there was too much inconsistency.	2	(2; 3)	3	(2; 3)	4	(3; 4)
Most people would learn to use this system very quickly.	3	(2; 3)	3	(3; 3)	4	(3; 4)
I found the system very cumbersome to use.	3	(2; 3)	3	(2; 3)	4	(3; 4)
I felt very confident using the system.	3	(2; 4)	3	(3; 3)	4	(3; 4)
I needed to learn a lot of things before I could get going with this system.	2	(1; 3)	3	(3; 3)	4	(3; 4)
Total SUS scores	65	(55; 82)	74	(65; 75)	90	(80; 95)

*Original values transformed to account for variations in the way the questions in the SUS were worded (higher values mean better usability).

IQR: interquartile range

Some usability issues persisted despite modifications made in the later versions of MedFC. One such issue was related to the use of colours in the app, which was mapped to the heuristics to "design a visually pleasing interface" (Chapter 3, Table 3). While participants' opinions on the visual appeal of the first version were related to its black and white appearance, the absence of colour variations was the central issue in the later versions. However, there was no consensus among participants regarding the use of colours in this analysis. App aesthetics are known to have significant influence over the initial adoption and continued utilization of apps (Bhandari, et al., 2015). Hence, one way to cater to the varied opinions on the use of colours would be to allow users to customize colours to their personal preferences.

Figure 11. Modifications to the different versions of MedFC to improve its usability.

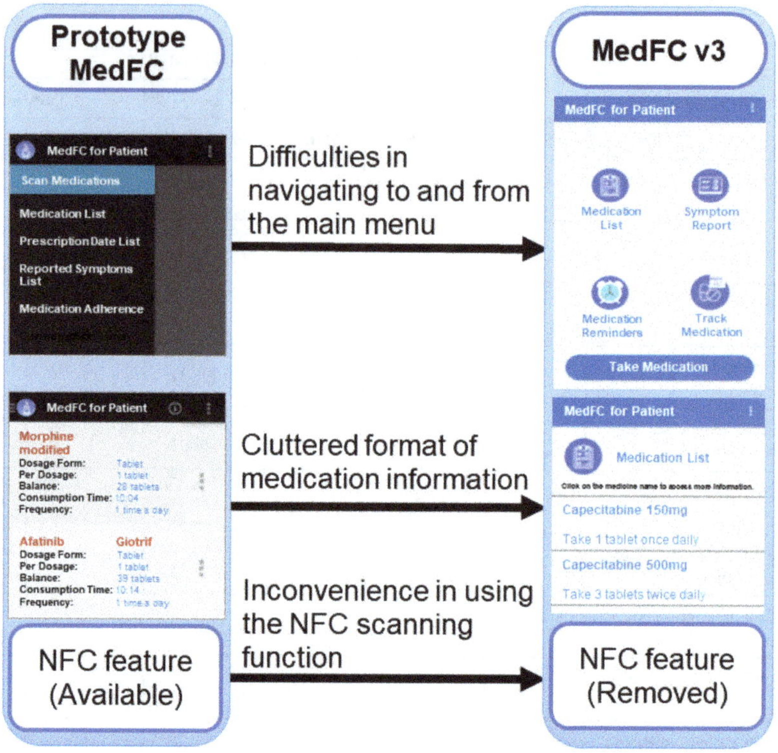

The current study found a high level of acceptance of MedFC among patients and caregivers. This was shown by the more than 80% of participants who agreed or strongly agreed to questions assessing their behavioral intentions to use MedFC (Table 7). Studies on the acceptance of technology-based health interventions suggested that users' perceptions of the interventions' usefulness, ease of use, and their perceived behavioral control and self-efficacy influenced their intentions to use the interventions (Lim et al., 2011; Sun, Wang, Guo, & Peng, 2013; Xue et al., 2012). Similar factors were found in this study to be significantly associated with participants' intentions to use MedFC (Table 8) These findings were also complemented by participants' opinions identified in the qualitative analysis. The relevance in medication management and suggested enhancement themes from the qualitative findings further clarified participants' perceptions on the usefulness of the different features of the app. Specifically, participants identified the symptom report and medication reminder features as their most preferred components of the MedFC app, which addressed the non-adherence reasons detailed in Table 1.

Table 7. Acceptability of MedFC among participants who evaluated the different versions of the app.

Intention to Use Items	Strongly Disagree		Disagree		Neither Agree/ Disagree		Agree		Strongly Agree	
	n	(%)	n	(%)	n	(%)	n	(%)	n	(%)
Assuming I have access to MedFC, I intend to use it.	4	(11.1)		--	3	(8.3)	21	(58.3)	8	(22.2)
If I have access to MedFC, I predict that I would use it.	2	(5.6)	1	(2.8)	3	(8.3)	23	(63.9)	7	(19.4)
Assuming I have access to MedFC, I plan to use it.	2	(5.6)	1	(2.8)	3	(8.3)	23	(63.9)	7	(19.4)

This finding further validated the findings of the patient surveys previously conducted (E. E. Ali, Leow, et al., 2018). The findings were also consistent with the existing literature on the importance of side-effect management and medication reminders in improving OAM adherence (Eskinder Eshetu Ali, et al., 2017; Graetz et al., 2018; Greer, et al., 2016; Moon, et al., 2017). Participants also suggested enhancements to MedFC to enable medical appointment reminders, provision of contact addresses, pharmacy queue status notifications and connection to support groups. The inclusion of these functionalities in the future iterations of MedFC would be important to enhance the acceptability of the app among patients.

MedFC Feasibility Evaluation

The pilot feasibility evaluation was conducted on the third version of MedFC (E. E. Ali, Leow, Chew, & Yap, 2019), and it involved 5 participants downloading the app to their smartphones and using it for 3 to 4 weeks, until their next clinic visit. MedFC was able to determine the adherence level based on users' logs on the app, and >80.0% adherence levels were seen in 60.0% of the participants. Overall, the system was able to capture at least 69.0% of the times the patients consumed their medication. When asked about their actual behavior during the follow-up period, 4 of the participants reported never missing a dose of their medication, while one participant was not able to recall. Three participants reported 2 or more side-effects or other symptoms in the course of the follow-up period.

Evaluation of the participants' symptom burden and adherence levels were adopted from the Memorial Symptom Assessment Scale – Short Form

Table 8. Relationship between participants' behavioral intention to use MedFC and their perceptions on factors influencing their intentions.

Construct	Median*	IQR*	Correlation With Intention to Use**	P-value
Intention to use MedFC	4.0	(4.0; 4.0)	1.0	--
Perceived usefulness	4.0	(4.0; 4.9)	0.73	< 0.001
Perceived ease of use	4.0	(4.0; 5.0)	0.63	< 0.001
Subjective norm	4.0	(3.0; 4.0)	0.30	0.074
Perceived behavioral control	4.0	(4.0; 4.7)	0.72	< 0.001
Self-efficacy	4.0	(3.8; 4.5)	0.78	< 0.001
Technology anxiety	1.4	(1.0; 2.0)	– 0.40	0.015
Perceived vulnerability	3.0	(2.0; 4.0)	0.27	0.112

* Scores were calculated based on an agreement scale of 1 (Strongly Disagree) to 5 (Strongly Agree).
** Correlation coefficients based on Spearman's rank-order test.
IQR: interquartile range

(MSAS-SF), the 12-item Adherence Starts with Knowledge (ASK-12) scale and the Medication Adherence Questionnaire (MAQ) (V. T. Chang, Hwang, Feuerman, Kasimis, & Thaler, 2000; Matza et al., 2009; Morisky, Green, & Levine, 1986). The ASK-12 tool was used to assess patients' overall adherence to all their medications in general, and the MAQ was used to assess OAM adherence. The combined use of these tools helped in assessing knowledge, motivation and skills associated with medication adherence in a way that corresponded with the IMB model.

The findings of this study indicated the usefulness of MedFC in reducing symptom burden and barriers to adherence. The symptom burden, based on the MSAS-SF median score, changed from 0.4 (IQR: 0.3–0.7) to 0.2 (IQR: 0.2–0.9), and the barriers to adherence as measured by the median ASK-12 score changed from 21.0 (IQR: 19.0–22.0) to 19.0 (IQR: 17.0–20.0). There was no difference in the median adherence score on MAQ from the pre- (4.0, IQR: 3.0–4.0) to post-intervention (4.0, IQR: 4.0–4.0) measurements. Regarding usability, MedFC scored a median value of 70.0 (IQR: 70.0–78.0) out of a maximum of 100. Acceptability of MedFC was measured based on participants' intention to continue using the app. The median score of the items, rated from 1 (strongly disagree) to 5 (strongly agree) on the behavioral intention construct of the TAM, was 4.0 (IQR: 4.0–4.0). These results further strengthened the case for the feasibility of using MedFC in routine clinical practice. However, more robust clinical evaluations of the app with longer follow-up periods should be done to demonstrate the longer-term efficacy of the app and facilitate recommendation by clinicians. The sample sizes in usability tests from the literature were generally between 8 to 12 evaluators (Brooke, 2013). Therefore, future studies evaluating MedFC should consider using larger sample sizes to fill this gap.

REFERENCES

Ahmed, I., Ahmad, N. S., Ali, S., Ali, S., George, A., Saleem Danish, H., ... Darzi, A. (2018). Medication adherence apps: Review and content analysis. *JMIR mHealth and uHealth*, *6*(3), e62. doi:10.2196/mhealth.6432 PMID:29549075

Ali, E. E., Chan, S. S. L., Leow, J. L., Chew, L., & Yap, K. Y. (2019). User acceptance of an app-based adherence intervention: Perspectives from patients taking oral anticancer medications. *Journal of Oncology Pharmacy Practice*, *25*(2), 390–397. doi:10.1177/1078155218778106 PMID:29792123

Ali, E. E., Chan, S. S. L., Poh, H. Y., Susanto, Y. A., Suganya, T., Leow, J. L., ... Yap, K. Y. (2019). Design considerations in the development of app-based oral anticancer medication management systems: A qualitative evaluation of pharmacists' and patients' perspectives. *Journal of Medical Systems*, *43*(3), 63. doi:10.100710916-019-1168-x PMID:30726518

Ali, E. E., Cheung, K. L., Lee, C. P., Leow, J. L., Yap, K. Y.-L., & Chew, L. (2017). Prevalence and determinants of adherence to oral adjuvant endocrine therapy among breast cancer patients in Singapore. *Asia-Pacific Journal of Oncology Nursing*, *4*(4), 283–289. doi:10.4103/2347-5625.212864 PMID:28966955

Ali, E. E., Leow, J. L., Chew, L., & Yap, K. Y. (2018). Patients' perception of app-based educational and behavioural interventions for enhancing oral anticancer medication adherence. *Journal of Cancer Education*, *33*(6), 1306–1313. doi:10.100713187-017-1248-x PMID:28707206

Ali, E. E., Leow, J. L., Chew, L., & Yap, K. Y. (2019). Usability and feasibility of a theory-based and user-centred oral anticancer medication adherence app. *Supportive Care in Cancer*, *27*(Suppl 1), 588.

Ali, E. E., Poh, H. Y., Susanto, Y. A., Pang, J., Chew, L., & Yap, K. Y. (2016, Oct 8-9). *Development of a m-health medication adherence prototype system using near field communication and text-to-speech technologies.* Paper presented at the 26th Singapore Pharmacy Congress, Suntec Convention and Exhibition Centre, Singapore.

Ali, E. E., Teo, A. K. S., Goh, S. X. L., Chew, L., & Yap, K. Y. (2018). MedAd-AppQ: A quality assessment tool for medication adherence apps on iOS and android platforms. *Research in Social & Administrative Pharmacy, 14*(12), 1125–1133. doi:10.1016/j.sapharm.2018.01.006 PMID:29402755

Atkins, L., & Fallowfield, L. (2006). Intentional and non-intentional non-adherence to medication amongst breast cancer patients. *European Journal of Cancer, 42*(14), 2271–2276. doi:10.1016/j.ejca.2006.03.004 PMID:16644208

Bangor, A., Kortum, P. T., & Miller, J. T. (2008). An empirical evaluation of the system usability scale. *International Journal of Human-Computer Interaction, 24*(6), 574–594. doi:10.1080/10447310802205776

Bartholomew, L. K., Parcel, G. S., Kok, G., Gottlieb, N. H., & Fernandez, M. E. (2011). *Planning Health Promotion Programs: An Intervention Mapping Approach* (3rd ed.). San Francisco, CA: Jossey-Bass.

Bernhard, G., Mahler, C., Seidling, H. M., Stützle, M., Ose, D., Baudendistel, I., ... Szecsenyi, J. (2018). Developing a shared patient-centered, web-based medication platform for Type 2 diabetes patients and their health care providers: Qualitative study on user requirements. *Journal of Medical Internet Research, 20*(3), e105. doi:10.2196/jmir.8666 PMID:29588269

Bhandari, U., Neben, T., & Chang, K. (2015). Understanding visual appeal and quality perceptions of mobile apps: An emotional perspective. In M. Kurosu (Ed.), Lecture Notes in Computer Science: Vol. 9169. *Human-Computer Interaction: Design and Evaluation. HCI 2015* (pp. 451–459). Cham: Springer.

Braun, V., & Clarke, V. (2006). Using thematic analysis in psychology. *Qualitative Research in Psychology, 3*(2), 77–101. doi:10.1191/1478088706qp063oa

Brooke, J. (2013). SUS: A retrospective. *Journal of Usability Studies, 8*(2), 29–40.

Cane, J., O'Connor, D., & Michie, S. (2012). Validation of the theoretical domains framework for use in behaviour change and implementation research. *Implementation Science; IS*, *7*(1), 37. doi:10.1186/1748-5908-7-37 PMID:22530986

Car, J., Tan, W. S., Huang, Z., Sloot, P., & Franklin, B. D. (2017). eHealth in the future of medications management: Personalisation, monitoring and adherence. *BMC Medicine*, *15*(1), 73. doi:10.118612916-017-0838-0 PMID:28376771

Chang, S. J., Choi, S., Kim, S.-A., & Song, M. (2014). Intervention strategies based on information-motivation-behavioral skills model for health behavior change: A systematic review. *Asian Nursing Research*, *8*(3), 172–181. doi:10.1016/j.anr.2014.08.002

Chang, V. T., Hwang, S. S., Feuerman, M., Kasimis, B. S., & Thaler, H. T. (2000). The memorial symptom assessment scale short form (MSAS-SF). *Cancer*, *89*(5), 1162–1171. doi:10.1002/1097-0142(20000901)89:5<1162::AID-CNCR26>3.0.CO;2-Y PMID:10964347

Charmaz, K. (2006). *Constructing Grounded Theory: A Practical Guide through Qualitative Analysis*. London: Sage Publications.

Darlow, S., & Wen, K.-Y. (2016). Development testing of mobile health interventions for cancer patient self-management: A review. *Health Informatics Journal*, *22*(3), 633–650. doi:10.1177/1460458215577994 PMID:25916831

Dayer, L., Heldenbrand, S., Anderson, P., Gubbins, P., & Martin, B. (2013). Smartphone medication adherence apps: Potential benefits to patients and providers. *Journal of the American Pharmacists Association*, *53*(2), 172–181. doi:10.1331/JAPhA.2013.12202 PMID:23571625

Dayer, L. E., Shilling, R., Van Valkenburg, M., Martin, B. C., Gubbins, P. O., Hadden, K., & Heldenbrand, S. (2017). Assessing the medication adherence app marketplace from the health professional and consumer vantage points. *JMIR mHealth and uHealth*, *5*(4), e45. doi:10.2196/mhealth.6582 PMID:28428169

Deloitte. (2015). *Mobile multiplies: Global mobile consumer survey*. Retrieved 7 Sep, 2019, from https://www2.deloitte.com/content/dam/Deloitte/sg/Documents/technology-media-telecommunications/sea-tmt-2014-global-mobile-consumer-survey-sea.pdf

Demonceau, J., Ruppar, T., Kristanto, P., Hughes, D. A., Fargher, E., Kardas, P., ... Vrijens, B. (2013). Identification and assessment of adherence-enhancing interventions in studies assessing medication adherence through electronically compiled drug dosing histories: A systematic literature review and meta-analysis. *Drugs*, *73*(6), 545–562. doi:10.100740265-013-0041-3 PMID:23588595

Fishbein, J. N., Nisotel, L. E., MacDonald, J. J., Amoyal Pensak, N., Jacobs, J. M., Flanagan, C., ... Greer, J. A. (2017). Mobile application to promote adherence to oral chemotherapy and symptom management: A protocol for design and development. *JMIR Research Protocols*, *6*(4), e62. doi:10.2196/resprot.6198 PMID:28428158

Fisher, W. A., Fisher, J. D., & Harman, J. (2003). The information-motivation-behavioral skills model: A general social psychological approach to understanding and promoting health behavior. In J. Suls & K. A. Wallston (Eds.), *Social Psychological Foundations of Health and Illness*. Malden, MA: Blackwell. doi:10.1002/9780470753552.ch4

Foo, J., Ali, E. E., Sia, H. L., Yap, K., & Chew, L. (2016, Oct 8-9). *Adherence to capecitabine therapy among patients of a tertiary cancer centre in Singapore.* Paper presented at the 26th Singapore Pharmacy Congress, Suntec Singapore Convention and Exhibition Centre, Singapore.

Fraccaro, P., Vigo, M., Balatsoukas, P., van der Veer, S. N., Hassan, L., Williams, R., ... Peek, N. (2018). Presentation of laboratory test results in patient portals: Influence of interface design on risk interpretation and visual search behaviour. *BMC Medical Informatics and Decision Making*, *18*(1), 11. doi:10.118612911-018-0589-7 PMID:29433495

Georgsson, M., & Staggers, N. (2016). Quantifying usability: An evaluation of a diabetes mHealth system on effectiveness, efficiency, and satisfaction metrics with associated user characteristics. *Journal of the American Medical Informatics Association*, *23*(1), 5–11. doi:10.1093/jamia/ocv099 PMID:26377990

Graetz, I., McKillop, C. N., Stepanski, E., Vidal, G. A., Anderson, J. N., & Schwartzberg, L. S. (2018). Use of a web-based app to improve breast cancer symptom management and adherence for aromatase inhibitors: A randomized controlled feasibility trial. *Journal of Cancer Survivorship: Research and Practice*, *12*(4), 431–440. doi:10.100711764-018-0682-z PMID:29492753

Greer, J. A., Amoyal, N., Nisotel, L., Fishbein, J. N., MacDonald, J., Stagl, J., ... Pirl, W. F. (2016). A systematic review of adherence to oral antineoplastic therapies. *The Oncologist*, *21*(3), 354–376. doi:10.1634/theoncologist.2015-0405 PMID:26921292

Groshek, M. R., Oldenburg, J., Sarasohn-Kahn, J., & Sitler, B. (2015). *mHealth app essentials: Patient engagement, considerations, and implementation.* Retrieved 18 Aug, 2019, from https://www.himss.org/mhealth-app-essentials-patient-engagement-considerations-and-implementation

Haase, J., Farris, K. B., & Dorsch, M. P. (2017). Mobile applications to improve medication adherence. *Telemedicine Journal and e-Health*, *23*(2), 75–79. doi:10.1089/tmj.2015.0227 PMID:27248315

Hsu, G. I.-H., Crawford, S. Y., Paolella, G., Cuellar, S., Wirth, S. M., Venepalli, N. K., ... Boyd, A. D. (2017). Design of customized mobile application for patient adherence to oral anticancer medications utilizing user-centered design. *The Journal of Biocommunication*, *41*(1), 5–14. doi:10.5210/jbc.v41i1.7499

Irwin, M., & Johnson, L. A. (2015). Factors influencing oral adherence: Qualitative metasummary and triangulation with quantitative evidence. *Clinical Journal of Oncology Nursing*, *19*(3Suppl), 6–30. doi:10.1188/15.S1.CJON.6-30 PMID:26030389

Kok, G. (2014). A practical guide to effective behavior change: How to apply theory- and evidence-based behavior change methods in an intervention. *European Health Psychologist, 16*(5), 156-170.

Krebs, P., & Duncan, D. T. (2015). Health app use among US mobile phone owners: A national survey. *JMIR mHealth and uHealth*, *3*(4), e101. doi:10.2196/mhealth.4924 PMID:26537656

Lacey, J., Cate, H., & Broadway, D. C. (2009). Barriers to adherence with glaucoma medications: A qualitative research study. *Eye (London, England)*, *23*(4), 924–932. doi:10.1038/eye.2008.103 PMID:18437182

Laing, B. Y., Mangione, C. M., Tseng, C. H., Leng, M., Vaisberg, E., Mahida, M., ... Bell, D. S. (2014). Effectiveness of a smartphone application for weight loss compared with usual care in overweight primary care patients: A randomized, controlled trial. *Annals of Internal Medicine*, *161*(10Suppl), S5–S12. doi:10.7326/M13-3005 PMID:25402403

Lavsa, S. M., Holzworth, A., & Ansani, N. T. (2011). Selection of a validated scale for measuring medication adherence. *Journal of the American Pharmacists Association, 51*(1), 90–94. doi:10.1331/JAPhA.2011.09154 PMID:21247831

Lim, S., Xue, L., Yen, C. C., Chang, L., Chan, H. C., Tai, B. C., ... Choolani, M. (2011). A study on Singaporean women's acceptance of using mobile phones to seek health information. *International Journal of Medical Informatics, 80*(12), e189–e202. doi:10.1016/j.ijmedinf.2011.08.007 PMID:21956003

Loy, J. S., Ali, E. E., & Yap, K. Y. (2016). Quality assessment of medical apps that target medication-related problems. *Journal of Managed Care & Specialty Pharmacy, 22*(10), 1124–1140. doi:10.18553/jmcp.2016.22.10.1124 PMID:27668561

Lyles, C. R., Sarkar, U., & Osborn, C. Y. (2014). Getting a technology-based diabetes intervention ready for primetime: A review of usability testing studies. *Current Diabetes Reports, 14*(10), 534. doi:10.100711892-014-0534-9 PMID:25173689

Matza, L. S., Park, J., Coyne, K. S., Skinner, E. P., Malley, K. G., & Wolever, R. Q. (2009). Derivation and validation of the ASK-12 adherence barrier survey. *The Annals of Pharmacotherapy, 43*(10), 1621–1630. doi:10.1345/aph.1M174 PMID:19776298

McCurdie, T., Taneva, S., Casselman, M., Yeung, M., McDaniel, C., Ho, W., & Cafazzo, J. (2012). mHealth consumer apps: The case for user-centered design. *Biomedical Instrumentation & Technology, 46*(s2), 49–56. doi:10.2345/0899-8205-46.s2.49 PMID:23039777

Michie, S., Richardson, M., Johnston, M., Abraham, C., Francis, J., Hardeman, W., ... Wood, C. E. (2013). The behavior change technique taxonomy (v1) of 93 hierarchically clustered techniques: Building an international consensus for the reporting of behavior change interventions. *Annals of Behavioral Medicine, 46*(1), 81–95. doi:10.100712160-013-9486-6 PMID:23512568

Mirkovic, J., Kaufman, D. R., & Ruland, C. M. (2014). Supporting cancer patients in illness management: Usability evaluation of a mobile app. *JMIR mHealth and uHealth, 2*(3), e33. doi:10.2196/mhealth.3359 PMID:25119490

Mohammed, H. B. M., Ibrahim, D., & Cavus, N. (2018). Mobile device based smart medication reminder for older people with disabilities. *Quality & Quantity, 52*(S2), 1329–1342. doi:10.100711135-018-0707-8

Moon, Z., Moss-Morris, R., Hunter, M. S., & Hughes, L. D. (2017). Understanding tamoxifen adherence in women with breast cancer: A qualitative study. *British Journal of Health Psychology*, *22*(4), 978–997. doi:10.1111/bjhp.12266 PMID:28850763

Morisky, D. E., & DiMatteo, M. R. (2011). Improving the measurement of self-reported medication nonadherence: Response to authors. *Journal of Clinical Epidemiology*, *64*(3), 255–257. doi:10.1016/j.jclinepi.2010.09.002 PMID:21144706

Morisky, D. E., Green, L. W., & Levine, D. M. (1986). Concurrent and predictive validity of a self-reported measure of medication adherence. *Medical Care*, *24*(1), 67–74. doi:10.1097/00005650-198601000-00007 PMID:3945130

Peters, G.-J. Y. (2014). A practical guide to effective behavior change: How to identify what to change in the first place. *European Health Psychologist, 16*(5), 142-155. doi: 10.31234/osf.io/hy7mj

Pew Research Center. (2016, Feb 18). *Smartphone ownership and Internet usage continues to climb in emerging economies*. Retrieved 31 Mar, 2020, from https://www.pewresearch.org/global/2016/02/22/smartphone-ownership-and-internet-usage-continues-to-climb-in-emerging-economies/technology-report-01-03/

Santo, K., Richtering, S. S., Chalmers, J., Thiagalingam, A., Chow, C. K., & Redfern, J. (2016). Mobile phone apps to improve medication adherence: A systematic stepwise process to identify high-quality apps. *JMIR mHealth and uHealth*, *4*(4), e132. doi:10.2196/mhealth.6742 PMID:27913373

Schneider, S. M., Hess, K., & Gosselin, T. (2011). Interventions to promote adherence with oral agents. *Seminars in Oncology Nursing*, *27*(2), 133–141. doi:10.1016/j.soncn.2011.02.005 PMID:21514482

Shen, Q., Ali, E. E., & Chew, L. (2017, Sep 23-24). *A survey on patient adherence to oral epidermal growth factor receptor tyrosine kinase inhibitor therapy.* Paper presented at the 27th Singapore Pharmacy Congress, Suntec Convention and Exhibition Centre, Singapore.

Spoelstra, S. L., & Sansoucie, H. (2015). Putting evidence into practice: Evidence-based interventions for oral agents for cancer. *Clinical Journal of Oncology Nursing*, *19*(3Suppl), 60–72. doi:10.1188/15.S1.CJON.60-72 PMID:26030394

Sun, Y., Wang, N., Guo, X., & Peng, Z. (2013). Understanding the acceptance of mobile health services: A comparison and integration of alternative models. *Journal of Electronic Commerce Research, 14*(2), 183–199.

Tan, G. (2017, Oct-Dec). New research methodology uncovers gene variations associated with breast cancer. *Salubris - A NCCS Quarterly Publication* Retrieved 31 Mar, 2020, from https://www.nccs.com.sg/Style%20Library/Images/Salubris/NCCS%20Salubris%20Issue%2043%20[Pages].pdf

Timmers, L., Boons, C. C., Kropff, F., van de Ven, P. M., Swart, E. L., Smit, E. F., ... Hugtenburg, J. G. (2014). Adherence and patients' experiences with the use of oral anticancer agents. *Acta Oncologica, 53*(2), 259–267. doi:10.3109/0284186X.2013.844353 PMID:24266637

Verbrugghe, M., Verhaeghe, S., Lauwaert, K., Beeckman, D., & Van Hecke, A. (2013). Determinants and associated factors influencing medication adherence and persistence to oral anticancer drugs: A systematic review. *Cancer Treatment Reviews, 39*(6), 610–621. doi:10.1016/j.ctrv.2012.12.014 PMID:23428230

Whiteley, L., Brown, L., Lally, M., Heck, N., & van den Berg, J. J. (2018). A mobile gaming intervention to increase adherence to antiretroviral treatment for youth living with HIV: Development guided by the information, motivation, and behavioral skills model. *JMIR mHealth and uHealth, 6*(4), e96. doi:10.2196/mhealth.8155 PMID:29685863

Whittaker, R., Merry, S., Dorey, E., & Maddison, R. (2012). A development and evaluation process for mHealth interventions: Examples from New Zealand. *Journal of Health Communication, 17*(Suppl 1), 11–21. doi:10.1080/10810730.2011.649103 PMID:22548594

Xue, L., Yen, C. C., Chang, L., Chan, H. C., Tai, B. C., Tan, S. B., ... Choolani, M. (2012). An exploratory study of ageing women's perception on access to health informatics via a mobile phone-based intervention. *International Journal of Medical Informatics, 81*(9), 637–648. doi:10.1016/j.ijmedinf.2012.04.008 PMID:22658778

Yagasaki, K., Komatsu, H., & Takahashi, T. (2015). Inner conflict in patients receiving oral anticancer agents: A qualitative study. *BMJ Open, 5*(4), e006699. doi:10.1136/bmjopen-2014-006699 PMID:25872938

Chapter 7
A Pharmaco-cybernetics Approach to Designing an Oncology Drug Interaction Database for Clinical Practice

ABSTRACT

This chapter describes how OncoRx-MI, a pharmaco-informatics platform for detecting chemotherapy interactions, was designed through a pharmaco-cybernetics approach targeting the 5 activities of the digital health innovation process. This is the first database of its kind that is able to provide interaction information for anticancer drugs and chemotherapy regimen cocktails. In order to identify the gap and determine the usefulness of this database in clinical oncology practice, the quality of online anticancer drug interactions was assessed, and the perceptions of oncology practitioners were sought. The results showed that the accuracy of drug interaction content and the clinical usefulness of the database was highly regarded by these practitioners. In addition, evidence of its relevance and credibility was demonstrated through user feedback on the database.

DOI: 10.4018/978-1-7998-3832-6.ch007

INTRODUCTION

In current practice, clinicians use a variety of resources for information on anticancer drug (ACD) interactions. These include primary literature, textbooks, compendia, conventional drug information texts, online databases, and websites. With the vast amounts of drug information sources that are available, they require accurate and effective methods for identifying relevant drug-drug interactions (DDIs), so that they can make better-informed decisions when confronted with such DDIs in their daily practice. The use of DDI databases is advantageous, since clinicians do not have to sieve through the large amounts of information from various sources to determine any suspected DDIs (P.D. Hansten, 2003). Furthermore, the use of such databases can also raise an alert to any potentially harmful drug combinations, and provide useful information about the detected DDI (Grönroos et al., 1997). A number of commercial drug information databases, such as Lexi-Interact®, Micromedex® and UpToDate®, are available electronically. Some databases provide detailed DDI information, including the effects, onset, severity and mechanisms of interaction (Kheshti, Aalipour, & Namazi, 2016). In contrast, there are also websites that only alert users to potential DDIs without giving other supporting details (Eysenbach, 2000). Databases that provide information about complementary and alternative medicines (CAMs) have limited information on ACD-CAM interactions, especially for traditional Chinese medicine (TCM) herbs. Additionally, major conflicts on DDI information exist among various commercial resources and compendia, especially with combination listings, consistency of interaction severities, and strengths of scientific evidences (Wong, Ko, & Chan, 2008). There is currently no oncology-specific drug database that is dedicated to ACD interactions based on both single-agent ACDs and multiple-agent chemotherapy cocktail searches. Most of the available drug databases require the input of individual drugs in a patient's prescription in order to search for DDIs. The closest oncology-specific interaction database was developed by Radboudumc and University of Liverpool, but the database was only able to detect the DDIs of individual ACDs and not chemoregimen cocktails (Radboudumc, n.d.).

As such, a pharmaco-informatics platform – called OncoRx – was built to address this clinical gap. OncoRx is an oncology-specific drug database that detects ACD interactions with *ONCO*logy drug prescriptions (*Rx*), so that DDI searches with ACDs and chemoregimen cocktails can be carried out. OncoRx was designed from a pharmaco-cybernetics perspective targeting the 5 activities described in the digital health innovation process (Figure 1, Chapter 3). These were:

Step 1: Identifying the healthcare problem in oncology practice;
Step 2: Research and innovation through engagement;
Step 3: Designing and developing the oncology drug interaction database;
Step 4: Evaluation and generating evidence of relevance and credibility; and
Step 5: Implementation of the oncology database in healthcare practice.

Core to its design were the four Pharmaco-cybernetic Maxims and user-centered design (UCD) principles, so that it could cater towards its target users who were clinicians dealing with cancer patients in their practices. The rest of this chapter describes how the development of OncoRx aligns to the digital health innovation process, and the considerations on how the issue of quality was addressed for this database.

USER INVOLVEMENT IN ONCORX DEVELOPMENT

As with the MedFC app, UCD was also applied in the design and development process of OncoRx. In the order to address the need for an oncology-specific drug-interaction database, a study was conducted to identify the drug information resources used by oncology pharmacy practitioners, the clinical gap in terms of ACD interactions and the essential interaction parameters to be included in such a database. Furthermore, feedback was also obtained from the database users to determine its usefulness and clinical relevance, as well as its usability and on the drug interaction content that was provided. In a study on drug prescribing patterns of ACDs by Cheung et al. (Cheung, Yap, Chui, & Chan, 2010), the authors had also used the interaction content from this database to determine the prevalence of potentially interacting co-prescribed drug combinations to cancer patients at their local ambulatory cancer center. The study showed that this database had the potential to aid oncology practitioners in reducing DDIs in clinical practice.

STEP 1: IDENTIFYING THE HEALTHCARE PROBLEM IN ONCOLOGY PRACTICE

Defining the Need for an Oncology-specific Database on ACD Interactions

In general, clinicians may not have the time or necessary skills to constantly update, critically evaluate and apply the enormous amount of published literature available to their clinical practice (Tan et al., 2006). Studies conducted on information sources used by oncology practitioners have concentrated on general cancer information instead of oncology DDIs (Dooley, Lee, & Marriott, 2004; Tan, et al., 2006). A higher percentage of practitioners has been reported to use electronic databases (51-79%) as sources for DDI information rather than printed references (9-24%) (Yu Ko et al., 2007); and approximately 53% and 25% of prescribers and pharmacists rely on a colleague for such DDI information (Yu Ko, et al., 2007). This phenomenon is worrying since healthcare professionals may lack the ability to identify potential DDIs (Cavuto, Woosley, & Sale, 1996; Glassman, Simon, Belperio, & Lanto, 2002; Langdorf, Fox, Marwah, Montague, & Hart, 2000; Nelson Jr., Hutchinson, Mahoney, & Ringstrom, 1976; Weideman, Bernstein, & McKinney, 1999). The practitioners' ability to identify DDIs is inversely affected by the number of drugs on patients' medication profiles (Weideman, et al., 1999). Thus, it is essential that clinicians find appropriate sources of ACD interaction information at the point of patient care. The practitioner's ability to keep abreast with the latest ACD-related information is likely to be hindered by inherent delays in traditional literature, such as book resources (Abernethy et al., 2009). In this aspect, online drug databases can be useful for obtaining up-to-date DDI information in a timely, efficient and accessible manner (Polen, Zapantis, Clauson, Jebrock, & Paris, 2008). In line with identifying the healthcare problem in clinical oncology practice and establishing the need for an oncology-specific database (Figure 1, Chapter 3), a study was developed to investigate the sources of DDI information among practitioners, the usefulness of such a database that targeted ACD interactions and the essential parameters for this database (K. Y. Yap, Chan, & Chui, 2010).

A qualitative, cross-sectional study was employed for this purpose. A structured questionnaire consisting of 10 questions obtained information regarding the respondents' practice characteristics, frequency of encountering ACD interactions in their daily practice, and their sources of DDI information.

The self-administered questionnaire was distributed to the participants of The 2nd Asia-Pacific Oncology Pharmacy Congress, who were healthcare professionals from the Asia-Pacific region, US and Australia. In addition, their opinions were sought regarding the usefulness of an online ACD interaction database, as well as the features that they deemed important for such a database, for example, the accuracy of DDI content, usefulness in clinical practice and user-friendliness. In addition, they had to rate the importance of several DDI parameters – pharmacokinetics of the ACDs and interacting drugs, mechanism of interaction, interaction severity, substantiation of the interaction and the presence of a management plan – using a five-point Likert scale ranging from "not essential at all" to "absolutely essential".

The response rate of the survey was 50% (105/209 returned questionnaires). Three (1%) were excluded from analysis as majority of the questions were not answered. Of the remaining questionnaires, only those that were completed by pharmacists working in Asia were included for analysis, since majority of the respondents were pharmacists by profession (96%) and practising in Asia (93%). As a result, a total of 91 completed questionnaires were analyzed. The rationale was to represent a clearer picture on the opinions of pharmacists in this part of the world regarding DDIs and the usefulness of such an oncology-specific interaction database. In terms of demographics, half practiced in inpatient (54 respondents, 59%) and outpatient settings (44 respondents, 48%), of which 31 (34%) and 21 (23%) were solely practising in either inpatient or outpatient settings. There were 2 respondents (2%) in community/retail, 5 respondents (6%) in hospice/home care and 1 respondent (1%) in private practice. Fifty-two respondents (57%) had 5 to 20 years of practice experience, while 36 (40%) had less than 5 years of practice. A quarter (23 respondents, 25%) frequently encountered ACD interactions (more than 25% of their time) in their daily practices. Electronic databases (e.g. PubMed, Medline, Scirus, Scopus, ScienceDirect, 70%), drug interaction textbooks (e.g. Drug Interaction Facts, Stockley's Drug Interactions, 69%) and drug compendia (e.g. AHFS Drug Information, British National Formulary, Drug Facts & Comparisons, Lexi-Comp's Drug Information Handbook, Martindale, Physician's Desk Reference, 64%) were the most common information resources used by the respondents to check for ACD interactions. On the other hand, medication package inserts (41%) and standard medical, pharmacology and pharmacotherapy textbooks (42%) were seldom used. Almost half (44 respondents, 48%) used specific drug information software (e.g. Clinical Pharmacology, Drugdex / Micromedex, Epocrates, Facts & Comparisons, Lexi-Comp, Martindale), while a minor proportion (16 respondents, 18%) did not use any computerized forms of information sources to check for ACD interactions. Interestingly, almost half of the pharmacists consulted their colleagues for ACD interaction information (44%), which was more than the proportion who used standard textbooks (42%) and product information (41%). Inpatient pharmacists were more likely than outpatient pharmacists to use standard textbooks as DDI sources for ACDs (52% versus 14% respectively, p=0.007).

An important finding was that there were lesser pharmacists practising in hospital inpatient (n=31) and outpatient settings (n=21) who used drug information software (45-57%) for ACD interaction information, compared to DDI textbooks (61-67%) and compendia (67-77%). A similar trend was observed with the inpatient pharmacists – more of them used DDI textbooks (61%) and compendia (77%) than electronic databases (58%). The authors attributed their results to several environmental barriers in hospital settings (K. Y. Yap, A. Chan, et al., 2010), such as connection or firewall issues in the hospitals, restricted access to the internet/intranet in clinical areas, limited number of computers in the wards and treatment areas, old or slow computers, and economic reasons like subscriptions to journals. These barriers have yet to be resolved in this day and age, where cybersecurity concerns have gained worldwide attention after the recent health data breaches in Singapore (Davis, 2018) and Australia (Ghioni, 2019; Henry, 2019).

Despite these environmental barriers, a large proportion of pharmacist respondents in the study still used e-databases (e.g. PubMed) and drug information software (e.g. Micromedex) as ACD interaction resources. In general, more pharmacy practitioners consulted electronic resources for DDI information compared to standard medical, pharmacology and pharmacotherapy textbooks. This is not surprising since clinicians tend to perceive these sources as being readily available and time-efficient at the point of patient care (Tan, et al., 2006). The advent of the internet and portable devices (e.g. portable digital assistants, tablets, iPads and various smartphones) have allowed clinicians to access online databases and drug information programs for evidence-based oncology information. The advantage of these electronic resources over hardcopy books is their timeliness of information.

In addition, the authors also observed that the proportion of pharmacists who used drug information software in their study (48%) was lower than what was reported in US practitioners (79%) (Yu Ko, et al., 2007). This difference in proportions was attributed to the fact that the US study was assessing sources of general DDI information used by prescribers in a variety of specialties instead (Yu Ko, et al., 2007). In addition, the drug information software used for evaluation, such as Micromedex, Lexi-Comp, and Facts and Comparisons, were not specific to ACD interactions. The lower proportions of pharmacy practitioners reported in the Asia-Pacific study who used these software to search for ACD interaction information was consistent with the high percentage of respondents (93%) who indicated a need for an online ACD interaction database. In summary, this study established that there was a need for an oncology-specific database that could target ACD interactions (K. Y. Yap, A. Chan, et al., 2010). Such a database would be a useful tool for pharmacy clinicians in the Asia-Pacific.

Determining the Interaction Parameters for an Oncology-specific Database

From the same study in pharmacy practitioners (n=91), the most important DDI parameters for the oncology-specific database, as indicated by ratings of "essential" and "absolutely essential", were the mechanism and severity of the detected interaction, as well as the presence of a management plan (98% each) (K. Y. Yap, A. Chan, et al., 2010). The high ratings for these parameters were probably because they were directly related to the interaction effects and how the interactions could be managed at the point of patient care. The respondents considered the presence of a proposed management plan to be more crucial than the other interaction parameters – this was reflected in their ratings of this parameter as "essential" and "absolutely essential". On the other hand, there were some respondents who rated the other interaction parameters with "not essential, but good to have". In addition, there were more outpatient (16/21, 76%) than inpatient (13/31, 42%) pharmacists who considered the interaction mechanism as an "absolutely essential" component of the database (p=0.014). This could probably be due to the difficulty of consulting DDI resources in outpatient settings in front of the customer/ patient; in contrast to inpatient pharmacists who could still refer to other DDI resources for supporting evidences of the interaction mechanisms. One inpatient pharmacist also felt that the mechanism of interaction was "not essential, but good to have" in the database.

Interestingly, the pharmacokinetic profiles of the drugs were seen as less important (95%) than the mechanism and severity of interaction, or the management plan (98% each). Substantiating studies for the interactions (85%) and reference source citations (90%) fared the most poorly. In fact, a small proportion of pharmacist respondents felt that the pharmacokinetic profiles

(2%) and substantiating studies (1%) were not needed at all. On the other hand, other than the necessity of having a proposed management plan; for the other parameters, there were small numbers of pharmacists who felt that those were either "good to have" or "not essential at all" (i.e. pharmacokinetics of interacting drugs, 4 pharmacists; mechanism and severity of interaction, 1 pharmacist each; references sources, 6 pharmacists).

Qualitative feedback by some of the respondents indicated that they would like to see additional DDI parameters in the database – these included the risk or incidence of interaction; interactions with combination chemotherapy regimens; interactions with TCMs, CAMs, parenteral and enteral nutritional products; and non-interacting alternative drugs.

The authors reported that a higher percentage of outpatient pharmacists rated the DDI parameters as "absolutely essential" compared to inpatient pharmacists, except for the severity of interaction, in which there were more inpatient than outpatient pharmacists who rated this parameter as "absolutely essential" (84% versus 76% respectively, p=0.495). The authors suggested that severity could have played a higher weightage in the clinical practices of inpatient pharmacists, probably because they viewed DDIs as being a preventable drug-related problem, and severity would play a more important role in their decisions to dispense or not dispense the affected drug combination. In addition, the authors quoted a study by Ducharme and Boothby, which had identified a substantially higher number of DDIs occurring in the outpatient setting compared to hospitalised inpatients (Ducharme & Boothby, 2007). Moreover, studies have shown the existence of inconsistent severity ratings among different drug compendia (Abarca et al., 2004; Chao & Maibach, 2005; Nikolic & Ilic, 2013; Vitry, 2007; Wong, et al., 2008). Hence, it was important that the oncology database could provide data on severity of the interaction, so that it could be reliable for clinical practice.

Consideration Factors for the Accuracy, Clinical Usefulness and User-friendliness Of The Oncology-specific Database

Majority of the pharmacists who completed the questionnaire (93%) indicated that it would be useful to have an online oncology-specific database catering towards DDIs. Only 2% disagreed. The rest felt that it was not essential, but a bonus, to have the database. The pharmacy respondents seemed to be more concerned about the accuracy of DDI content (98%) and clinical usefulness of the database (97%) than its user-friendliness (88%).

Almost all the pharmacy practitioners considered DDI content accuracy as an important factor for the database. Using the assumption that respondents who rated the factors as "absolutely essential" would consider these factors to be of higher priority than "essential", the authors reported that there were more outpatient pharmacists (n=19/21, 91%) who considered DDI content accuracy to be of higher priority than inpatient pharmacists (n=20/31, 65%, p=0.013). The trend was similar for clinical usefulness of the database, whereby more outpatient (n=16/21, 76%) than inpatient pharmacists (n=16/31, 52%, p=0.043) rated it as "absolutely essential". Interestingly, one respondent who was not working in either inpatient or outpatient settings had indicated that clinical usefulness was "not essential, but good to have". Nonetheless, the authors hypothesized that these 2 factors played more important roles for outpatient practitioners and could be related to the ease-of-access to the various DDI resources in inpatient and outpatient settings. Studies have suggested that pharmacists in outpatient settings may be suitable for improving the quality of patient care (Austwick, Brown, Goodyear, & Brooks, 2002; Boddy, 2001; Tucker, 2004). However, outpatient pharmacists could be subjected to time constraints and greater difficulty in accessing drug information resources because of their contact with patients at the point of dispensing. The outpatient pharmacist respondents in the study could have viewed the database as their main source of ACD interactions at the point of dispensing, and thus considered these factors to be of higher priority, while those in inpatient practice would probably have viewed the database as being complementary to other available resources.

On the other hand, user-friendliness of the database was considered to be less important by pharmacists working in both inpatient and outpatient practices (n=4/23, 17%) than those who were in other practice settings (n=0, p=0.006), as indicated by their response of "not essential, but good to have". In fact, all the pharmacists who were practising in other settings felt that user-friendliness was an "essential" or "absolutely essential" (n=8/16, 50% each) component of the database. In contrast, there were 9 out of 75 pharmacists in inpatient and outpatient settings (10%) who were either neutral or considered this factor to only be of added value to the database.

Even though user-friendliness is a subjective factor and depends on the practitioner's familiarity with the database, there was still a large proportion of respondents (n=80/91, 88%) who considered this as an important factor. User-friendliness was more highly desirable among pharmacists who were working in other settings (e.g. academia, retail, home care, and private practice), probably because they relied heavily on electronic databases (81%) and software (44%) as resources for DDI information, but had to work independently in their workplace. A user-friendly database would have enabled them to be more efficient in terms of time-management when searching for DDIs. Some desirable features of a good online database are ease-of-use and good navigation features (Clauson, Marsh, Polen, Seamon, & Ortiz, 2007). Database usability is also becoming increasingly important in clinical practice with the availability of software programs for handheld devices (e.g. portable digital assistants, mobile apps). One respondent had indicated that a software program was preferred over an online DDI database. However, ease-of-use comes at a price which may compromise the scope and completeness of drug information (Clauson, Polen, & Marsh, 2007), thus it was no surprise that content accuracy and clinical usefulness still edged over user-friendliness as being more important.

While the authors noted that the respondents in their study were mainly pharmacists practising in Asia, hence their results might not reflect the views of pharmacists in other parts of the world or other healthcare professionals; they indicated that their results were still useful because patients would generally be seen by pharmacists as the last line of practitioners during their consultations with the healthcare team for dispensing and medication counseling. Hence, the opinions of this subgroup of healthcare professionals could provide an insight to the development of future digital health and drug information systems aimed at providing a "slice" to the Swiss cheese model of safety incidents (Perneger, 2005), in order to enhance patient safety (Figure 1).

In addition, the authors acknowledged their limitation of assuming that some of their conclusions regarding the usefulness of the database with ratings of "absolutely essential" would consistently be a notch higher in terms of priority than "essential". Due to the nature of the Likert-scaled questions in the survey and the different practice settings of the surveyed pharmacists, the interpretations of the "absolutely essential" and "essential" anchor points could vary among the respondents, leading to subtle differences in their responses. However, they attempted to control for this difference by arranging the parameters for each of the sections as separate parts of a single question. For example, the importance of the 3 different factors of the database (information accuracy, usefulness in clinical practice, and user-friendliness) were designed as one full question with the same set of Likert scales, so that participants could compare the factors in terms of importance. An "essential" rating for both clinical usefulness and user-friendliness would imply that

Figure 1. The Swiss Cheese Model of safety incidents showing digital health systems providing a "slice of cheese" to enhance patient safety.

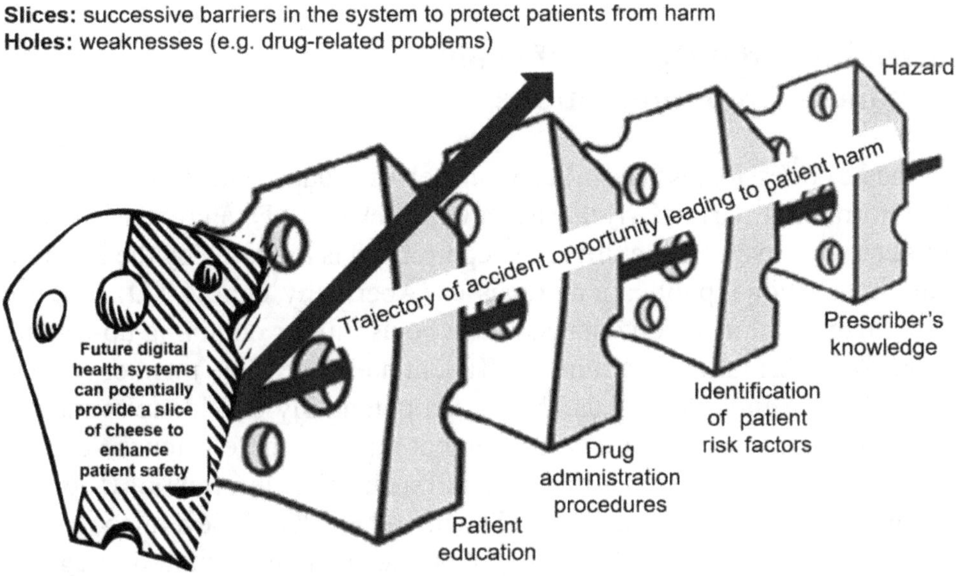

these factors were equally important, while an "absolutely essential" rating for information accuracy would imply that this factor was considered to be more crucial than the other 2 factors.

Lastly, another limitation of the study was the "ceiling effect" of their respondents who might have skewed their results toward a higher priority end of the spectrum. The authors suggested that future studies should obtain opinions from healthcare professionals in other specialisations, such as psychiatrists and neurologists, since cancer patients tend to also suffer from depression due to the emotional impact of the cancer diagnosis (Lim, 2007; Newport & Nemeroff, 1998; Spiegel & Giese-Davis, 2003), and from epilepsy due to metastases of the tumor to the brain (Lassman & DeAngelis, 2003; Newton, Goldlust, & Pearl, 2006). The opinions of these healthcare specialists would be valuable since they might hold different points of view from the oncology pharmacists surveyed in the study.

STEP 2: RESEARCH AND INNOVATION THROUGH ENGAGEMENT

Determining the Quality of Online Anticancer Drug Interactions

Healthcare professionals need to keep themselves updated with the most current DDI information, particularly those involving newer ACDs and chemotherapy regimens. However, their ability to keep updated is hindered by the inherent delays in traditional publication processes (Abernethy, et al., 2009). The use of online drug information databases can be useful for obtaining up-to-date interaction information in a timely, efficient and accessible manner (Polen, et al., 2008). Although drug databases can potentially provide relevant and up-to-date DDI information in a convenient manner, there is much concern regarding the wide variation in the quality of such online information (Provost, Koompalum, Dong, & Martin, 2006; Sheehan et al., 2003). Several tools have been developed to evaluate the quality of online health information and guide healthcare professionals and patients to the best sources (Gagliardi & Jadad, 2002). Some manifest as codes of conduct for voluntary compliance, while others provide guidance to users in the form of a questionnaire or checklist. Six available assessment tools are described in Table 1 with a summary of their evaluation criteria.

Although these tools are useful in appraising online drug databases, they also possess limitations in terms of utility. Tools such as Netscoring (Darmoni, 2001) are more comprehensive than others (e.g. eEurope (Commission of the European Communities (Brussels), 2002) and DARTS (Närhi et al., 2008)), but are time-consuming to use. On the other hand, tools with fewer questions provide a fast and user-friendly way to evaluate health information websites. These tools also differ in terms of their quality assessment criteria. For example, DISCERN (Charnock & Shepperd, 2004) and eEurope (Commission of the European Communities (Brussels), 2002) do not include the presence of disclaimers and biasness as part of their evaluation criteria. In contrast, the Health on the Net code (HONcode) (Boyer, Selby, Scherrer, & Appel, 1998), DARTS (Närhi, et al., 2008) and Quality Evaluation Scoring Tool (QUEST) (Robillard, Jun, Lai, & Feng, 2018) do not consider editorial review and target audiences as part of their quality assessment. Some tools like HONcode, eEurope and DARTS also do not provide a scoring system, which makes objective comparisons among databases difficult.

More importantly, a common limitation among these tools is the absence of assessment criteria for evaluating the accuracy of health-related content. Furthermore, these tools do not cater toward any specific clinical specialty and can only be used to evaluate general health information websites. Despite the high potential risk of cancer patients suffering from ACD interactions, based on the author's knowledge, there was no quality assessment tool that evaluated drug databases for information on ACD interactions. Therefore, an assessment tool, called OncoRx-IQ, was developed to evaluate the *I*nformation *Q*uality of DDI information from *Onco*logy drug prescriptions (*Rx*), including the content accuracy of the online ACD interaction information. Akin to the operationalized quality definition for health-related websites put forth by Provost et al. (Provost, et al., 2006), the quality of online drug databases assessed by OncoRx-IQ was defined as the level of excellence which characterized an online drug database in terms of its ability to satisfy DDI information needs.

Based on a review of the quality assessment tools described above (Table 1), OncoRx-IQ was developed in the form of a questionnaire which consisted of 25 questions separated into two sections (K. Y. Yap, Raaj, & Chan, 2010) (Table 2). The first section evaluated the accuracy and comprehensiveness of the details of a DDI provided by a drug database for an ACD and a combination chemotherapy regimen cocktail (27 points). In this section, summaries of the studies and reference citations for the identified DDIs were provided for verification of the interaction evidences. These included in-vitro and animal studies, case reports and human studies, as well as product information of the interacting drugs.

The second section evaluated the overall quality of the drug database (40 points) in terms of two aspects – ease-of-use (12 points) and reliability (28 points). Database usability was assessed based on whether it had certain tools and features which allowed for easy navigation, such as a help function, site map or menu and the loading speed of the database. Conversely, database reliability was determined through quality aspects such as its credibility (e.g. authorship, presence of bias), the types of drug-related information and resources it provided, its target audiences, user privacy policy and how its drug-related content should be interpreted by users (e.g. disclaimers).

OncoRx-IQ was reviewed by 4 pharmacy undergraduate students to ensure its user-friendliness. Alterations to the tool were made according to their feedback. However, their responses were not considered for a pilot study on the evaluation of drug databases, described in the next section.

Table 1. Comparison of the characteristics and evaluation criteria of 6 available quality assessment tools.

Characteristics	DARTS	DISCERN	eEUROPE	HONcode	Netscoring	QUEST
Aims	To allow users to identify good quality information.	To provide users with a valid and reliable way of assessing the quality of information on treatment choices.	To help users distinguish valid and reliable information from those which are inaccurate or misleading.	To standardize the reliability of medical and health information available on the World-Wide Web.	To provide a set of criteria that can be used to assess the quality of health information on the internet.	To provide a quantitative measure of six aspects of quality of online health information.
Specific to a clinical speciality	X	X	X	X	X	X
Quantitative assessment (score/ weight)	X	✓	X	X	✓	✓
Content accuracy evaluation	X	X	X	X	X	X
Evaluation Criteria						
Authorship	✓	✓	✓	✓	✓	✓
Disclaimer/ Complementarity	X	X	X	✓	✓	✓
Editorial review	X	X	✓	X	✓	X
Financial disclosure	✓	X	✓	✓	✓	X
Presence of bias	X	X	X	✓	✓	✓
User privacy	X	X	✓	✓	✓	X
Purpose of database	✓	✓	✓	✓	✓	X
Referencing/ Attribution	✓	✓	✓	✓	✓	✓
Target audience	X	✓	✓	X	✓	X
Navigation tools	✓	X	✓	✓	✓	X
Links to other databases	X	✓	X	✓	✓	X
User support features	X	X	✓	X	✓	X
Loading speed	X	X	✓	X	✓	X

✓ The assessment tool contains the characteristic or criteria.
X The assessment tool does not contain the characteristic or criteria.

Assessing the Quality of Drug Databases Through Oncorx-IQ

The OncoRx-IQ tool was used by a panel of 6 pre-registration pharmacists in Singapore to evaluate 4 drug databases in a pilot study. The top 3 databases that were selected appeared most frequently in a Google search of keywords

Table 2. Evaluation criteria in the OncoRx-IQ tool.

Sections of OncoRx-IQ	Evaluation Criteria	Explanation of Criteria
A) Content Accuracy (27 points)		
Interaction details for an anticancer drug and a chemotherapy regimen cocktail	Effects of interaction	Provision of the drug interaction effects and/or clinical manifestations
	Mechanism of interaction	Provision of the mechanism of drug interaction
	Evidence of interaction	Provision of evidences that substantiate the drug interaction (e.g. case reports, in-vitro / animal / human studies, package inserts)
	Management strategies	Provision of appropriate recommendations to manage a drug interaction
B) Overall Quality (40 points)		
Ease-of-use	Navigation tools	Presence of a site map, index or menu system
	User support features	Presence of a help feature or frequently asked questions (FAQ) section
	Loading speed	Acceptability of the time taken for the database to load
Reliability	Authorship	Presence of the names and credentials of authors
	Purpose of database	Indication of the database's objectives
	Target audience	Indication of who the database is intended for
	Editorial review	Explanation of the database's content verification procedure
	Financial disclosure	Indication of the database's sources of funding
	Presence of bias	Presence of advertisements and/or affiliations
	Disclaimer	Presence of a statement indicating that information should not replace a healthcare professional's advice
	User privacy	Presence of a privacy policy statement pertaining to users
	Drug interaction risk information	Indication of the likelihood of a drug interaction occurring
	Drug interaction severity information	Indication of the severity of a drug interaction
	Referencing	Presence of citations for the editorial content
	Links to other databases	Presence of hyperlinks to other drug databases for verification of drug information

related to chemotherapy, ACDs and drug interactions, and were accessible by direct links. These were Drugs.com (www.drugs.com), Medscape (www.medscape.com) and Drug Digest (www.drugdigest.org/wps/portal/ddigest). In addition, Micromedex Healthcare Series was also included for evaluation as it was a commonly used database by healthcare professionals (Clauson, Marsh, et al., 2007).

Among the 4 databases, Micromedex was rated the best in terms of overall quality with the highest composite score of 66.9%, followed by Drugs.com (50.5%) and Medscape (42.3%). Drug Digest had the lowest composite score at 35.8%, and this was also reflected by its low scores in content accuracy (8.0%) and reliability (48.2%). In contrast, Micromedex scored the highest in all the 3 domains of content accuracy (56.3%), ease-of-use (75.0%) and reliability (73.6%). Micromedex (56.3%) was the only database that scored above 50% in terms of content accuracy, compared to the other databases (Drugs.com 34.0%, Medscape 17.9%, Drug Digest 8.0%). The statistical difference in content accuracy (p=0.008) and reliability (p=0.046) scores of the databases led to a statistical variance in their composite scores (p=0.007).

Content accuracy in OncoRx-IQ was evaluated based on the interactions between the chemotherapy regimen cocktail EP (consisting of 2 ACDs – etoposide and cisplatin) with valproic acid, causing increased risks of etoposide and hematological toxicities, as well as loss of seizure control (Bourg, Lebrun, Chichmanian, Thomas, & Frenay, 2001; Ikeda, Murakami, Takano, Usui, & Kihira, 2005; Neef & de Voogd-van der Straaten, 1988). The interaction between the ACD vorinostat and valproic acid (an antiepileptic) leading to increased risks of severe thrombocytopenia and gastrointestinal bleeding was also evaluated (Eyal et al., 2004; Göttlicher et al., 2001; Merck & Co. Inc., 2020; Phiel et al., 2001). Interestingly, among all the evaluated databases, Micromedex was the only database which scored higher than 50%. Although both Micromedex and Drugs.com managed to identify interacting pairs of drugs between valproic acid with cisplatin and vorinostat, the information in Micromedex was more detailed and specific, thus leading to the higher scores in this domain. Closer inspection of the DDI content in the databases showed that there were deficiencies in the DDI information – Micromedex, Drugs.com and Drug Digest only managed to identify one of the interaction effects between cisplatin and valproic acid, that is, a decrease in plasma valproic acid concentrations resulting in loss of seizure control. The other interaction effect of an increased risk of hematological toxicity due to inhibition of the cytochrome P450 (CYP450) 2C9 metabolism of cisplatin (Bourg, et al., 2001; Ikeda, et al., 2005; Neef & de Voogd-van der Straaten, 1988), which necessitates monitoring of signs and symptoms of bleeding as a management plan (Bourg, et al., 2001; Vecht, Wagner, & Wilms, 2003a, 2003b), was not detected by any of the drug databases. Moreover, even though management plans to monitor for seizure control were suggested by the databases, none of them indicated alternative non-interacting anti-epileptic drugs, such as gabapentin or levetiracetam, as part of managing the drug interaction (Vecht, et al., 2003b).

Similarly, none of the online databases managed to identify the interaction between etoposide and valproic acid due to inhibition of CYP3A4-mediated etoposide metabolism (Bourg, et al., 2001; Vecht, et al., 2003a). However, an evaluator who used the CD-ROM version of Micromedex indicated that he managed to identify this interaction pair. Medscape (17.9%) and Drug Digest (8.0%) were the lowest scorers for content accuracy, obtaining less than one-third the score of Micromedex (56.3%). These low scores could be due to Medscape only identifying one out of the 3 DDI pairs (vorinostat and valproic acid), while Drug Digest did not manage to identify any of the interactions at all. A quick search had showed that vorinostat was not in the list of drugs in Drug Digest.

The authors reported that all the evaluators in this study agreed that content accuracy was an important component of determining quality of a DDI database. The inter-rater agreement for content accuracy was the highest (W=0.79) compared to reliability (W=0.54) and usability (W=0.12). Although Micromedex fared the best among all the evaluated databases in terms of content accuracy, the authors noted that the comprehensiveness of the interaction data in such a professional subscription database that was commonly used among healthcare professionals could be improved from its average content accuracy score of 56.3%.

In OncoRx-IQ, reliability of databases was differentiated from content accuracy through determining the level of trustworthiness of the drug databases through criteria such as authorship information, editorial review processes and the possible presence of bias. Interestingly, even though Micromedex was deemed to be the most reliable among all the databases (average reliability score of 73.6% versus Drugs.com 58.9%, Medscape 55.4%, Drug Digest 48.2%), the authors also reported that there were 2 evaluators who rated Drugs.com as being more reliable than Micromedex. The authors attributed these ratings to be due to the presence of the HONcode approval seal in the Drugs.com website. However, the reliability score of Drug Digest was not as high as Drugs.com, even though it was also HONcode certified. The reason could be due to Drugs.com displaying an additional "TRUSTe certified privacy" logo on its homepage. TRUSTe is an independent organization that ensures online privacy and protection of confidential user information on certified websites so as to instil the trust and confidence in visitors and users of these websites (TRUSTe, 2008). This feature could have been an additional indicator of the reliability of a drug database in OncoRx-IQ and thus might have influenced the responses of the evaluators.

As part of evaluating reliability, OncoRx-IQ also assessed whether the drug databases contained a disclaimer specifying that the drug information provided was not meant to replace the advice of a healthcare professional. All but one of the evaluators agreed that Drugs.com clearly displayed such a disclaimer, but only half indicated that this disclaimer was clearly displayed in Medscape. This discrepancy between the 2 databases could be due to the way in which the information was displayed to users – users of Drugs.com were required to read and agree to a set of terms and conditions, which includes the disclaimer, before being allowed access to the interaction checker. In contrast, this disclaimer was only available if users clicked on the "Terms of Use" in Medscape. For online databases that offer access to information to the public, the presence of such a disclaimer is important for patients who may alter their dosing regimens themselves based on the information that they find in these databases.

Although equivalent scoring weightages were allocated to the parameters of content accuracy and reliability in OncoRx-IQ, for databases whereby content accuracy played a major role in correlating to their overall quality, such as Drugs.com (r^2=0.89), its reliability played a secondary role. On the other hand, the reliability scores of the other databases, such as Medscape and Drug Digest, had a higher correlation and impact to their overall quality assessments (r^2=0.89 for Medscape, r^2=0.82 for Drug Digest) compared to their content accuracy. Consequently, the lower ratings in both of the parameters of these 2 databases led to their lower composite scores.

OncoRx-IQ assessed the user-friendliness of the databases with questions on various aspects, such as a help feature or frequently asked questions section, website navigation tools, and on loading times and overall expediencies of the drug databases. In contrast to the other quality domains of content accuracy and database reliability, ease-of-use of the databases was less of a determining factor in their overall quality. This domain was allocated the lowest weightage in OncoRx-IQ because its scores could be affected by users' prior experiences and familiarity with the databases. One of the questions in this domain asked about the databases' ability to detect interactions with combination chemotherapy regimen cocktails based on their acronyms, since cancer patients would often be administered with such regimen cocktails. Certain regimens might consist of as many as 7 to 8 drugs, for example, BEACOPP (bleomycin, etoposide, doxorubicin, cyclophosphamide, vincristine, procarbazine and prednisone) (Tesch et al., 1998) and the double-delayed intensification regimen for pediatrics (vincristine, dexamethasone, doxorubicin, L-asparaginase, cyclophosphamide, cytarabine, thioguanine and methotrexate) (Lange et al., 2002). It would not only be time-consuming and inconvenient for clinicians to search for DDIs of each individual drug within the regimen, especially during clinic visits, but if they are in a rush for time, they might accidentally omit an interaction search with a particular ACD in the regimen, which might lead to a possibility of DRPs and adverse outcomes in patients. The ability for a database to detect DDIs of combination regimen cocktails would minimize the probability of accidental omissions in interaction searches, since there would not be a need to enter each individual drug in the cocktail in the interaction search. However, none of the databases that were evaluated had such a feature, suggesting that this feature could potentially be useful for drug databases targeted at cancer chemotherapy. The scores for ease-of-use were similar among the databases. Micromedex achieved the highest score (75.0%), while Medscape obtained the lowest score (66.7%, p=0.631). The authors postulated that the high score of Micromedex was due to the evaluators' familiarity with this database, since it was a common resource for drug information in hospital settings. In contrast, the low score for Medscape could be due to the additional required login step before users could access the interaction checker. Since this step was not a prerequisite to use the interaction checkers from Drugs.com and Drug Digest, the hassle and inconvenience of spending time to register for an account was avoided.

A disadvantage of the quality assessment tool was the length of time required for each evaluator to assess the 4 drug databases. Evaluation of the databases was a laborious task. Feedback from the evaluators indicated that each person took an approximate 45 minutes to an hour to fully complete the evaluations, which might have caused them to be more fatigued and less meticulous in their evaluations. It was for this reason that pre-registration pharmacists were recruited into the study instead of clinicians, since they were already practising in the clinical setting and would also be familiar with the area of DDIs. Nonetheless, the authors acknowledged that OncoRx-IQ should also be tested by clinicians, but with fewer numbers of databases being assigned for evaluation.

Another limitation was the use of Likert-scaled questions, which imparted some subjectivity in the quality assessment of the databases. Certain quality aspects, such as the convenience of using a database and loading within an acceptable time frame, were perhaps more efficiently and exhaustively determined by the perceptions of users, especially if the database was unfamiliar to them. Furthermore, evaluating the databases without these questions would lead to a less comprehensive assessment of quality. In order to cater for time and resource limitations in conducting the quality assessments using OncoRx-IQ, a compromise of the top 3 databases that appeared most frequently in the Google search were chosen, with the assumption that these databases would be the most frequently encountered and utilised by users. However, the authors acknowledged that larger scale studies could involve using OncoRx-IQ to assess a wider variety of online DDI databases.

STEP 3: DESIGNING AND DEVELOPING THE ONCOLOGY DRUG INTERACTION DATABASE

OncoRx was an oncology interaction database developed with the aim of creating awareness and providing knowledge to healthcare professionals about the harmful effects of DDIs that were relevant to ACDs and chemoregimen cocktails. This database was developed in modular format and is currently able to detect interactions with psychotropic agents and CAMs. With the advancement of 3rd and 4th generation (3G and 4G) networks and new mobile devices, a mobile web app (called OncoRx-MI for the *M*obile *I*nternet) was developed for users to access on their smartphones. In contrast to popular drug reference guides (e.g. Epocrates Rx (Epocrates Inc., 2020) and Lexi-Comp ON-HAND (Lexi-Comp Inc., 2020)) that tended to be less comprehensive in terms of completeness and scope when made available as applications on smartphones, compared to their online versions, the information in OncoRx-MI was not compromised because both the mobile and online versions retrieved the DDI information from the same Structured Query Language (SQL) database, albeit via different platforms. Furthermore, many of the drug databases, such as those mentioned above, only allowed for DDI searches among individual drugs, but not for DDIs of chemoregimen cocktail prescriptions. A mobile web app that drew on the utility of 3G/4G and Wireless Fidelity (Wi-Fi) networks would be useful to healthcare professionals in both the hospital and clinic settings, who might need to check for DDIs "on-the-spot" during patient consultations.

At the time of development, the OncoRx-MI application was the first of its kind that allowed for DDI searches of chemoregimens on smartphones. Coupled to its parent online database, it could be accessed 3G/4G or Wi-Fi connection. Users could search for DDIs on their smartphone browsers. Relevant information on the DDI would be extracted and presented on the results page, which consisted of 4 sections: information about the selected chemotherapy regimen, pharmacokinetic profiles of the individual ACDs in the chemoregimen, information about the selected psychotropic agent or CAM, as well as data on the detected interaction (Figure 2).

Figure 2. Example of an interaction search in OncoRx-MI.

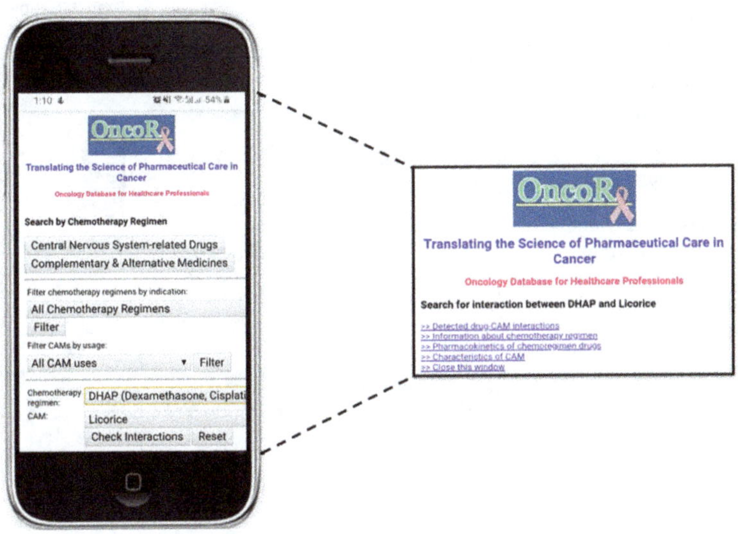

The interface of OncoRx-MI was designed to fit the smaller resolutions of smartphones so as to allow for better usability among users. The data in OncoRx-MI was organized in longitudinal format, so that users could scroll in an up-down fashion instead of panning sideways to read the DDI information. In addition, users did not need to frequently zoom in and out of the smartphone screen to read the DDI content.

When the user accessed OncoRx-MI on their smartphone browser, the gateway would pass the request to the web server via the standard http-protocol, and the request would be handled by the server as a normal request for a web page. However, if the user did an action (e.g. searching for a DDI), the hypertext preprocessor (PHP) scripts would first be processed by the server-side page.

The DDI search query would then be handled, the output formatted, and the result returned to the gateway as a new hypertext markup language (HTML) web page, which would then be passed back to the smartphone browser. The processing logic would reside in the internet server, and the whole process involving this request (i.e. DDI search) and response (i.e. results of the detected DDI) would be known as a server round trip (Figure 3).

The creation of OncoRx-MI involved 3 main steps: (a) collation and compilation of drug, chemoregimen and interaction information from published literature, (b) creation of the database and graphical user interface, and (c) mounting of the database and web documents on the internet cloud. The next few sections describe these steps in detail. A flowchart illustrating the process of creation is also shown in Figure 4.

Figure 3. Steps of a server round trip, showing how data flows through server-side technology when a drug interaction (DDI) search query is performed.

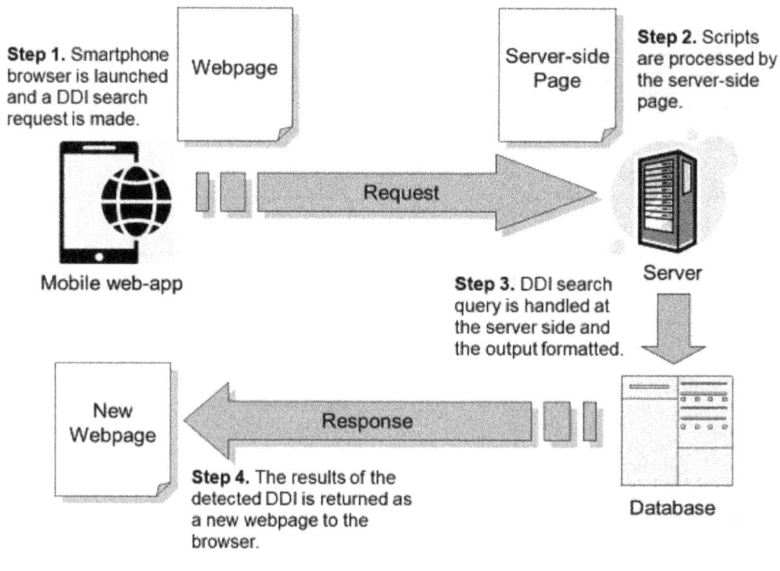

Drug information on ACDs, psychotropic agents, and DDIs were collated from a variety of online and hardcopy resources. These included drug manuals, textbooks, monographs and databases, such as the American Hospital Formulary Service (AHFS) Drug Information (2007 ed.) (American Society of Health-System Pharmacists, 2007), British Columbia Cancer Agency (BCCA) Cancer Drug Manual (BC Cancer Agency, n.d.), British

Figure 4. Flowchart showing the process of creating OncoRx-MI.

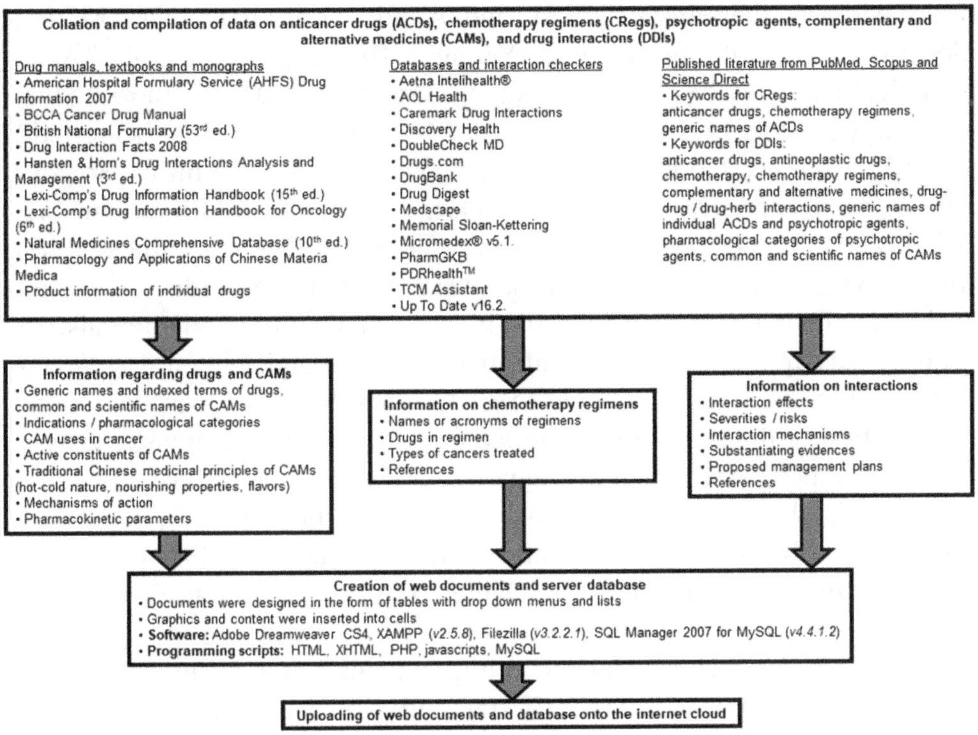

National Formulary (53rd ed.) (British Medical Association & Pharmaceutical Society of Great Britain, 2007), Drug Interaction Facts (2008 ed.) (Tatro, 2008), Hansten and Horn's Drug Interactions Analysis and Management (3rd ed.) (Philip D. Hansten & Horn, 2008), Lexi-Comp's Drug Information Handbook (15th ed.) (Lacy, Armstrong, Goldman, & Lance, 2007-2008) and Drug Information Handbook for Oncology (6th ed.) (Solimando, 2007). In addition, the databases that were included were DrugBank (Wishart et al., 2006), PharmGKB (Klein et al., 2001), Micromedex Healthcare Series (v5.1) (Thomson Healthcare, n.d.), and Up To Date (v16.2) (UpToDate Inc., n.d.). Interaction checkers were also utilized for the compilation of DDIs. These comprised of AOL Health (Healthwise Incorporated, 2006), Caremark (Gold Standard Inc., 2010), Discovery Health (Discovery Communications LLC, 2007), DoubleCheckMD (Enhanced Medical Decisions Inc., 2007), Drugs.com (Drugsite Trust, 2000), Drug Digest (Express Scripts Inc., 2008), Physician's Desktop Reference (PDRhealth) (Thomson Reuters, 2010), and Medscape (WebMD Inc., 2010). Furthermore, information was acquired from the package inserts of the various ACDs and psychotropic drugs. Data on the characteristics and clinical uses of CAMs and their interactions were compiled from the Pharmacology and Applications of Chinese Materia Medica (Chang, But, Yao, Wang, & Yeung, 2001), Aetna Intelihealth (Aetna InteliHealth Inc., 2010), TCM Assistant (e-MS Inc., 2004), Memorial Sloan Kettering (Gerstner Jr., 2008), Micromedex (v5.1) (Thomson Healthcare, n.d.), Natural Medicines Comprehensive Database (10th ed.) (Jellin & Gregory, 2007), Drugs.com (Drugsite Trust, 2000), Caremark (Gold Standard Inc., 2010), and DoubleCheckMD (Enhanced Medical Decisions Inc., 2007). Alternative therapies (e.g. Ayurveda), substances with limited documentation on their medicinal properties (e.g. alkaline water), vitamins and minerals, and commercial supplements (e.g. Centrum) were excluded. Literature searches on DDIs were conducted in PubMed, Scopus and Science Direct based on a combination of the keywords – "anticancer drugs", "antineoplastic drugs", "chemotherapy", "chemotherapy regimens", "complementary and alternative medicines", "drug-drug interactions", "drug-herb interactions", the generic names of the individual ACDs and psychotropic agents, pharmacological categories of the psychotropics, as well as common and scientific names of the CAMs.

Information on single-agent and multiple-agent chemoregimens that were positively evaluated in Phase II or III trials and published in English-language journals, or regimens approved by the US Food and Drug Administration (FDA), were also collated with substantiating references in scientific literature, using the keywords "anticancer drugs", "chemotherapy regimens" and the generic names of the ACDs. Due to the varying doses and frequencies of administering the chemotherapy combinations among institutions, these parameters were not included in the database.

Drug information that was compiled included the generic names and indexed terms of the drugs, their pharmacological categories, mechanisms of action and pharmacokinetic properties (e.g. percentage bound protein, metabolism, elimination and enzymatic parameters). CAM-related information included their common and scientific names, active constituents, uses in cancer, pharmacokinetic properties and TCM principles (e.g. hot-cold nature, nourishing properties and flavours). Chemotherapy-related information included the chemoregimen acronyms, drugs in the regimens, the types of cancers they treat and substantiating references.

On the other hand, interaction-related information consisted of the interaction effects, interaction mechanisms, substantiating evidences and references, and proposed management plans. DDI information included in-vitro studies, animal models, human case reports, clinical studies and other relevant abstracts and review articles that were published in English. When the DDI documented in various resources was found to be different, this information would be presented to the user with the appropriate substantiating evidences and reference citations.

Creation of the Database and Graphical User Interface

The compiled data was distributed into inter-related tables in Microsoft Excel. The program structure of the user search interface was designed around the generic names of the ACDs and the chemoregimen acronyms. Users could search for specific ACDs, or ACDs within a chemoregimen based on its acronym. A Structured Query Language (known as MySQL) was used to build the backend database and store the data based on the structure of the Excel tables. An example of the scripting layer is shown in Figure 5.

Figure 5. Example scripts for table creation and data input into a MySQL database.

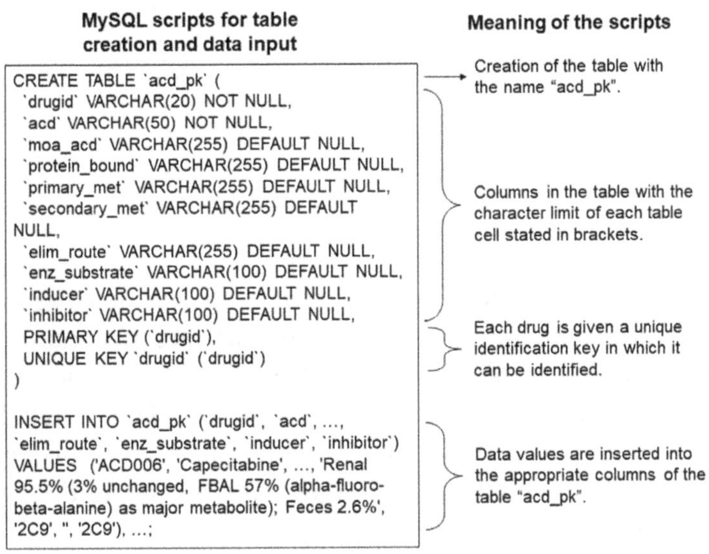

Web documents were created using Adobe Dreamweaver CS4 (Adobe Systems Incorporated, San Jose, California), and were associated with a combination of HTML, extensible HTML (XHTML) and javascripts. Cascading style sheets were used to provide a consistent look for the website.

The web documents were served from a web server associated with a Multi-Purpose Internet Mail Extension type, so that the browser could determine how the file should be processed, for example, handled by a helper application or rendered as a HTML file. An example of the code used to create a HTML document is shown in Figure 6.

Figure 6. Example of the code used to create a HTML document.

```
<!DOCTYPE HTML PUBLIC "-//W3C//DTD HTML 4.01
Transitional//EN">
<html>
<head>
<title>Search for Interactions by Chemotherapy
Regimens</title>
<meta http-equiv="Content-Type" content="text/html;
charset=iso-8859-1">
<link href="../style.css" rel="stylesheet" type="text/css">
<style type="text/css">
...
</style>

  <script language="javascript" src="../togglesearch.js">
                                   </script>
  <script type="text/JavaScript">
...</script>
</head>
<body>...
<span><strong><a id="xcategory"
href="javascript:Toggle('category');">[+]</a>Click here to see
the chemoregimens based on the cancers they
treat</strong></span><br>
...</body>
</html>
```

Example of HTML code used in designing a web document.

This code links a cascading style sheet to the document so as to provide a consistent look for the documents in the website.

Example of JavaScript code used to toggle a list of chemoregimens based on the cancers they treat.

The graphical user interfaces were created using various elements, such as forms, drop-down menus and lists. The software programs XAMPP (version 7.4.2) and Filezilla (version 3.46.3) for the Windows platform were used to upload the documents onto the server. The collated data on ACDs, psychotropics, CAMs and their interactions were transferred from the Microsoft Excel tables into the MySQL database using the EMS SQL Manager for MySQL.

Mounting of Database on the Internet Cloud

The database was programmed with the server-side scripting language PHP running as a common gateway interface application. A domain was bought from a local web hosting company and PHP was embedded in the HTML documents to handle the MySQL administration over the web. Database queries were handled through SQL access to the database, and the contents of the database would be returned to the user's smartphone browser. The choice of scripting language was somewhat arbitrary. PHP was used in this project due to its ease of implementation, compared to other languages available at the time of implementation, such as Active Server Pages and Perl. An example of a PHP script that connects to the MySQL server and selects the OncoRx database is shown in Figure 7.

Figure 7. Example of the PHP script used to connect to the MySQL server and select the OncoRx database.

```
<?PHP
// open connection to MySQL server
   $hostname = "xxx";
   $username = "xxx";
   $password = "xxx";
   $connection = mysql_connect($hostname,
$username, $password)
or die ('Our website is temporarily unavailable.
Please check back soon.');
//unable to connect!

// select database for use
   $dbname = "oncorx";
   mysql_select_db($dbname) or die ('The OncoRx
database is temporarily unavailable. Please check
back soon.');
//Unable to select database!
...
//close connection to MySQL server
   mysql_close ($connection);
?>
```

Opens a connection to the server. An error shows when a connection cannot be made.

Selects the OncoRx database. An error shows when the database cannot be selected.

Closes the connection to the server.

User Search Strategies for Interactions in OncoRx-MI

The structure of OncoRx-MI was designed around ACDs and chemoregimens. Its graphical user interface was designed for ease of navigation and searching of DDIs. Instructions on how to search for a DDI were provided above the search box. Users could search for DDIs with either psychotropic agents or CAMs from two search interfaces – generic ACD names or chemoregimen acronyms. In the sections that follow, the search for the different interactions are described.

Search Strategy Using Generic Anticancer Drug Names

When a user searches for a DDI by the generic name of the ACD, for example between doxorubicin and valproic acid, the relevant data will be extracted from the database and the results displayed for the user. The information is presented in tabular format and consists of 3 parts: the pharmacokinetic parameters of the ACD and the psychotropic drug, which in this case is an antiepileptic drug, and parameters of the detected DDI (Figure 8).

The generic names of the user choice of drugs are displayed at the top of the results page, together with other indexed terms of the drugs. Pharmacokinetic data include the absorption, protein-binding information, metabolism and elimination routes of the drugs, as well as enzymatic parameters such as substrate, inducer and/or inhibitor information. In addition, the pharmacological category of the ACD, its indication in cancer therapy, and mechanism of action are also shown. The last section of the results page provides the DDI effects, severities and/or risks, mechanisms of interaction, substantiating evidences, and proposed management plans where appropriate. In the given example, a decrease in plasma valproic acid concentrations is expected, which may lead to decreased effectiveness of the antiepileptic drug and possible loss of seizure control (Neef & de Voogd-van der Straaten, 1988). The clinician should monitor the patient for seizure control when using these drugs concurrently or consider an alternative antiepileptic drug. Alternative non-interacting antiepileptics identified by the database are listed as well.

Additional information that is provided to users if they search for an interaction with a CAM include the common, scientific and pinyin names of the CAMs, their uses in cancer and supportive care therapy, mechanisms of actions, pharmacokinetic data and data on adverse reactions, unless there is no documented data available (Figure 9). Furthermore, the active constituents and other characteristics related to TCM principles, such as their hot-cold nature, nourishing properties (e.g. nourishing yin, yang, qi, or blood) and flavours (e.g. sweet, sour, pungent, salty, or bitter) are also shown. For example, American ginseng, also known as *Panax quinquefolius*, is used for cancer prevention and treatment, or immuno-stimulation. It has a sweet, yet slightly bitter property, and its active constituents are the ginsenosides, which are primarily excreted unchanged in the urine (Chang, et al., 2001; Chen, Sawchuk, & Staba, 1980; Gerstner Jr., 2008; Jellin & Gregory, 2007; Shin, Kim, Yun, Morgan, & Vainio, 2000).

Figure 8. Results of the interaction search between doxorubicin and valproic acid.

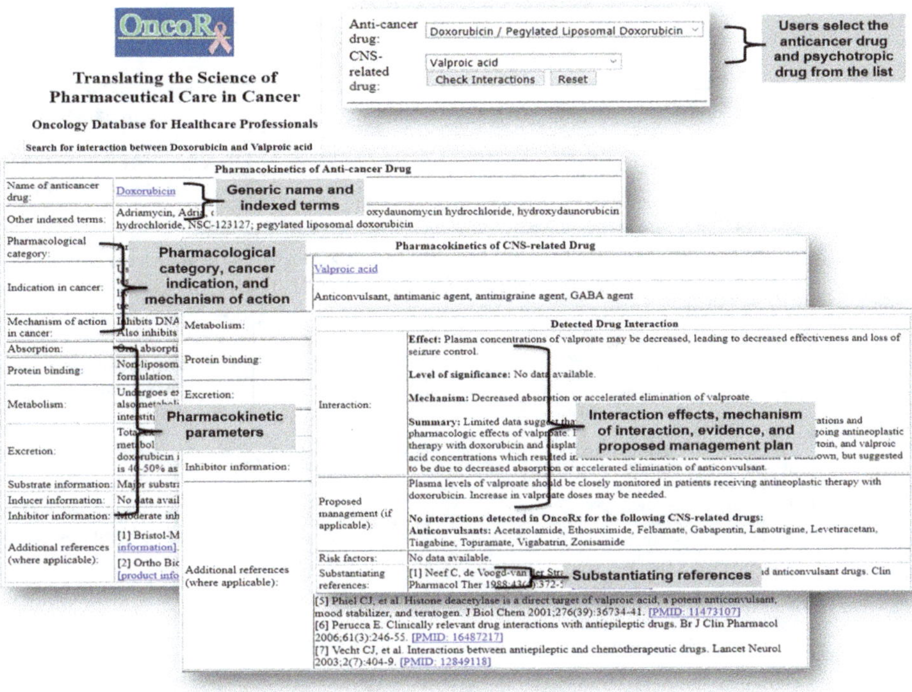

Search Strategy Using Acronyms of Chemotherapy Regimens

Users can also search for DDIs of combination chemoregimens. A section providing information on the regimen will be displayed, showing the acronym and type of regimen, the type of cancer in which it can be used, the drugs in the regimen, as well as substantiating references for the use of the regimen for that particular cancer type. Figure 10 shows the interaction between the chemoregimen AC (used for the treatment of breast cancer) (Fisher et al., 1997; Fisher et al., 1990) and its interaction with fluvoxamine (an antidepressant). The interaction details of each drug in the regimen (doxorubicin and cyclophosphamide) are provided together with an overall management plan for the interaction. Increases in plasma concentrations of the ACDs are expected due to inhibition of their CYP3A4-mediated metabolism (Anttila, Rasanen, & Leinonen, 2001; Apotex Corp., 2020; Spina, Santoro, & D'Arrigo, 2008). Clinical and laboratory monitoring of plasma ACD levels is advised during concurrent administration of AC with fluvoxamine, and dosage adjustments

Figure 9. Results showing the characteristics of the complementary and alternative medicine, with American ginseng as example.

Characteristics of CAM	
Name of CAM:	Ginseng (American)
Scientific name(s):	Panax quinquefolius
Other common names:	Xi yang shen, western ginseng, five-fingers, hua qi shen
Main constituents:	Saponin glycosides (panaquilon, ginsenosides)
Flavors and properties according to TCM practice:	Flavor: Sweet, slightly bitter Property: Data not available.
CAM use in cancer:	Cancer prevention, cancer treatment, immunostimulation Mode of action: The exact mechanism of action is unknown. Ginsenoside Rg1 is associated with improvements in humoral and cell-mediated immune response in mice. Anticancer activity has been shown in vitro for several ginsenosides.
Metabolism:	Data not available.
Elimination:	All ginsenosides are primarily eliminated unchanged in the urine. Elimination half-lives range from 20-500 minutes.
Substrate information:	Data not available.
Inducer information:	Data not available.
Inhibitor information:	Data not available.
CAM data references:	[1] Chen SE, et al. American ginseng. III. Pharmacokinetics of ginsenosides in the rabbit. Eur J Drug Metab Pharmacokinet 1980;5(3):161-8. [PMID: 7202434] [2] Ginseng (American). Memorial Sloan-Kettering Cancer Center. http://www.mskcc.org/mskcc/html/69236.cfm. [3] Shin HR, et al. The cancer-preventive potential of Panax ginseng: a review of human and experimental evidence. Cancer Causes Control 2000;11(6):565-76. [PMID: 10880039]
Adverse reactions:	No significant reactions reported.
Adverse reaction references:	[1] Ginseng (American). Memorial Sloan-Kettering Cancer Center. http://www.mskcc.org/mskcc/html/69236.cfm.

Common, scientific and pinyin names

Active constituents and TCM characteristics

CAM use in cancer

Pharmacokinetic parameters

Adverse reactions and references

of the ACDs may also be needed. Alternative non-interacting antidepressants are also provided.

Hierarchical Development of the Oncorx Search Engine

The search engine of OncoRx was developed in a hierarchical format so that users could narrow their searches for DDIs with ACDs or chemoregimens. Users would begin by either searching for an ACD interaction or a chemoregimen interaction by clicking on the links of collapsible menus coded in javascript. They could then narrow their searches by selecting the interacting agent from either drugs used in central nervous system (CNS)-related disorders, or CAMs. Although users would have the option to search for DDIs based on all psychotropic drugs or all CAMs, OncoRx-MI also provided a further breakdown of these modules by allowing users to search based on their specific indications and uses. The psychotropic drugs were categorized into 4 classes: CNS stimulants and attention-deficit hyperactivity disorder (ADHD), depression, epilepsy, and substance dependence. Similarly, the CAMs were categorized into 8 classes: alopecia, cancer prevention and treatment,

Figure 10. Results of an interaction search between the chemoregimen AC and fluvoxamine.

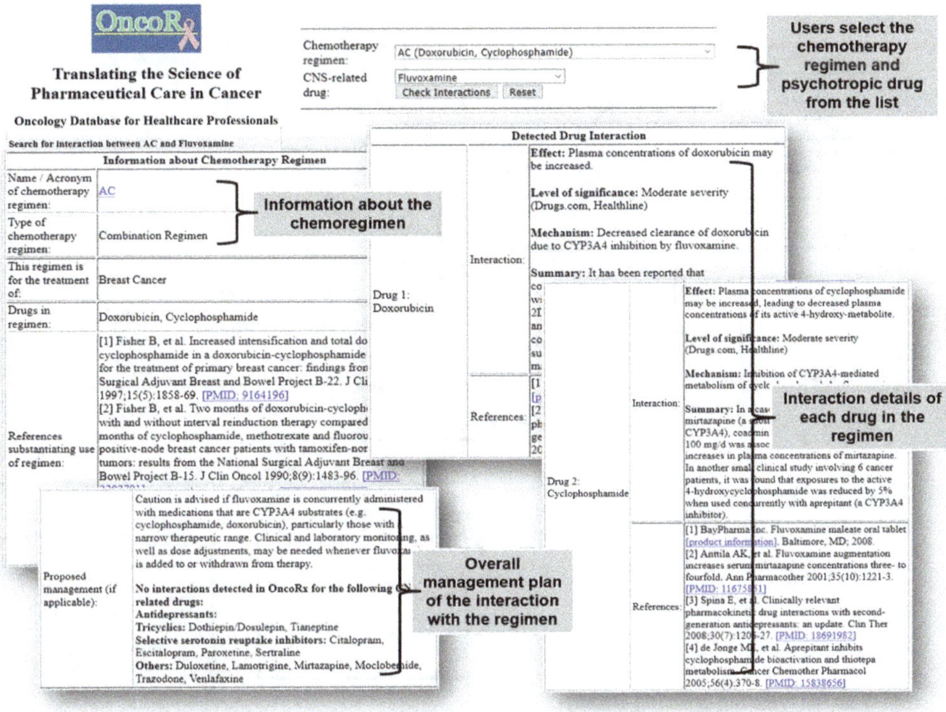

fatigue, immune-system-related, inflammation, nausea and vomiting, pain and neuropathy, and non-cancer-related.

To allow for easy searching of regimens by oncology specialty (e.g. breast and gynecologic cancers, gastrointestinal and colorectal cancers, CNS and brain cancers) and by clinician users who might otherwise be unfamiliar with the chemoregimens, OncoRx also provided an additional option to narrow the chemoregimen searches by cancer types. There were 15 categories of chemoregimens that users could choose from (Figure 11). Furthermore, regimens for the treatment of pediatric cancers were also categorized as a separate class on its own in order to cater for clinicians who encounter this group of special population in their practices. This hierarchical structure of the search engine made the database more user-friendly as it allowed clinicians to narrow their regimen searches to only those that were relevant to them in their practices.

Figure 11. Hierarchical system development of the OncoRx-MI search engine.

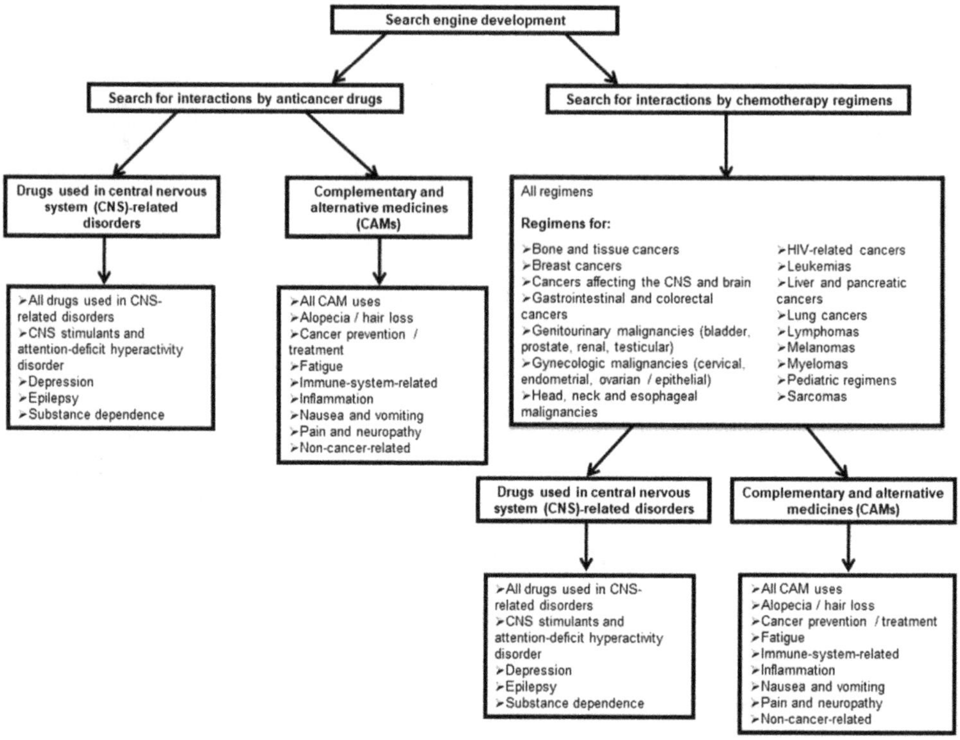

Database Statistics

The OncoRx database consisted of 117 ACDs, which made up 256 single-agent and multiple-agent combination regimens. This database covered all the major ACDs and their frequently prescribed chemoregimen combinations used in the treatment of patients with cancer, and it focused primarily on pharmacokinetic and pharmacodynamic interactions. Leukemias (16.8%), lymphomas and myelomas (16.0%) had the largest number of regimens, while CNS and brain cancers (5.1%) and bone and tissue cancers (4.7%) had the lowest numbers of regimens. Table 3 shows a breakdown of the classifications of ACDs based on their pharmacological categories and the chemoregimens based on the types of cancers they treat.

The database was developed to detect DDIs with 51 psychotropic drugs (Table 4). Antiepileptics and antidepressants made up the majority of the psychotropics in the database (over 90%), while CNS stimulants and ADHD drugs, and substance dependence agents made up 3.9% and 7.8% respectively.

Table 3. Statistics of anticancer drugs and chemotherapy regimens in the OncoRx database.

Pharmacological Categories of Anticancer Drugs	**Number of Drugs in the Category (%)+**
Alkylating agents	15 (12.8)
Antimetabolites	15 (12.8)
Antimicrotubules	7 (6.0)
Biological modifiers	7 (6.0)
Corticosteroids	5 (4.3)
Hormone agonists / antagonists	19 (16.2)
Platinum compounds	3 (2.6)
Topoisomerase inhibitors	9 (7.7)
Tyrosine kinase inhibitors and monoclonal antibodies	16 (13.7)
Other categories of anticancer drugs	21 (17.9)
Chemotherapy Regimens by Types of Cancers	**Number of Regimens in the Category (%)+**
Bone and tissue cancers	12 (4.7)
Breast cancers	36 (14.1)
Central nervous system and brain cancers	13 (5.1)
Gastrointestinal, colorectal, liver and pancreatic cancers	24 (9.4)
Genitourinary cancers	30 (11.7)
Leukemias	43 (16.8)
Lung cancers	25 (9.8)
Lymphomas and myelomas	41 (16.0)
Other types of cancers	32 (12.5)

+Percentages may not add to 100% due to rounding of data.

On the other hand, the database also comprised of 166 CAMs categorized based on their uses in cancer therapy. Much of the focus in this module had been on TCMs. CAMs for cancer treatment and prevention (39.8%), inflammation (23.5%), and immune-system-related (12.0%), made up the highest proportions in the database. In contrast, fatigue syndrome (3.0%), alopecia (1.8%), and nausea and vomiting (1.2%) had the lowest proportions of CAMs. In addition, over a third of the CAMs were for non-cancer-related purposes.

Table 4. Statistics of psychotropic agents and complementary and alternative medicines in the OncoRx database.

Pharmacotherapeutic Indications of Psychotropic Agents	Number of Drugs in the Category (%)+
Agents for depression	21 (41.2)
Agents for epilepsy	26 (51.0)
Central nervous system stimulants and agents for attention-deficit hyperactivity disorder	2 (3.9)
Substance dependence agents	4 (7.8)
Uses of CAMs	**Number of CAMs in the Category (%)+**
Alopecia	3 (1.8)
Cancer treatment and prevention	66 (39.8)
Fatigue syndrome	5 (3.0)
Immune-system-related	20 (12.0)
Inflammation	39 (23.5)
Nausea and vomiting	2 (1.2)
Peripheral neuropathy and pain	15 (9.0)
Non-cancer-related	64 (38.6)

+Percentages may not add to 100% due to rounding of data and inclusion of agents into multiple categories based on their indications and uses.

CAM: complementary and alternative medicine

Interaction Statistics With Psychotropic Agents

A total of 737 and 4,800 drug-pair interactions were identified between ACDs and chemoregimens with psychotropics, which translated to over 520 interacting chemoregimen-psychotropic drug pairs (Table 5).

The drugs in all the psychotropic classes had interactions with ACDs, except for the antiepileptic drugs, whereby no interactions were identified for piracetam and vigabatrin. In general, the majority of the DDIs were pharmacokinetic (60.0-69.2%), with the highest proportion occurring with antiepileptics (82.5-88.7%). The antiepileptics also had higher overall numbers of total interactions with both ACDs and chemoregimens. In contrast, the other psychotropics had more pharmacodynamic interactions. Substance dependence agents (77.1-83.1%) and CNS stimulants and ADHD drugs (75.0-93.3%) had higher proportions of pharmacodynamic interactions than antidepressants (50.3-63.0%). This inflation in proportions could be due to the lower numbers of drugs in the former 2 psychotropic classes. Nonetheless, a substantial

Table 5. Interaction statistics among the classes of psychotropics.

Interaction Parameters	Classes of Psychotropics				All Psychotropic Agents+
	Antiepileptics	**Antidepressants**	**Substance Dependence Agents**	**CNS Stimulants and ADHD Drugs**	
Number of interacting PSYs	24 out of 26	21 out of 21	4 out of 4	2 out of 2	49 out of 51
Interactions With Anticancer Drugs					
Proportion of PK DDIs (%)	82.5	37.0	16.9	25.0	60.0
Proportion of PD DDIs (%)	17.5	63.0	83.1	75.0	40.0
Total number (%) of DDIs	416 (54.6)	273 (35.8)	65 (8.5)	8 (1.0)	737
Interactions With Chemotherapy Regimens					
Proportion of PK DDIs (%)	88.7	49.7	22.9	6.7	69.2
Proportion of PD DDIs (%)	11.3	50.3	77.1	93.3	30.8
Total number (%) of ACD-PSY DDIs	2915 (57.9)	1573 (31.3)	498 (9.9)	45 (0.9)	4800
Total number (%) of interacting chemoregimen-PSY pairs	230 (34.2)	200 (29.8)	206 (30.7)	36 (5.4)	521

+Numbers may not add up due to some psychotropics in multiple classes.

ACD: anticancer drug, ADHD: attention-deficit hyperactivity disorder, CNS: central nervous system, Chemoregimen: chemotherapy regimen, DDI: drug-drug interaction, PK: pharmacokinetic, PD: pharmacodynamic, PSY: psychotropic agent

amount of pharmacodynamic interactions occurred with psychotropic drugs (30.8-40.0%), thus caution is advised when extrapolating these interactions to other psychotropics agents.

Among the pharmacokinetic interactions, induction of CYP450 isozymes was the most significant, explaining more than one-third of the interactions with ACDs and chemoregimens (Table 6). In contrast, enzyme inhibition only explained about one-fifth of the psychotropic interactions. The higher proportions of enzyme induction activity were accounted for by over half of the DDIs with antiepileptics, which were mainly inducers of the CYP450 isozymes. The older generation antiepileptics such as carbamazepine, phenytoin, phenobarbital and primidone were strong isozyme inducers, while valproic acid was predominantly enzyme-inhibiting. On the other hand, the enzyme-inhibiting effects of the other psychotropic classes are more evident, with the highest proportions observed with antidepressants (33.7% with ACDs, 46.5% with chemoregimens). Lower proportions of other types of pharmacokinetic interactions between psychotropics with ACDs and chemoregimens included

Table 6. Types and proportions of interactions between anticancer drugs and chemotherapy regimens with psychotropic agents.

Type of Interaction Effect	Proportion of PSY Interactions With ACDs (%)+	Proportion of PSY Interactions With Chemoregimens (%)+
Pharmacokinetic Interactions		
Altered bioavailability and/or protein displacement	3.8	8.3
Altered volume of distribution and/or elimination	1.0	6.4
Induction of metabolism / CYP isozymes (1A2, 2B6, 2C8/9/10, 3A4/5)	34.3	34.5
Inhibition of metabolism / CYP isozymes (1A2, 2B6, 2C8/9/19, 2D6, 3A4) and/or PGP	20.3	20.0
Pharmacodynamic Interactions		
Cardiotoxicity, QT prolongation and torsades de pointes	11.4	9.5
CNS / respiratory effects (e.g. depression, mood problems, sedation, seizures)	9.0	4.5
CNS toxicity (e.g. peripheral neuropathy) and serotonin syndrome	4.7	5.7
Hematological effects (e.g. altered platelet function, anemia, leucopenia, neutropenia, thrombocytopenia, gastrointestinal bleeding)	7.2	2.3
Hepatotoxicity	7.3	7.1
Other pharmacodynamic effects	0.9	1.5

+Percentages may not add up to 100% due to rounding of data.

ACD: anticancer drug, Chemoregimen: chemotherapy regimen, CNS: central nervous system, CYP: cytochrome P450, PGP: p-glycoprotein, PSY: psychotropic agent

altered bioavailabilities of the drugs, protein displacement reactions and altered volumes of distribution and/or eliminations.

Pharmacodynamic interactions that were most frequently recorded with the psychotropics were increased risks of cardiotoxicity, QT prolongation and torsades de pointes (9.5-11.4%). Antidepressants accounted for majority of the cardiotoxic effects (30.3-30.8%), in contrast to substance dependence agents, CNS stimulants and ADHD drugs, which did not account for this effect at all. Increased risks of hepatotoxicity (7.1-7.3%) and CNS/respiratory effects (e.g. CNS/respiratory depression, mood disorders, sedation and occurrence of seizures, 4.5-9.0%) were also among the detected DDIs. On the contrary, CNS toxicity (e.g. peripheral neuropathy) and serotonin syndrome (4.7-5.7%), and hematological effects (e.g. altered platelet function, anemia, leucopenia, neutropenia, thrombocytopenia, gastrointestinal bleeding) only accounted for only a small percentage (2.3-7.2%) of the DDIs.

Interaction Statistics With Complementary And Alternative Medicines

The numbers of ACD and chemoregimen interactions with CAMs were 584 and 2,750 respectively, with the latter making up a total of 4,408 drug-CAM interacting pairs (Table 7). The proportion of pharmacokinetic interactions (75.9-79.1%) was higher than pharmacodynamic interactions (20.9-24.1%). Among CAMs for cancer-related uses, those for nausea and vomiting (90.5-98.0%) had the highest proportions of pharmacokinetic herb-drug interactions (HDIs). On the other hand, CAMs used for non-cancer-related uses had almost similar proportions of pharmacokinetic HDIs (88.7-95.7%). In contrast, only one CAM for alopecia (fenugreek) had HDIs with ACDs, and these HDIs were pharmacodynamic in nature. Among CAMs for cancer-related uses, those for cancer treatment and prevention had the highest amounts of HDIs (38.9-39.0%), followed by those for inflammation (17.6-17.9%), since these categories had the largest numbers of CAMs.

Table 7. Interaction statistics among the categories of complementary and alternative medicines.

Interaction Parameters	Classes of CAMs								All CAMs
	Cancer Treatment and Prevention	Alopecia	Fatigue Syndrome	Immune-System-Related	Inflammation	Nausea and Vomiting	Peripheral Neuropathy and Pain	Non-Cancer-Related	
Number of interacting CAMs	18 out of 66	1 out of 3	5 out of 5	7 out of 20	7 out of 39	2 out of 2	5 out of 15	3 out of 64	29 out of 166
Interactions With Anticancer Drugs									
Proportion of PK HDIs (%)	69.7	0.0	65.3	69.3	65.3	90.5	76.2	95.7	75.9
Proportion of PD HDIs (%)	30.3	100.0	34.7	30.7	34.7	9.5	23.8	4.3	24.1
Total number (%) of HDIs	356 (39.0)	4 (0.4)	62 (6.8)	101 (11.1)	163 (17.9)	42 (4.6)	103 (11.3)	82 (9.0)	584
Interactions With Chemotherapy Regimens									
Proportion of PK HDIs (%)	73.2	0.0	66.9	67.9	68.9	98.0	84.3	88.7	79.1
Proportion of PD HDIs (%)	26.8	100.0	33.1	32.1	31.1	2.0	15.7	11.3	20.9
Total number (%) of ACD-CAM HDIs	2684 (38.9)	6 (0.1)	447 (6.5)	826 (12.0)	1212 (17.6)	296 (4.3)	690 (10.0)	732 (10.6)	4408
Total number (%) of interacting chemoregimen-CAM pairs	1692 (39.0)	5 (0.1)	306 (7.1)	550 (12.7)	730 (16.8)	178 (4.1)	418 (9.6)	456 (10.5)	2750

ACD: anticancer drug, CAM: complementary and alternative medicine, Chemoregimen: chemotherapy regimen, HDI: herb-drug interaction, PK: pharmacokinetic, PD: pharmacodynamic

Inhibition of CYP450-mediated metabolism accounted for more than half of the ACD-CAM interactions, while induction of CYP450 isozymes and p-glycoprotein accounted for approximately one-quarter (Table 8). Hepatotoxicity was the most commonly observed pharmacodynamic HDI (8.2-10.4%), especially among CAMs for inflammation and cancer treatment and prevention. Altered immunomodulatory effects accounted for ~6.0% of the HDIs and these effects mainly occurred with co-administration of corticosteroids, leading to altered efficacies of the drugs. A small proportion of HDI effects were due to hematological effects (1.1-3.9%), which generally resulted in increased risks of bleeding. Interestingly, rituximab-induced hypoglycemia was identified as a HDI that was not detected with the psychotropics. The least common HDIs were increased risks of CNS effects (e.g. sedation, CNS depression, peripheral neuropathy, paraesthesias and serotonin syndrome, 0.5-0.7%) and toxic skin reactions (0.05-0.7%).

Table 8. Types and proportions of interactions between anticancer drugs and chemotherapy regimens with complementary and alternative medicines.

Type of Interaction Effect	Proportion of CAM Interactions With ACDs (%)+	Proportion of CAM Interactions With Chemoregimens (%)+
Pharmacokinetic Interactions		
Induction of metabolism / CYP isozymes (2B, 2C9/19, 2D6, 3A4) and/or PGP	23.4	23.9
Inhibition of metabolism / CYP isozymes (1A2, 2B6, 2C9/19, 2D6, 2E1, 3A4)	52.5	55.2
Pharmacodynamic Interactions		
Altered immunomodulatory effects	6.0	6.2
CNS effects (sedation, CNS depression, peripheral neuropathy, paraesthesias, serotonin syndrome)	0.5	0.7
Hematological effects (hypertensive crisis, anti-platelet, anti-coagulation)	3.9	1.1
Hepatotoxicity	10.4	8.2
Hypoglycemia	1.4	0.7
Skin reactions	0.7	0.05
Other pharmacodynamic effects	1.4	3.9

+Percentages may not add up to 100% due to rounding of data.

ACD: anticancer drug, CAM: complementary and alternative medicine, Chemoregimen: chemotherapy regimen, CNS: central nervous system, CYP: cytochrome P450, PGP: p-glycoprotein

STEP 4: EVALUATION AND GENERATING EVIDENCE OF RELEVANCE AND CREDIBILITY

Certification of the Database

Since the target audiences of the OncoRx database were mainly healthcare professionals, it would be mandatory to show that the application was committed to providing trustworthy drug-related information. Hence, certification of the website's quality was obtained from the Health On the Net (HON) Foundation. Despite a few shortcomings with regards to the lack of certain quality indicators (previously described in Table 1), the HON Foundation and the HON Code of Conduct (also known as the HONcode) is one of the oldest and most widely recognized third-party quality evaluators in the healthcare world. This non-profit organization accredited to the Economic and Social Council of the United Nations was first launched in July 1996, and it provides a voluntary certification system that is based on an "active quality seal" concept to show that health-related websites comply with the HONcode principles, and that the information provided is useful, reliable and up to the appropriate ethical standards.(Boyer, et al., 1998; Health On the Net Foundation, 2019, 2020)

The OncoRx database has been certified to be compliant to the HONcode and the HONcode quality seal indicates that this database provides objective and reliable drug information to its users. As a guide, Table 9 also shows a summary of the HONcode principles and how this database complies with these principles.

Catering the Design of OncoRx-MI Towards the Pharmaco-cybernetic Maxims

OncoRx-MI is the first application of its kind where practitioner users can search for DDIs of combination chemoregimen cocktails by their acronyms. Healthcare professionals not only save time and effort when searching for chemotherapy interactions "on-the-spot" as and when they encounter such DDIs in their practice, but is also practical since cancer patients are often on combination chemo-cocktails in which the individual ACDs within the regimen are usually standard. OncoRx-MI further substantiates this advantage by drawing on the popularity of smartphones and other handheld devices, as well as the widespread availability of 3G/4G and Wi-Fi networks to deliver

Table 9. The HONcode principles and how the OncoRx database complies with these principles.

HONcode Principles	Descriptions of Principles	How the OncoRx Database Complies With the Principles
Authority	Details about the editorial team and the site/app team are clearly stated.	• Authors' names and credentials are clearly listed.
Complementarity	Clear mention of the limitations of the site/app and that it does not replace the doctor-patient relationship.	• Disclaimer is provided to declare that information is not meant to replace a healthcare professional's advice.
Confidentiality	Statement explaining all legal requirements regarding the confidentiality of personal data.	• A privacy policy is provided as part of the terms and conditions of use.
Attribution/ Validity	The site/app and all legal and medical/health pages/content have a date of last update. The sources of health content are given.	• Drug information is referenced to published references with a hyperlink where appropriate. • Date of last modification of the content are provided.
Justifiability and Objectivity	Health information is complete, has references and provided in an objective, balanced and transparent manner	• Claims relating to the drugs and complementary and alternative medicines are supported by clear references to scientific literature.
Transparency/ User's Practice	The site/app is easy to use, its mission is clear, and the team is easily reachable.	• The intended objectives of the database and its target audiences are clearly stated. • A valid email address of the webmaster is provided. • A feedback form is provided and easily accessible.
Financial Disclosure	All sources of funding and paid services are identified and transparent.	• Funding is clearly stated as part of the terms and conditions of use.
Advertising Policy	All advertisements are identified and clearly separated from content.	• A clear statement explaining that the database does not host or accept advertisements is provided.

the DDI content to healthcare professionals "on-the-go". Unlike other native mobile apps, the drug information provided by the OncoRx-MI web app is not compromised regardless of the type of platform used, be it from a laptop browser or the smartphone browser, since its content is drawn from the same backend database.

The unique feature that allows users to search for chemoregimen interactions through their acronyms also lowers the risk of accidental omissions by providing the interactions of all the ACDs within the regimen. For example, if a clinician wants to search for a DDI with the RCHOP regimen for non-Hodgkin's lymphoma, which consists of 5 drugs (cyclophosphamide, doxorubicin, vincristine, prednisone and rituximab) (Coiffier et al., 2002);

instead of entering each individual drug within the regimen in his interaction search, he can just search for all DDIs based on the "RCHOP" acronym. A proposed plan for the overall management of the patient on this chemoregimen is also provided if an interaction is detected. Users can then get a holistic view of the chemoregimen interactions instead of collating and extracting the information for each individual ACD by themselves. If they are in a rush for time, searching for multiple drug-pair interactions in a chemo-cocktail may also predispose them to a risk of accidental omissions of a DDI search with a particular ACD within the regimen, especially when dealing with the small resolutions of mobile touch-screen interfaces, which may lead to a possibility of DRPs and adverse outcomes in patients.

Some drug information databases (e.g. Micromedex, AHFS Drug Information) provide detailed information about an interaction. However, it is time-consuming for a clinician to thoroughly read through the details in order to sieve out relevant information in the practice setting. On the other hand, other databases (e.g. Caremark, PDRhealth) only provide a summarized paragraph of the interaction effects and precautions to take. Clinicians who want to know more details regarding the interactions have to do additional searches on other information resources. The content in OncoRx-MI is summarized and placed under relevant sections and headings so that healthcare professionals can rapidly sieve out the information they need.

Some resources do not provide interactions of individual drugs, but of drug classes or drugs with certain common parameters instead (e.g. Lexi-comp's Drug Information Handbook, British National Formulary). This requires some specialized knowledge on the part of the clinicians regarding the drug and may be time consuming if they need to look up additional information in the practice setting. For example, the increased risk of carboplatin toxicity when used concurrently with nephrotoxic drugs (Lacy, et al., 2007-2008) implies that clinicians need to know whether the interacting drug is nephrotoxic, or otherwise look up for this piece of information on the interacting drug. OncoRx-MI enables users to search for interactions between specific drug-pairs, since it extrapolates these class effects to the individual drugs, thus minimizing the chances of ambiguity. This feature is especially important for interactions involving CAMs, since their interactions, particularly for TCMs, have not been well-documented in literature. Furthermore, such information may not be consistent for the less well-established CAMs. It is important for clinicians to gain better understanding on the interactions between ACDs and TCMs because TCMs are gaining increasing acceptance in the West as a therapeutic option, particularly for the treatment of chronic diseases such as cancer (Parekh, Liu, & Wei, 2009). Therefore, OncoRx-MI aims to bridge this gap by combining information from CAM- and TCM-specific sources in addition to the typical DDI resources used by clinicians.

Lastly, as the content in OncoRx-MI is compiled from a variety of drug information and interaction sources, and published literature, it is able to provide users with any contradictory information regarding a detected interaction. For example, corticosteroids such as dexamethasone, which are commonly used as antiemetic agents in treating chemotherapy-induced nausea and vomiting (Lohr, 2008), have been reported to cause both increases and decreases in plasma phenytoin concentrations. OncoRx-MI is able to provide this piece of information as a summary of the evidence with substantiating references, so that clinician users have the flexibility of deciding how to manage their patients based on their clinical judgement. Table 10 provides a summary of how the features of OncoRx-MI cater towards the design principles of the Pharmaco-cybernetic Maxims.

Potential of the Database in Clinical Practice

There had been few studies that determined the occurrence of DDIs for ACDs and chemoregimens. In a retrospective prevalence study conducted by Cheung et al. (Cheung, et al., 2010) to determine a 3-year prescribing pattern of ACDs and antiepileptic drugs at a local ambulatory cancer center in Singapore, the authors identified a prescription pool of "co-prescribed medications" (an ACD and antiepileptic drug jointly prescribed by the same prescriber and dispensed on the same day) and "concomitant medications" (concurrent use of an ACD and antiepileptic drug prescribed by one or more prescribers, but not necessarily dispensed on the same day) from their institutional electronic prescription database. The study utilized the interaction information from OncoRx-MI to identify potentially interacting ACD-antiepileptic drug pairs in their institution. Of the 42,810 prescriptions that were identified with at least one ACD, 274 (0.64%) prescriptions were combined with an antiepileptic drug, with majority (82.8%) of the drug pairs being co-prescribed, while the remaining 17.2% were concomitant prescriptions. Among the 274 identified prescriptions, 51 drug pairs (18.6%) were potentially interacting in a total of 22 patients. More than one potentially interacting pair was observed in 2 patients. These interactions only occurred with 4 antiepileptic drugs – carbamazepine, clonazepam, phenytoin and valproic acid. The most common interactions were associated with lomustine and valproic acid (7 patients),

Table 10. Summary of how OncoRx-MI caters towards the design principles of the Pharmaco-cybernetic Maxims.

Design Principle in the Pharmaco-Cybernetic Maxims	Explanation of Principle	Summary of How OncoRx-MI Caters Towards Design Principle
Quality	• Content should be accurate. • There should be appropriate resources for evidence-based therapies.	• Content is based on a variety of drug manuals, textbooks, drug monographs, drug databases, interaction checkers and published literature from PubMed, Scopus and Science Direct. • All content is cited, and reference sources are provided to target users.
Quantity	• Adequate information is provided so that the likelihood of drug-related problems is minimized.	• Content in OncoRx-MI is not compromised regardless of the type of platform used (e.g. laptop browser versus mobile web app) as the information is extracted from the same backend database and shown to users. • Users can search for chemoregimen cocktails by their acronyms instead of collating information for each individual drug by themselves, thus minimizing the risk of accidental omissions of an interaction search. • Contradictory information regarding a detected drug interaction is provided to users together with substantiating references.
Relation	• Content is relevant to what target audience needs to know • Content should clarify doubts instead of making the target audience more confused.	• Content provided is based on a cross-sectional study conducted among oncology clinicians to identify the relevant drug interaction parameters for the database. • Database is designed in a hierarchical format so that users can narrow their searches by different categories of ACDs, psychotropics and CAMs.
Manner	• Content is conveyed clearly and avoids ambiguity and misinterpretation.	• Content is phrased so that it is understandable by both clinicians in general practice and in oncology practice. • Content is summarized and placed under relevant sections with prominent headers for easy interpretation by users. • Interaction effects of drug classes are extrapolated to individual drug-pair interactions, so that chances of ambiguity are minimized.

ACD: anticancer drug, CAM: complementary and alternative medicine, Chemoregimen: chemotherapy regimen

and with capecitabine and phenytoin (5 patients). The authors of the study postulated from the high proportion of co-prescribed medications that most of the interacting drug pairs prescribed by clinicians were given intentionally because they could have been unaware of the potential for DDIs. Moreover, another study suggested that specialists were less likely to identify DDIs than clinicians in general practice (Y. Ko et al., 2008). The results of the prevalence study by Cheung and colleagues indicated that OncoRx-MI had a great potential to aid clinicians, particularly oncology practitioners, in reducing DRPs such as DDIs in clinical practice.

STEP 5: IMPLEMENTATION OF THE ONCOLOGY DATABASE IN HEALTHCARE PRACTICE

In a span of one year, OncoRx-MI had a total of 90 users. Their demographics are shown in Table 11. Most of the users were from the US and Canada (38%), followed by Australia (19%). Large proportions were also from Germany and France (9%), as well as Italy, the UK and Ireland (7% each). The Singaporean population made up 6%, while other users included those from Europe, such as Spain (2%), Belgium, Sweden and Switzerland (1% each); the Asia-Pacific region (China, Hong Kong, India, Japan, Korea and New Zealand, 1% each); as well as the Middle East (Israel and Turkey, 1% each).

Approximately 40% of the users were from academia or affiliated with an academic institution, and nearly half were working in hospitals, cancer/medical centres and health service provider organizations. One user (1%) was in private practice, and a small minority was from non-profit governmental organizations (2%), as well as pharmacies and the pharmaceutical industry (3%).

Approximately 60% of users were healthcare professionals. These included pharmacists (24%), physicians (20%), nurses (13%) and other allied health professionals (2%). The latter comprised of a clinical social worker and a psychologist. Among the first 3 groups of healthcare professionals, a large percentage specialised in oncology (41% pharmacists, 50% physicians and 75% nurses). The proportion of naturopaths was also high (16%), edging over that of nurses. Researchers and trainees/students made up one-fifth of the users, with the latter including those from the medicine, pharmacy, life sciences and biomedical engineering fields.

Users were asked to indicate how they got to know about the database when they signed up for an account. Over a quarter of them found out about the database through word-of-mouth from their colleagues. This finding could probably explain the large numbers of users who were from network hospitals and health service providers (28%). Other major sources of knowledge about the database included the publications on the database (31%), as well as through searches in PubMed or through institutional libraries (11%). Among those who knew about the database through its publications, ~75% of them had read about its ability to identify oncology interactions with CAMs (K. Y.-L. Yap, Kuo, Lee, Chui, & Chan, 2010). Hence, many of the users were naturopaths (16%).

Table 11. Demographics of OncoRx-MI users. (N=90)

Demographics	Number of Users (%)+
Countries	
Australia	17 (19%)
France and Germany	8 (9%)
Italy	6 (7%)
Singapore	5 (6%)
Spain	2 (2%)
UK and Ireland	6 (7%)
US and Canada	34 (38%)
Others	12 (13%)
Organizations	
Academic institutions	29 (32%)
Academic-affiliated / teaching hospitals	7 (8%)
Cancer / medical centres	6 (7%)
Governmental organizations	2 (2%)
Hospitals	12 (13%)
Natural medicine clinics	2 (2%)
Network hospitals / health service providers	25 (28%)
Pharmacies / pharmaceutical industries	3 (3%)
Others	4 (4%)
Occupations	
Naturopaths	14 (16%)
Nurses	12 (13%)
Pharmacists	22 (24%)
Physicians	18 (20%)
Other allied health professionals	2 (2%)
Researchers	8 (9%)
Trainees / students	10 (11%)
Other non-healthcare professionals	4 (4%)
Knowledge of the database	
Publications on the database	28 (31%)
Citations of other published articles	4 (4%)
Searches from PubMed and institutional libraries	10 (11%)
Internet, search engines and listserves	8 (9%)
Word-of-mouth	23 (26%)

+Percentages may not add up to 100% due to missing values and rounding of data.
UK: United Kingdom, US: United States

A specific online form was created to seek feedback from users about the usefulness of the database and its relevance to their clinical practices. For usefulness, they were asked to rate the database in terms of information on the drugs, chemoregimens and CAMs, interaction-related content, management plans, non-interacting alternatives, and usability through a 5-point Likert scale (a lot better, a little better, makes no difference, a little worse, a lot worse). For clinical relevance, users were asked whether the database increased their knowledge on managing oncology DDIs, improved their drug-related decision making, and if it was a useful tool in practice. Users could agree, disagree or remain neutral to these questions. Users were also encouraged to provide suggestions for improvement of the database.

A total of 16 users completed the feedback form. Majority of them agreed that this database was better than their current sources of oncology DDI information (Table 12), with 13 of them (81%) indicating that the content on drugs, regimens and CAMs were better than their current sources of information. The same number of users also felt that the interaction-related data provided by OncoRx-MI was better. However, one user indicated that its content was "a lot worse" because he could not find interactions with a curcumin product, but curcumin was indexed under a different name (turmeric) in the database. In his comments, he stated that he would like to see more CAMs in the database so that more HDIs could be identified, but nevertheless, he agreed that this database would be useful in the future if the list of interactions could be further expanded.

Nearly 70% of the users (11 users) indicated that the management plans provided by OncoRx-MI were better than their current information sources, but only a little more than half (9 users) indicated the same for the non-interacting alternatives. This could be because the non-interacting alternatives were provided in the same paragraph as the management plans, and if the users did not read the management plans in detail, they could have missed out on these alternatives, especially at the point of patient consultations. An improvement would be to provide a separate section for non-interacting drugs/CAMs that is distinct from the rest of the management plan, so that users could see it even when they were in a rush for time. Although majority of the users (11 users) indicated that the ease-of-use of the database was better, one user also indicated that its usability was "a little worse". This user felt confused due to the many drug and CAM categories that he could choose from. He said that he would have preferred to just select the ACD and the interacting drug/CAM instead. In fact, this option was provided for users as the default search

Table 12. Ratings of OncoRx-MI parameters based on user feedback.

Parameters	Number of Users Who Provided Ratings (%)+				
	A Lot Better	A Little Better	Makes No Difference	A Little Worse	A Lot Worse
Content on drugs, regimens and CAMs	5 (31)	8 (50)	2 (13)	0 (0)	1 (6)
Interaction-related content	7 (44)	6 (38)	2 (13)	0 (0)	1 (6)
Management plans	5 (31)	6 (38)	5 (31)	0 (0)	0 (0)
Non-interacting alternatives	2 (13)	7 (44)	7 (44)	0 (0)	0 (0)
Ease-of-use	5 (31)	6 (38)	4 (25)	1 (6)	0 (0)

+Percentages may not add up to 100% due to rounding of data.
CAMs: complementary and alternative medicines

interface. A statement describing this default search interface as part of the instructions might clarify users' doubts on how to conduct a DDI search.

In terms of clinical relevance, 12 users (75%) indicated that the database was a useful tool in their practices, and that it helped increase their knowledge on managing oncology DDIs. Fourteen of them (88%) also indicated that it helped to improve their drug-related decision making. One user, who was an oncology practitioner, had found this database useful when handling a patient query about DDIs. Despite several neutral ratings, many of the users still gave positive comments saying that the database was an "awesome resource" and it was "much more complete for oncology regimens and CAMs". Some users stated that this database was "very good as it is, as long as the current information can be maintained". In fact, one user said that "more practitioners should know about it", while another complimented on its ability to suggest alternative medications and wished that "all patients had clear instructions on drugs to take and drugs to avoid". A limitation of the feedback results was the small number of respondents, which might not be representative of all users of the database. Nevertheless, the following comment by a user clearly summarized how those who responded to the survey felt about the database and its usefulness to healthcare professionals:

"I have found the level of detail with regard to the interaction to surpass that in most other databases. In fact, there are a couple interactions identified in your database that are completely lacking in other databases. As well, the referencing is excellent. When searching for drug interaction information I usually check more than a single database and I have added [this database] to my list of routinely searched databases. Good job!" – Feedback by a user

The users also provided detailed suggestions on what they would like to see as improvements. Many of the suggestions included expanding the database to include other natural remedies (e.g. amino acids, vitamins and minerals, other natural supplements), and other drug classes. Some users suggested inclusions of more specific monitoring plans and DDI identifications based on the pharmacological classes of the ACDs. Others wanted ways to carry out multiple DDI searches, and also a list of non-interacting ACDs when a DDI was identified with a CAM or non-ACD. Lastly, one user suggested updates in the form of letters or newsletters. Some of these feedbacks would be considered as updates in future work.

Limitations of the Database

The main limitation of OncoRx-MI is its ability to only detect interactions with certain classes of psychotropics and CAMs. Future modules on DDIs with other drug classes of prescription medicines and CAMs is intended to make the database more comprehensive. The database is also limited to searching one interaction at a time. Separate searches have to be conducted for multiple DDIs, which can be troublesome for users. Furthermore, users can only search for HDIs based on the common names of the CAMs. Some CAMs are known by various names (e.g. Asian, Chinese, Korean and Oriental ginsengs all fall under the *Panax* genus). It can be difficult for users to search for a CAM if they are not familiar with the name that is currently indexed in the database. Enabling multiple DDI searches and the ability to search based on various drug or CAM names can improve its usability.

In terms of the graphical user interface, the links provided can be small and difficult for users to tap or "click" with their fingers. Technical disparities with the screen resolution and interface designs may differ when viewed with different mobile devices. However, OncoRx-MI is still useful since it leverages on 3G/4G and Wi-Fi networks to operate. Hence, it can be used on any mobile web browser. OncoRx-MI is able to identify a substantial number of interactions with single-agent and combination regimens in its current stage; thus it will be useful to clinicians in a variety of clinical settings and who are always on-the-go.

REFERENCES

Abarca, J., Malone, D. C., Armstrong, E. P., Grizzle, A. J., Hansten, P. D., Van Bergen, R. C., & Lipton, R. B. (2004). Concordance of severity ratings provided in four drug interaction compendia. *Journal of the American Pharmacists Association*, *44*(2), 136–141. doi:10.1331/154434504773062582 PMID:15098847

Abernethy, A. P., Raman, G., Balk, E. M., Hammond, J. M., Orlando, L. A., Wheeler, J. L., ... McCrory, D. C. (2009). Systematic review: Reliability of compendia methods for off-label oncology indications. *Annals of Internal Medicine*, *150*(5), 336–343. doi:10.7326/0003-4819-150-5-200903030-00107 PMID:19221366

Aetna InteliHealth Inc. (2010, Jun 28). *Index of herbal medicines and supplements*. Retrieved 10 January, 2011, from http://www.intelihealth.com/IH/ihtIH/WSIHW000/8513/31402.html

American Society of Health-System Pharmacists. (2007). *AHFS Drug Information* (2007 ed.). Bethesda, MD: American Society of Health-System Pharmacists Inc.

Anttila, A. K., Rasanen, L., & Leinonen, E. V. (2001). Fluvoxamine augmentation increases serum mirtazapine concentrations three- to fourfold. *The Annals of Pharmacotherapy*, *35*(10), 1221–1223. doi:10.1345/aph.1A014 PMID:11675851

Apotex Corp. (2020). *Fluvoxamine maleate tablet*. Retrieved from https://dailymed.nlm.nih.gov/dailymed/drugInfo.cfm?setid=6eeb14df-6fcf-a737-5359-5744eb4accea

Austwick, E. A., Brown, L. C., Goodyear, K. H., & Brooks, D. J. (2002). Pharmacist's input into a palliative care clinic. *The Pharmaceutical Journal*, *268*(7190), 404–406.

BC Cancer Agency. (n.d.). *BCCA cancer drug manual*. Retrieved 10 January, 2020, from http://www.bccancer.bc.ca/health-professionals/clinical-resources/cancer-drug-manual

Boddy, C. (2001). Pharmacist involvement with warfarin dosing for inpatients. *Pharmacy World & Science*, *23*(1), 31–35. doi:10.1023/A:1011289304437 PMID:11344589

Bourg, V., Lebrun, C., Chichmanian, R. M., Thomas, P., & Frenay, M. (2001). Nitroso-urea-cisplatin-based chemotherapy associated with valproate: Increase of haematologic toxicity. *Annals of Oncology: Official Journal of the European Society for Medical Oncology*, *12*(2), 217–219. doi:10.1023/A:1008331708395 PMID:11300327

Boyer, C., Selby, M., Scherrer, J. R., & Appel, R. D. (1998). The Health On the Net Code of Conduct for medical and health websites. *Computers in Biology and Medicine*, *28*(5), 603–610. doi:10.1016/S0010-4825(98)00037-7 PMID:9861515

British Medical Association & Pharmaceutical Society of Great Britain. (2007). *British National Formulary* (53rd ed.). London, UK: BMJ Publishing Group Ltd & RPS Publishing.

Cavuto, N. J., Woosley, R. L., & Sale, M. (1996). Pharmacies and prevention of potentially fatal drug interactions. *Journal of the American Medical Association*, *275*(14), 1086–1087. doi:10.1001/jama.1996.03530380028022 PMID:8601923

Chang, H.-M., But, P. P.-H., Yao, S.-C., Wang, L.-L., & Yeung, S. C.-S. (2001). Pharmacology and Applications of Chinese Materia Medica (S.-C. Yao, L.-L. Wang & S. C.-S. Yeung, Trans.; Vols. 1-2). Singapore: World Scientific Publishing Co.

Chao, S. D., & Maibach, H. I. (2005). Lack of drug interaction conformity in commonly used drug compendia for selected at-risk dermatologic drugs. *American Journal of Clinical Dermatology*, *6*(2), 105–111. doi:10.2165/00128071-200506020-00005 PMID:15799682

Charnock, D., & Shepperd, S. (2004). Learning to DISCERN online: Applying an appraisal tool to health websites in a workshop setting. *Health Education Research*, *19*(4), 440–446. doi:10.1093/her/cyg046 PMID:15155597

Chen, S. E., Sawchuk, R. J., & Staba, E. J. (1980). American ginseng. III. Pharmacokinetics of ginsenosides in the rabbit. *European Journal of Drug Metabolism and Pharmacokinetics*, *5*(3), 161–168. doi:10.1007/BF03189460 PMID:7202434

Cheung, Y. T., Yap, K. Y., Chui, W. K., & Chan, A. (2010). Drug-drug interactions between oral antiepileptics and oral anticancer drugs: Implications to clinicians. *European Neurology*, *64*(2), 88–94. doi:10.1159/000315031 PMID:20606454

Clauson, K. A., Marsh, W. A., Polen, H. H., Seamon, M. J., & Ortiz, B. I. (2007). Clinical decision support tools: Analysis of online drug information databases. *BMC Medical Informatics and Decision Making*, *7*(1), 7. doi:10.1186/1472-6947-7-7 PMID:17346336

Clauson, K. A., Polen, H. H., & Marsh, W. A. (2007). Clinical decision support tools: Performance of personal digital assistant versus online drug information databases. *Pharmacotherapy*, *27*(12), 1651–1658. doi:10.1592/phco.27.12.1651 PMID:18041886

Coiffier, B., Lepage, E., Brière, J., Herbrecht, R., Tilly, H., Bouabdallah, R., ... Gisselbrecht, C. (2002). CHOP chemotherapy plus rituximab compared with CHOP alone in elderly patients with diffuse large B-cell lymphoma. *The New England Journal of Medicine*, *346*(4), 235–242. doi:10.1056/NEJMoa011795 PMID:11807147

Commission of the European Communities (Brussels). (2002). eEurope 2002: Quality criteria for health related websites. *Journal of Medical Internet Research*, *4*(3), e15. doi:10.2196/jmir.4.3.e15 PMID:12554546

Darmoni, S. (2001, Jul 18). *Net Scoring®: criteria to assess the quality of health internet information.* Retrieved 10 January, 2011, from https://www.chu-rouen.fr/netscoring/netscoringeng.html

Davis, J. (2018, Jul 21). *Hackers breach 1.5 million Singapore patient records, including the prime minister's.* Retrieved 20 Jan, 2020, from https://www.healthcareit.com.au/article/hackers-breach-15-million-singapore-patient-records-including-prime-ministers

Discovery Communications LLC. (2007). *Discovery Health Drug Interaction Checker*. Retrieved 10 Jan, 2011, from http://health.discovery.com/webapps/drugchecker.do%3FjspLetter=A

Dooley, M. J., Lee, D. Y., & Marriott, J. L. (2004). Practitioners' sources of clinical information on complementary and alternative medicine in oncology. *Supportive Care in Cancer*, *12*(2), 114–119. doi:10.100700520-003-0570-5 PMID:14655043

Drugsite Trust. (2000). *Drugs.com™: drug interactions checker*. Retrieved 10 Jan, 2020, from https://www.drugs.com/drug_interactions.html

Ducharme, M. M., & Boothby, L. A. (2007). Analysis of adverse drug reactions for preventability. *International Journal of Clinical Practice*, *61*(1), 157–161. doi:10.1111/j.1742-1241.2006.01130.x PMID:17229189

e-MS Inc. (2004). *TCM Assistant*. Retrieved 10 Jan, 2011, from http://www.tcmassistant.com/index.html

Enhanced Medical Decisions Inc. (2007). *DoublecheckMD.com™*. Retrieved 10 Jan, 2011, from http://www.doublecheckmd.com

Epocrates Inc. (2020). *Epocrates*. Retrieved 10 Jan, 2020, from http://www.epocrates.com/products/rx/

Express Scripts Inc. (2008). *Drug Digest interactions checker*. Retrieved 10 Jan, 2020, from http://www.drugdigest.org/wps/portal/ddigest

Eyal, S., Yagen, B., Sobol, E., Altschuler, Y., Shmuel, M., & Bialer, M. (2004). The activity of antiepileptic drugs as histone deacetylase inhibitors. *Epilepsia*, *45*(7), 737–744. doi:10.1111/j.0013-9580.2004.00104.x PMID:15230695

Eysenbach, G. (2000). Consumer health informatics. *British Medical Journal*, *320*(7251), 1713–1716. doi:10.1136/bmj.320.7251.1713 PMID:10864552

Fisher, B., Anderson, S., Wickerham, D. L., DeCillis, A., Dimitrov, N., Mamounas, E., ... Deckers, P. (1997). Increased intensification and total dose of cyclophosphamide in a doxorubicin-cyclophosphamide regimen for the treatment of primary breast cancer: Findings from National Surgical Adjuvant Breast and Bowel Project B-22. *Journal of Clinical Oncology*, *15*(5), 1858–1869. doi:10.1200/JCO.1997.15.5.1858 PMID:9164196

Fisher, B., Brown, A. M., Dimitrov, N. V., Poisson, R., Redmond, C., Margolese, R. G., ... Kardinal, C. G. (1990). Two months of doxorubicin-cyclophosphamide with and without interval reinduction therapy compared with 6 months of cyclophosphamide, methotrexate and fluorouracil in positive-node breast cancer patients with tamoxifen-nonresponsive tumors: Results from the National Surgical Adjuvant Breast and Bowel Project B-15. *Journal of Clinical Oncology*, *8*(9), 1483–1496. doi:10.1200/JCO.1990.8.9.1483 PMID:2202791

Gagliardi, A., & Jadad, A. R. (2002). Examination of instruments used to rate quality of health information on the internet: Chronicle of a voyage with an unclear destination. *British Medical Journal*, *324*(7337), 569–573. doi:10.1136/bmj.324.7337.569 PMID:11884320

Gerstner, L. V., Jr. (2008). *Memorial Sloan-Kettering Cancer Center - cancer information (about herbs, botanicals and other products)*. Retrieved 10 Jan, 2020, from https://www.mskcc.org/mskcc/html/11570.cfm

Ghioni, A. (2019, Oct 9). *A summary of healthcare data breaches in Australia*. Retrieved 21 Jan, 2020, from https://www.stanfieldit.com/data-breaches-in-australia/

Glassman, P. A., Simon, B., Belperio, P., & Lanto, A. (2002). Improving recognition of drug interactions: Benefits and barriers to using automated drug alerts. *Medical Care*, *40*(12), 1161–1171. doi:10.1097/00005650-200212000-00004 PMID:12458299

Gold Standard Inc. (2010). *Caremark Drug Interactions*. Retrieved 10 Jan, 2020, from http://cpref.goldstandard.com/inter.asp?r=8084

Göttlicher, M., Minucci, S., Zhu, P., Krämer, O. H., Schimpf, A., Giavara, S., ... Heinzel, T. (2001). Valproic acid defines a novel class of HDAC inhibitors inducing differentiation of transformed cells. *The EMBO Journal*, *20*(24), 6969–6978. doi:10.1093/emboj/20.24.6969 PMID:11742974

Grönroos, P. E., Irjala, K. M., Huupponen, R. K., Scheinin, H., Forsström, J., & Forsström, J. J. (1997). A medication database - a tool for detecting drug interactions in hospital. *European Journal of Clinical Pharmacology*, *53*(1), 13–17. doi:10.1007002280050330 PMID:9349924

Hansten, P. D. (2003). Drug interaction management. *Pharmacy World & Science*, *25*(3), 94–97. doi:10.1023/A:1024077018902 PMID:12840961

Hansten, P. D., & Horn, J. R. (2008). *Hansten and Horn's Drug Interactions Analysis and Management* (3rd ed.). Vancouver, WA: Lippincott Williams & Wilkins.

Health On the Net Foundation. (2019, Nov). *Discover the 8 principles of the HONcode in 35 languages*. Retrieved 10 Jan, 2020, from https://www.hon.ch/cgi-bin/HONcode/principles.pl?English

Health On the Net Foundation. (2020, Jan). *Health On the Net*. Retrieved 10 Jan, 2020, from http://www.hon.ch/

Healthwise Incorporated. (2006). *AOL Health Drug Interaction Checker*. Retrieved 10 Jan, 2011, from http://drugchecker.aol.com/

Henry, J. (2019, Oct 1). *Victorian hospitals go offline after ransomware attack*. Retrieved 21 Jan, 2020, from https://www.itnews.com.au/news/victorian-hospitals-go-offline-after-ransomware-attack-531696

Ikeda, H., Murakami, T., Takano, M., Usui, T., & Kihira, K. (2005). Pharmacokinetic interaction on valproic acid and recurrence of epileptic seizures during chemotherapy in an epileptic patient. *British Journal of Clinical Pharmacology*, *59*(5), 593–597. doi:10.1111/j.1365-2125.2005.02339.x PMID:15842559

Jellin, J. M., & Gregory, P. J. (2007). *Natural Medicines Comprehensive Database* (10th ed.). Stockton, CA: Therapeutic Research Faculty.

Kheshti, R., Aalipour, M., & Namazi, S. (2016). A comparison of five common drug-drug interaction software programs regarding accuracy and comprehensiveness. *Journal of Research in Pharmacy Practice*, *5*(4), 257–263. doi:10.4103/2279-042X.192461 PMID:27843962

Klein, T. E., Chang, J. T., Cho, M. K., Easton, K. L., Fergerson, R., Hewett, M., ... Altman, R. B. (2001). Integrating genotype and phenotype information: An overview of the PharmGKB project. *The Pharmacogenomics Journal*, *1*(3), 167–170. doi:10.1038j.tpj.6500035 PMID:11908751

Ko, Y., Abarca, J., Malone, D. C., Dare, D. C., Geraets, D., Houranieh, A., ... Wilhard, M. (2007). Practitioners' views on computerized drug-drug interaction alerts in the VA system. *Journal of the American Medical Informatics Association*, *14*(1), 56–64. doi:10.1197/jamia.M2224 PMID:17068346

Ko, Y., Malone, D. C., D'Agostino, J. V., Skrepnek, G. H., Armstrong, E. P., Brown, M., & Woosley, R. L. (2008). Potential determinants of prescribers' drug-drug interaction knowledge. *Research in Social & Administrative Pharmacy*, *4*(4), 355–366. doi:10.1016/j.sapharm.2007.10.004 PMID:19064242

Lacy, C. F., Armstrong, L. L., Goldman, M. P., & Lance, L. L. (2007-2008). *Drug Information Handbook with International Trade Names Index* (15th ed.). Hudson, OH: Lexi-comp Inc.

Langdorf, M. I., Fox, J. C., Marwah, R. S., Montague, B. J., & Hart, M. M. (2000). Physician versus computer knowledge of potential drug interactions in the emergency department. *Academic Emergency Medicine*, *7*(11), 1321–1329. doi:10.1111/j.1553-2712.2000.tb00483.x PMID:11073486

Lange, B. J., Bostrom, B. C., Cherlow, J. M., Sensel, M. G., La, M. K., Rackoff, W., ... Sather, H. N. (2002). Double-delayed intensification improves event-free survival for children with intermediate-risk acute lymphoblastic leukemia: A report from the Children's Cancer Group. *Blood, 99*(3), 825–833. doi:10.1182/blood.V99.3.825 PMID:11806983

Lassman, A. B., & DeAngelis, L. M. (2003). Brain metastases. *Neurologic Clinics, 21*(1), 1-23. doi:10.10160733-8619(02)00035-x

Lexi-Comp Inc. (2020). *Lexi-Comp®*. Retrieved 10 Jan, 2020, from https://www.wolterskluwercdi.com/drug-reference/apps/

Lim, L. (2007). Diagnosis and management of depression in terminal cancer. *Singapore General Hospital Proceedings, 16*(2), 88–96.

Lohr, L. (2008). Chemotherapy-induced nausea and vomiting. *Cancer Journal (Sudbury, Mass.), 14*(2), 85–93. doi:10.1097/PPO.0b013e31816a0f07 PMID:18391612

Merck & Co. Inc. (2020). *Zolinza™ (vorinostat) capsules*. Retrieved from https://www.merck.com/product/usa/pi_circulars/z/zolinza/zolinza_pi.pdf

Närhi, U., Pohjanoksa-Mäntylä, M., Karjalainen, A., Saari, J. K., Wahlroos, H., Airaksinen, M. S., & Bell, S. J. (2008). The DARTS tool for assessing online medicines information. *Pharmacy World & Science, 30*(6), 898–906. doi:10.100711096-008-9249-9 PMID:18791806

Neef, C., & de Voogd-van der Straaten, I. (1988). An interaction between cytostatic and anticonvulsant drugs. *Clinical Pharmacology and Therapeutics, 43*(4), 372–375. doi:10.1038/clpt.1988.45 PMID:3128415

Nelson, A. A. Jr, Hutchinson, R. A., Mahoney, D., & Ringstrom, J. (1976). Evaluation of the utilization of medication profiles for the purpose of drug-drug interaction surveillance by pharmacists in a community setting. *Drug Intelligence & Clinical Pharmacy, 10*(5), 274–281. doi:10.1177/106002807601000503 PMID:10236241

Newport, D. J., & Nemeroff, C. B. (1998). Assessment and treatment of depression in the cancer patient. *Journal of Psychosomatic Research, 45*(3), 215–237. doi:10.1016/S0022-3999(98)00011-7 PMID:9776368

Newton, H. B., Goldlust, S. A., & Pearl, D. (2006). Retrospective analysis of the efficacy and tolerability of levetiracetam in brain tumor patients. *Journal of Neuro-Oncology*, *78*(1), 99–102. doi:10.100711060-005-9070-4 PMID:16541329

Nikolic, B. S., & Ilic, M. S. (2013). Assessment of the consistency among three drug compendia in listing and ranking of drug-drug interactions. *Bosnian Journal of Basic Medical Sciences*, *13*(4), 253–258. doi:10.17305/bjbms.2013.2334 PMID:24289762

Parekh, H. S., Liu, G., & Wei, M. Q. (2009). A new dawn for the use of traditional Chinese medicine in cancer therapy. *Molecular Cancer*, *8*(1), 21. doi:10.1186/1476-4598-8-21 PMID:19298677

Perneger, T. V. (2005). The Swiss cheese model of safety incidents: Are there holes in the metaphor? *BMC Health Services Research*, *5*(1), 71. doi:10.1186/1472-6963-5-71 PMID:16280077

Phiel, C. J., Zhang, F., Huang, E. Y., Guenther, M. G., Lazar, M. A., & Klein, P. S. (2001). Histone deacetylase is a direct target of valproic acid, a potent anticonvulsant, mood stabilizer, and teratogen. *The Journal of Biological Chemistry*, *276*(39), 36734–36741. doi:10.1074/jbc.M101287200 PMID:11473107

Polen, H. H., Zapantis, A., Clauson, K. A., Jebrock, J., & Paris, M. (2008). Ability of online drug databases to assist in clinical decision-making with infectious disease therapies. *BMC Infectious Diseases*, *8*(1), 153. doi:10.1186/1471-2334-8-153 PMID:18990224

Provost, M., Koompalum, D., Dong, D., & Martin, B. C. (2006). The initial development of the WebMedQual scale: Domain assessment of the construct of quality of health web sites. *International Journal of Medical Informatics*, *75*(1), 42–57. doi:10.1016/j.ijmedinf.2005.07.034 PMID:16169770

Radboudumc. (n.d.). *Cancer Drug Interactions – Drug Interaction Checker*. Retrieved 20 Jan, 2020, from https://cancer-druginteractions.org/checker

Robillard, J. M., Jun, J. H., Lai, J. A., & Feng, T. L. (2018). The QUEST for quality online health information: Validation of a short quantitative tool. *BMC Medical Informatics and Decision Making*, *18*(1), 87. doi:10.118612911-018-0668-9 PMID:30340488

Sheehan, N. L., Kelly, D. V., Tseng, A. L., van Heeswijk, R. P. G., Béïque, L. C., & Hughes, C. A. (2003). Evaluation of HIV drug interaction web sites. *The Annals of Pharmacotherapy*, *37*(11), 1577–1586. doi:10.1345/aph.1D039 PMID:14565802

Shin, H. R., Kim, J. Y., Yun, T. K., Morgan, G., & Vainio, H. (2000). The cancer-preventive potential of Panax ginseng: A review of human and experimental evidence. *Cancer Causes & Control*, *11*(6), 565–576. doi:10.1023/A:1008980200583 PMID:10880039

Solimando, D. A. J. (2007). *Drug Information Handbook for Oncology* (6th ed.). Hudson, OH: Lexi-comp.

Spiegel, D., & Giese-Davis, J. (2003). Depression and cancer: Mechanisms and disease progression. *Biological Psychiatry*, *54*(3), 269–282. doi:10.1016/S0006-3223(03)00566-3 PMID:12893103

Spina, E., Santoro, V., & D'Arrigo, C. (2008). Clinically relevant pharmacokinetic drug interactions with second-generation antidepressants: An update. *Clinical Therapeutics*, *30*(7), 1206–1227. doi:10.1016/S0149-2918(08)80047-1 PMID:18691982

Tan, E. L., Stark, H., Lowinger, J. S., Ringland, C., Ward, R., & Pearson, S. A. (2006). Information sources used by New South Wales cancer clinicians: A qualitative study. *Internal Medicine Journal*, *36*(11), 711–717. doi:10.1111/j.1445-5994.2006.01171.x PMID:17040357

Tatro, D. S. (2008). *Drug Interaction Facts: The Authority on Drug Interactions* (2008 ed.). St. Louis, MO: Facts & Comparisons.

Tesch, H., Diehl, V., Lathan, B., Hasenclever, D., Sieber, M., Ruffer, U., ... Loeffler, M. (1998). Moderate dose escalation for advanced stage Hodgkin's disease using the bleomycin, etoposide, adriamycin, cyclophosphamide, vincristine, procarbazine, and prednisone scheme and adjuvant radiotherapy: A study of the German Hodgkin's Lymphoma Study Group. *Blood*, *92*(12), 4560–4567. doi:10.1182/blood.V92.12.4560 PMID:9845521

Thomson Healthcare. (n.d.). *Micromedex® (intranet database).* Retrieved 10 January 2020 https://www.micromedexsolutions.com/

Thomson Reuters. (2010). *Physicians' Desktop Reference (PDRhealth™) Drug Interaction Tool.* Retrieved 10 Jan, 2011, from http://pdrhealth.com/health/health-tools-drug-interactions.aspx

TRUSTe. (2008, Jul 15). *TRUSTe responds to consumer privacy threats with major expansion*. Retrieved 10 Jan, 2020, from http://www.jpubb.com/en/press/8840/

Tucker, R. (2004). Pharmacist-led dermatology clinics can improve prisoners' quality of life. *The Pharmaceutical Journal*, *272*(7298), 577–579.

UpToDate Inc. (n.d.). *UpToDate® (Intranet Database)*. Retrieved 10 January 2020, from UpToDate Inc. http://www.uptodateonline.com

Vecht, C. J., Wagner, G. L., & Wilms, E. B. (2003a). Interactions between antiepileptic and chemotherapeutic drugs. *Lancet Neurology*, *2*(7), 404–409. doi:10.1016/S1474-4422(03)00435-6 PMID:12849118

Vecht, C. J., Wagner, G. L., & Wilms, E. B. (2003b). Treating seizures in patients with brain tumors: Drug interactions between antiepileptic and chemotherapeutic agents. *Seminars in Oncology Nursing*, *30*(6Suppl 19), 49–52. doi:10.1053/j.seminoncol.2003.11.030 PMID:14765386

Vitry, A. I. (2007). Comparative assessment of four drug interaction compendia. *British Journal of Clinical Pharmacology*, *63*(6), 709–714. doi:10.1111/j.1365-2125.2006.02809.x PMID:17166171

Web, M. D. Inc. (2010). *Medscape® drug interaction checker*. Retrieved 10 Jan, 2020, from https://www.medscape.com/druginfo/druginterchecker

Weideman, R. A., Bernstein, I. H., & McKinney, W. P. (1999). Pharmacist recognition of potential drug interactions. *American Journal of Health-System Pharmacy*, *56*(15), 1524–1529. doi:10.1093/ajhp/56.15.1524 PMID:10478990

Wishart, D. S., Knox, C., Guo, A. C., Shrivastava, S., Hassanali, M., Stothard, P., ... Woolsey, J. (2006). DrugBank: A comprehensive resource for in silico drug discovery and exploration. *Nucleic Acids Research*, *34*(Database issue), D668–D672. doi:10.1093/nar/gkj067 PMID:16381955

Wong, C. M., Ko, Y., & Chan, A. (2008). Clinically significant drug-drug interactions between oral anticancer agents and nonanticancer agents: Profiling and comparison of two drug compendia. *The Annals of Pharmacotherapy*, *42*(12), 1737–1748. doi:10.1345/aph.1L255 PMID:19033481

Yap, K. Y., Chan, A., & Chui, W. K. (2010). Opinions on drug interaction sources in anticancer treatments and parameters for an oncology-specific database by pharmacy practitioners in Asia. *Health Services Insights*, *3*, 1–12. doi:10.4137/HSI.S3679

Yap, K. Y., Raaj, S., & Chan, A. (2010). OncoRx-IQ: A tool for quality assessment of online anticancer drug interactions. *International Journal for Quality in Health Care*, *22*(2), 93–106. doi:10.1093/intqhc/mzq004 PMID:20172863

Yap, K. Y.-L., Kuo, E. Y., Lee, J. J. J., Chui, W. K., & Chan, A. (2010). An onco-informatics database for anticancer drug interactions with complementary and alternative medicines used in cancer treatment and supportive care: An overview of the OncoRx project. *Supportive Care in Cancer*, *18*(7), 883–891. doi:10.100700520-009-0729-9 PMID:19756775

Conclusion

This book has provided an overview of the various pharmaco-cybernetic frameworks and quality considerations for developing mHealth apps for medication management. Of relevance are the digital health innovation process, Pharmaco-cybernetic Maxims, user-centered (UCD), experience-centered (ECD) and activity-centered designs (ACD), and the Ecological Systems Theory. Additionally, the Intervention Mapping (IM) framework provides an understanding of how behavioral change techniques can be applied in the holistic design of mHealth systems. Concepts on the Technology Acceptance Model (TAM) and the Unified Theory of Acceptance and Use of Technology (UTAUT) model have been introduced to understand the factors that influence patients' acceptance of mHealth apps for medication adherence. Furthermore, the quality consideration factors for designing and evaluating medication management apps have been put forward to encourage the design and development of better-quality apps. Besides, a chronological evolution timeline of mHealth research has been described, together with two relevant case studies to illustrate how the various frameworks can be applied through the designing of an oral anticancer medication adherence app and an oncology drug interaction database.

It is envisaged that the maturing digital health market will lead to several trends in mHealth research, which will have enormous implications in health and patient care. In a survey by The Economist on 400 global business leaders in the healthcare sector, technologies that will become widespread realities in the future include portable medical devices for healthcare professionals, health sensors for consumers, telemedicine, Internet-of-Things (IoT), as well as precision medicine, among others (The Economist, 2017). There will be a paradigm shift in the patient-practitioner relationship. For example, with the advancement in technologies such as portable diagnostics, wearables, sensors and drones, the focus on the point-of-care will shift from hospital institutions to the patients' homes (Meskó, Drobni, Bényei, Gergely, &

Győrffy, 2017). Medication therapies will shift from being population-focused to individual-focused where the individual's health parameters will enable personalization of therapies and treatments (Meskó, et al., 2017). The patient-practitioner relationship will shift from a hierarchical model where the physician has the sole responsibility of clinical decision-making to a more collaborative model where the patient is empowered to make decisions about their own care; and health-related data that is currently owned by healthcare institutions and insurance systems will shift towards ownership and control by patients themselves (Meskó, et al., 2017). In short, healthcare will evolve from being patient-centered to person-directed (Lines, Lepore, & Wiener, 2015; Starfield, 2011).

With wearables, portable devices and other health sensors going mainstream into the health consumer market, there will also be a seismic shift towards big data in health. Information from wearable health sensors and the vast amounts of health-related and drug-related information on the internet means that medical knowledge will no longer be limited to healthcare professionals, but patients will also be able to gain access to these information anytime and anywhere (Meskó, et al., 2017). Hence, there is a need to conduct more robust studies to generate a strong evidence base for mHealth systems and validate wearables as effective tools in healthcare practices.

These technological trends will give rise to two major phenomena – the first builds on the concept of the "Internet-of-Things" (IoT) and is known as the "Internet-of-Patients" (IoP) (Mishra & Chakraborty, 2020). In the hospital setting, the IoT relies on a network of medical devices and sensor systems that are connected to the electronic medical records of patients via Internet Protocol (IP) communications. By integrating medical devices with an enterprise service bus with IP, data exchange is enabled so that clinicians can access health information and medical resources in a timely fashion at the point of care – resulting in the "Internet-of-Medical-Things" (IoMT). Integrating this network of intercommunicating devices with a secure mHealth system that facilitates cost-effective interactions between patients and health service providers leads to the IoP, also known as the "Internet-of-Healthcare-Things" (IoHT) (Mishra & Chakraborty, 2020). Not surprisingly, there are over 20 billion devices connected to the IoT (Andriopoulou, Dagiuklas, & Orphanoudakis, 2017; Mishra & Chakraborty, 2020). It is not uncommon to see patients using mHealth apps to manage their healthcare needs on a regular basis. However, the IoP brings with it challenges in terms of data interoperability and exchange, as well as security and privacy (Andriopoulou, et al., 2017). In order to address these challenges, many organizations are adopting blockchain technologies to enhance interoperability, strengthen health data integrity and protect patient's digital identities (Krawiec et al., 2016).

Other upcoming innovations that involve big data analytics, artificial intelligence (AI), robotics, genomic medicine and digimeds will also largely influence the future trend in mHealth research and practice. AI chatbots are now a reality with apps such as Babylon (Babylon, 2020; Lunden, 2020) and Ada (Ada Health GmbH, 2020; O'Brien, 2019). The use of machine learning and AI for clinical diagnostics, risk predictions and in public health are also becoming a reality through Google's DeepMind Health's AI system for breast cancer screening (Hao, 2020; McKinney et al., 2020), and Apple Watch's ability to detect risks of falls and atrial fibrillation and soon, the risks of respiratory or cardiac arrest with its blood oxygen monitoring capabilities (Apple Inc., 2020; Chin, 2020). Interestingly, AI has also been used in public health for preventing suicides (Berrouiguet et al., 2019) and for predicting the spread of the novel coronavirus (COVID-19) pandemic (Long & Ehrenfeld, 2020; Wu, Leung, & Leung, 2020). Furthermore, the combination of AI with robotics have led to robot companions to help with medication management (e.g. Pillo (Muoio, 2019; Pillo Inc., 2019)) and healthy aging (e.g. ElliQ (Ackerman, 2019; Intuition Robotics, 2020)). The use of AI in genomic diagnostics is a foreseeable future (Dias & Torkamani, 2019), and Proteus Digital Health has developed the world's first "digital pill" for enhancing medication adherence in a myriad of medical conditions (Alan, 2019; Beekley, 2019; Muoio, 2018; Robbins, 2019).

All these technological innovations will result in a diverse "forest" of health-related data (Yap, 2012) that can be harnessed by the "data-driven healthcare professional" – the second major phenomenon. In a recent survey of 523 US physicians and 210 medical residents and students conducted by the Stanford Medicine and Brunswick Insight (Lloyd, 2020), majority of physicians, medical residents and students had indicated that they were insufficiently prepared to deal with digital health innovations in practice, even though they recognized these innovations as being of great benefit to patients. The rapid pace in which digital health technologies are evolving means that clinicians will need both patient skills and digital literacy, as well as new technological knowledge and skills in order to catch up with the digital health revolution (Meskó, 2019). As such, many of them (47% physicians, 73% medical students) are seeking out additional training in order to prepare themselves to handle such innovations in healthcare. In fact, a quarter of physicians will consider classes in advanced statistics and data science (23%), population health management (31%), artificial intelligence (34%), clinical genomics (27%) and genetic counselling (38%).

In the midst of the rapidly changing digital health world, one thing is certain. Patients need to be assured that their health is monitored by accurate, reliable and robust technology, and healthcare professionals need to be well-prepared to implement these emerging technologies in clinical practices. mHealth will play a major role in the healthcare of the future. As such, clinicians, designers and developers will need to work collaboratively through the whole digital health innovation process – from identifying the healthcare problem to implementing and supporting the mHealth innovation in clinical practice – so that useful and efficacious mHealth systems can be co-designed to enhance medication management, patient care and safety.

REFERENCES

Ackerman, E. (2019, Jan 9). *ElliQ, a social home robot for older adults, now available for pre-order.* Retrieved 17 Mar, 2020, from https://spectrum.ieee.org/automaton/robotics/home-robots/elliq-a-social-home-robot-for-older-adults-now-available-for-preorder

Ada Health GmbH. (2020). *Ada: Your health companion.* Retrieved 17 Mar, 2020, from https://ada.com/

Alan. (2019, Nov 12). *Digital meds boost hepatitis C drug adherence.* Retrieved 17 Mar, 2020, from https://sciencebusiness.technewslit.com/?p=37725

Andriopoulou, F., Dagiuklas, T., & Orphanoudakis, T. (2017). Integrating IoT and fog computing for healthcare service delivery. In G. Keramidas, N. Voros, & M. Hübner (Eds.), *Components and Services for IoT Platforms: Paving the Way for IoT Standards* (pp. 213–232). Cham: Springer International Publishing. doi:10.1007/978-3-319-42304-3_11

Apple Inc. (2020). *Use fall detection with Apple Watch.* Retrieved 17 Mar, 2020, from https://support.apple.com/en-au/HT208944

Babylon. (2020). *Babylon Health.* Retrieved 17 Mar, 2020, from https://www.babylonhealth.com/

Beekley, K. L. (2019, Nov 13). *Proteus Digital Health® DigiMeds data demonstrates 99% of hepatitis C patients at high risk for nonadherence achieved a cure*. Retrieved 17 Mar, 2020, from https://www.bloomberg.com/press-releases/2019-11-12/proteus-digital-health-digimeds-data-demonstrates-99-of-hepatitis-c-patients-at-high-risk-for-nonadherence-achieved-a-cure

Berrouiguet, S., Barrigón, M. L., Castroman, J. L., Courtet, P., Artés-Rodríguez, A., & Baca-García, E. (2019). Combining mobile-health (mHealth) and artificial intelligence (AI) methods to avoid suicide attempts: The Smartcrises study protocol. *BMC Psychiatry*, *19*(1), 277. doi:10.118612888-019-2260-y PMID:31493783

Chin, M. (2020, Mar 9). Apple Watches may soon detect blood oxygen levels. *The Verge*. Retrieved from https://www.theverge.com/2020/3/9/21171483/apple-watch-ios-14-code-blood-oxygen-features-update

Dias, R., & Torkamani, A. (2019). Artificial intelligence in clinical and genomic diagnostics. *Genome Medicine*, *11*(1), 70. doi:10.118613073-019-0689-8 PMID:31744524

Hao, K. (2020, Jan 3). *Google's AI breast cancer screening tool is learning to generalize across countries*. Retrieved 17 Mar, 2020, from https://www.technologyreview.com/f/615004/googles-ai-breast-cancer-screening-tool-is-learning-to-generalize-across-countries/

Intuition Robotics. (2020). *ElliQ*. Retrieved 17 Mar, 2020, from https://elliq.com

Krawiec, R., Housman, D., White, M., Filipova, M., Quarre, F., Barr, D., . . . Tsai, L. (2016). *White paper - Blockchain: Opportunities for health care*. Retrieved from https://www2.deloitte.com/content/dam/Deloitte/us/Documents/public-sector/us-blockchain-opportunities-for-health-care.pdf

Lines, L. M., Lepore, M., & Wiener, J. M. (2015). Patient-centered, person-centered, and person-directed care: They are not the same. *Medical Care*, *53*(7), 561–563. doi:10.1097/MLR.0000000000000387 PMID:26067878

Lloyd, B. M. (2020). *Stanford Medicine 2020 Health Trends Report: The rise of the data-driven physician*. Retrieved 15 Mar, 2020, from http://med.stanford.edu/dean/healthtrends.html

Long, J. B., & Ehrenfeld, J. M. (2020). The role of augmented intelligence (AI) in detecting and preventing the spread of novel coronavirus. *Journal of Medical Systems*, *44*(3), 59. doi:10.100710916-020-1536-6 PMID:32020374

Lunden, I. (2020, Jan 23). Babylon Health is building an integrated, AI-based health app to serve a city of 300K in England. *Tech Crunch*. Retrieved from https://techcrunch.com/2020/01/22/babylon-health-is-building-an-integrated-ai-based-health-app-to-serve-a-city-of-300k-in-england/

McKinney, S. M., Sieniek, M., Godbole, V., Godwin, J., Antropova, N., Ashrafian, H., ... Shetty, S. (2020). International evaluation of an AI system for breast cancer screening. *Nature*, *577*(7788), 89–94. doi:10.103841586-019-1799-6 PMID:31894144

Meskó, B. (2019). *The Technological Future of Medical Specialties* Retrieved from https://leanpub.com/future-of-medical-specialties

Meskó, B., Drobni, Z., Bényei, É., Gergely, B., & Győrffy, Z. (2017). Digital health is a cultural transformation of traditional healthcare. *mHealth*, *3*(9), 38. doi:10.21037/mhealth.2017.08.07 PMID:29184890

Mishra, K. N., & Chakraborty, C. (2020). A novel approach towards using big data and IoT for improving the efficiency of m-Health systems. In D. Gupta, A. Hassanien, & A. Khanna (Eds.), *Advanced Computational Intelligence Techniques for Virtual Reality in Healthcare. Studies in Computational Intelligence* (Vol. 875, pp. 123–139). Cham: Springer. doi:10.1007/978-3-030-35252-3_7

Muoio, D. (2018, Oct 15). Proteus, Otsuka expand their digital medicine collaboration with five-year, $88M deal. *MobiHealthNews*. Retrieved from https://www.mobihealthnews.com/content/proteus-otsuka-expand-their-digital-medicine-collaboration-five-year-88m-deal

Muoio, D. (2019, May 29). Pillo Health raises $11M Series A for conversational adherence, engagement platforms. *MobiHealthNews*. Retrieved from https://www.mobihealthnews.com/content/north-america/pillo-health-raises-11m-series-conversational-adherence-engagement-platforms

O'Brien, C. (2019, Dec 19). Ada Health cofounder on AI: Focus on solving problems, not technology. *VentureBeat*. Retrieved from https://venturebeat.com/2019/12/19/ada-health-cofounder-on-ai-focus-on-solving-problems-not-technology/

Pillo Inc. (2019). *PilloHealth - Bringing health home*. Retrieved 17 Mar, 2020, from https://pillohealth.com/

Robbins, R. (2019, Jan 17). *A 'digital pill' for cancer patients is rolled out for the first time, in hopes of improving outcomes*. Retrieved 17 Mar, 2020, from https://www.statnews.com/2019/01/17/a-digital-pill-for-cancer-patients-is-rolled-out-for-the-first-time-in-hopes-of-improving-outcomes/

Starfield, B. (2011). Is patient-centered care the same as person-focused care? *The Permanente Journal*, *15*(2), 63–69. doi:10.7812/TPP/10-148 PMID:21841928

The Economist. (2017). *Infographic: Realities or science fiction?* Retrieved 16 Mar, 2020, from https://thefutureishere.economist.com/healthcare/thefutureofheathcare-infographic.html

Wu, J. T., Leung, K., & Leung, G. M. (2020). Nowcasting and forecasting the potential domestic and international spread of the 2019-nCoV outbreak originating in Wuhan, China: A modelling study. *Lancet*, *395*(10225), 689–697. doi:10.1016/S0140-6736(20)30260-9 PMID:32014114

Yap, K. Y.-L. (2012). The evolving role of pharmacoinformatics in targeting drug-related problems in clinical oncology practice. In T. M. Gasmelseid (Ed.), *Pharmacoinformatics and Drug Discovery Technologies: Theories and Applications* (pp. 130–177). Hershey, PA: IGI Global. doi:10.4018/978-1-4666-0309-7.ch009

Related Readings

To continue IGI Global's long-standing tradition of advancing innovation through emerging research, please find below a compiled list of recommended IGI Global book chapters and journal articles in the areas of green cities, environmental management, and sustainable urban development. These related readings will provide additional information and guidance to further enrich your knowledge and assist you with your own research.

Aarnoutse, F., Renes, C., Batenburg, R., & Spruit, M. (2016). STRIPA: The Potential Usefulness of a Medical App. In T. Gasmelseid (Ed.), *Advancing Pharmaceutical Processes and Tools for Improved Health Outcomes* (pp. 114–135). Hershey, PA: IGI Global. doi:10.4018/978-1-5225-0248-7.ch005

Abu Seman, S. A., & Ramayah, T. (2017). Are We Ready to App?: A Study on mHealth Apps, Its Future, and Trends in Malaysia Context. In J. Pelet (Ed.), *Mobile Platforms, Design, and Apps for Social Commerce* (pp. 69–83). Hershey, PA: IGI Global. doi:10.4018/978-1-5225-2469-4.ch005

Adjin-Tettey, T. D. (2020). Healthcare Gets Smarter: Smart and Digital Technology Usage by Maternal and Neo-Natal Healthcare Providers. In S. Umair (Ed.), *Mobile Devices and Smart Gadgets in Medical Sciences* (pp. 39–55). Hershey, PA: IGI Global. doi:10.4018/978-1-7998-2521-0.ch003

Advinha, A. M., Nunes, C., Lopes, M. J., & Oliveira-Martins, S. (2020). Ability Assessment of the Elders to Manage Their Own Medication: A First Step for the Empowerment of the Geriatric Population. In C. Fonseca, M. Lopes, D. Mendes, F. Mendes, & J. García-Alonso (Eds.), *Handbook of Research on Health Systems and Organizations for an Aging Society* (pp. 128–151). Hershey, PA: IGI Global. doi:10.4018/978-1-5225-9818-3.ch010

Ahmad, M., Khan, M. A., Bibi, M., Ullah, Z., & Shah, S. T. (2020). Mobile Apps for Human Nutrition: A Review. In S. Umair (Ed.), *Mobile Devices and Smart Gadgets in Medical Sciences* (pp. 121–147). Hershey, PA: IGI Global. doi:10.4018/978-1-7998-2521-0.ch007

Al Mustafa, S. A., Khan, M., & Hussain, M. (2018). Implementing Barcode Medication Administration Systems in Public Sector Medical Units. *International Journal of Decision Support System Technology, 10*(2), 23–39. doi:10.4018/IJDSST.2018040102

Ali, N., Ullah, S., & Musa, Z. (2020). The Effect of List-Liner-Based Interaction Technique in a 3D Interactive Virtual Biological Learning Environment. In S. Umair (Ed.), *Mobile Devices and Smart Gadgets in Medical Sciences* (pp. 297–317). Hershey, PA: IGI Global. doi:10.4018/978-1-7998-2521-0.ch014

Alsalamah, S., Alsalamah, H., Gray, A. W., & Hilton, J. (2016). Information Security Threats in Patient-Centred Healthcare. In A. Moumtzoglou (Ed.), *M-Health Innovations for Patient-Centered Care* (pp. 298–318). Hershey, PA: IGI Global. doi:10.4018/978-1-4666-9861-1.ch015

Altinpulluk, H., & Kurubacak, G. (2016). MoBip Project: To Raise Awareness about Bipolar Disorder through an 3D Pop-Up Book. In A. Moumtzoglou (Ed.), *M-Health Innovations for Patient-Centered Care* (pp. 147–169). Hershey, PA: IGI Global. doi:10.4018/978-1-4666-9861-1.ch008

Anastasiou, A., Giokas, K., Koutsouri, G., & Iliopoulou, D. (2017). Intelligent Medication Adherence Monitoring System. In A. Moumtzoglou (Ed.), *Design, Development, and Integration of Reliable Electronic Healthcare Platforms* (pp. 72–85). Hershey, PA: IGI Global. doi:10.4018/978-1-5225-1724-5.ch004

Antunes, A. C., & Silva, C. (2020). Designing for Blind Users: Guidelines for Developing Mobile Apps for Supporting Navigation of Blind People on Public Transports. In T. Álvarez Robles, F. Álvarez Rodríguez, & E. Benítez-Guerrero (Eds.), *User-Centered Software Development for the Blind and Visually Impaired: Emerging Research and Opportunities* (pp. 1–25). Hershey, PA: IGI Global. doi:10.4018/978-1-5225-8539-8.ch001

Archondakis, S., Vavoulidis, E., Nasioutziki, M., Oustampasidou, O., Daniilidis, A., Vatopoulou, A., ... Dinas, K. (2019). Mobile Health Applications and Cloud Computing in Cytopathology: Benefits and Potential. In A. Moumtzoglou (Ed.), *Mobile Health Applications for Quality Healthcare Delivery* (pp. 165–202). Hershey, PA: IGI Global. doi:10.4018/978-1-5225-8021-8.ch008

Azaria, B., Kaye, R., Ron, R., Chen, O., Bar-Ilan, M., Zlatkin, A. S., ... Lahr, M. (2020). Use of a Mobile App by Older People in an Integrated Care Setting. In R. McHaney, I. Reychev, J. Azuri, M. McHaney, & R. Moshonov (Eds.), *Impacts of Information Technology on Patient Care and Empowerment* (pp. 291–321). Hershey, PA: IGI Global. doi:10.4018/978-1-7998-0047-7.ch015

Baihan, M. S., Sánchez, Y. K., Shao, X., Gilman, C., Demurjian, S. A., & Agresta, T. P. (2018). A Blueprint for Designing and Developing M-Health Applications for Diverse Stakeholders Utilizing FHIR. In R. Rajkumar (Ed.), *Contemporary Applications of Mobile Computing in Healthcare Settings* (pp. 85–124). Hershey, PA: IGI Global. doi:10.4018/978-1-5225-5036-5.ch006

Baker, A., Iqbal, F., Laila, M., & Waheed, A. (2020). Psychology With Mahnoor App: Android-Based Application for Self Assessment, Psychology Dictionary, and Notes. In S. Umair (Ed.), *Mobile Devices and Smart Gadgets in Medical Sciences* (pp. 214–231). Hershey, PA: IGI Global. doi:10.4018/978-1-7998-2521-0.ch010

Baker, A., Iqbal, F., & Rukh, L. (2020). UBERGP: Doctor Home Consultancy App. In S. Umair (Ed.), *Mobile Devices and Smart Gadgets in Medical Sciences* (pp. 253–269). Hershey, PA: IGI Global. doi:10.4018/978-1-7998-2521-0.ch012

Bangash, J. I., Khan, A. W., Sheraz, A., Khan, A., & Umair, S. (2020). QoS-Aware Data Dissemination Mechanisms for Wireless Body Area Networks. In S. Umair (Ed.), *Mobile Devices and Smart Gadgets in Medical Sciences* (pp. 74–96). Hershey, PA: IGI Global. doi:10.4018/978-1-7998-2521-0.ch005

Barigou, B. N., Barigou, F., Benchehida, C., Atmani, B., & Belalem, G. (2018). The Design of a Cloud-based Clinical Decision Support System Prototype: Management of Drugs Intoxications in Childhood. *International Journal of Healthcare Information Systems and Informatics*, *13*(4), 28–48. doi:10.4018/IJHISI.2018100103

Barroca, I., Aquino, G., & Lima, M. A. (2018). Promoting Better Healthcare for Patients in Critical Condition: An IoT-Based Solution to Integrate Patients, Physicians, and Ambulance Services. In J. Machado, A. Abelha, M. Santos, & F. Portela (Eds.), *Next-Generation Mobile and Pervasive Healthcare Solutions* (pp. 1–21). Hershey, PA: IGI Global. doi:10.4018/978-1-5225-2851-7.ch001

Barry, M., Doherty, K., & Doherty, G. (2020). Communicating "What's Not Said": Mobile Apps for Psychological Wellbeing. In I. Management Association (Ed.), Innovations in Global Maternal Health: Improving Prenatal and Postnatal Care Practices (pp. 355-368). Hershey, PA: IGI Global. doi:10.4018/978-1-7998-2351-3.ch015

Barua, R., Datta, S., Chowdhury, A. R., & Datta, P. (2018). Advances in MEMS and Micro-Scale Technologies for Application in Controlled Drug-Dosing Systems: MEMS-Based Drug Delivery Systems. In A. Bit (Ed.), *Design and Development of Affordable Healthcare Technologies* (pp. 165–179). Hershey, PA: IGI Global. doi:10.4018/978-1-5225-4969-7.ch007

Bellina, L., & Nucatola, I. (2017). Overcoming the Quality Gap and Ethics in M-Health: MobileDiagnosis-Innovation and Quality to All. *International Journal of Reliable and Quality E-Healthcare*, *6*(4), 17–26. doi:10.4018/IJRQEH.2017100103

Brunet, T., & Ramachandran, P. G. (2017). Accessible and Inclusive Content and Applications. In S. Mukherjea (Ed.), *Mobile Application Development, Usability, and Security* (pp. 54–67). Hershey, PA: IGI Global. doi:10.4018/978-1-5225-0945-5.ch003

Carvalho, I., & Almeida, F. (2020). Promoting Healthy Food Habits Through an mHealth Application. In S. Umair (Ed.), *Mobile Devices and Smart Gadgets in Medical Sciences* (pp. 1–21). Hershey, PA: IGI Global. doi:10.4018/978-1-7998-2521-0.ch001

Chakraborty, C. (2019). Mobile Health (M-Health) for Tele-Wound Monitoring: Role of M-Health in Wound Management. In A. Moumtzoglou (Ed.), *Mobile Health Applications for Quality Healthcare Delivery* (pp. 98–116). Hershey, PA: IGI Global. doi:10.4018/978-1-5225-8021-8.ch005

Chakraborty, C., Gupta, B., & Ghosh, S. K. (2016). Mobile Telemedicine Systems for Remote Patient's Chronic Wound Monitoring. In A. Moumtzoglou (Ed.), *M-Health Innovations for Patient-Centered Care* (pp. 213–239). Hershey, PA: IGI Global. doi:10.4018/978-1-4666-9861-1.ch011

Chan, L., & Liu, D. (2016). Policy Planning to Support Technological Innovation in the Pharmaceutical Industry. In T. Gasmelseid (Ed.), *Advancing Pharmaceutical Processes and Tools for Improved Health Outcomes* (pp. 1–23). Hershey, PA: IGI Global. doi:10.4018/978-1-5225-0248-7.ch001

Das, P. K., Ghosh, D., Jagtap, P., Joshi, A., & Finin, T. (2017). Preserving User Privacy and Security in Context-Aware Mobile Platforms. In S. Mukherjea (Ed.), *Mobile Application Development, Usability, and Security* (pp. 166–193). Hershey, PA: IGI Global. doi:10.4018/978-1-5225-0945-5.ch008

DeBenedetti, G., Kuru, K., Picton, P., Monico, L., & Shaw-Verbic, T. (2018). Virtual Community Engagement to Advance Interoperability in Digital Health. In C. El Morr (Ed.), *Novel Applications of Virtual Communities in Healthcare Settings* (pp. 148–170). Hershey, PA: IGI Global. doi:10.4018/978-1-5225-2958-3.ch006

Donmez, B., & Seneler, C. (2019). Locating Gender Differences in Mobile Use and Habits. In X. Xu (Ed.), *Impacts of Mobile Use and Experience on Contemporary Society* (pp. 37–52). Hershey, PA: IGI Global. doi:10.4018/978-1-5225-7885-7.ch003

Edoh, T. O. (2018). Towards Secure Off-Label Drug Prescribing and Improved Drug Supply. In *Advanced Systems for Improved Public Healthcare and Disease Prevention: Emerging Research and Opportunities* (pp. 101–134). Hershey, PA: IGI Global. doi:10.4018/978-1-5225-5528-5.ch003

Ekambaram, V., Sharma, V., & Rajput, N. (2017). Mobile Application Testing. In S. Mukherjea (Ed.), *Mobile Application Development, Usability, and Security* (pp. 25–53). Hershey, PA: IGI Global. doi:10.4018/978-1-5225-0945-5.ch002

Eken, I., & Gezmen, B. (2020). Accessibility for Everyone in Health Communication Mobile Application Usage. In Y. Demir Uslu, H. Dinçer, & S. Yüksel (Eds.), *Multidimensional Perspectives and Global Analysis of Universal Health Coverage* (pp. 152–181). Hershey, PA: IGI Global. doi:10.4018/978-1-7998-2329-2.ch006

Ekkirala, C. (2016). Application of Metadata Repository and Master Data Management in Clinical Trial and Drug Safety. In P. Chakraborty & A. Nagal (Eds.), *Software Innovations in Clinical Drug Development and Safety* (pp. 33–46). Hershey, PA: IGI Global. doi:10.4018/978-1-4666-8726-4.ch003

El Halabieh, R., Beaudry, A., & Tamblyn, R. (2018). From E-Prescribing to Drug Management System: Impacts of Stress on Usage Continuance. *International Journal of Healthcare Information Systems and Informatics*, *13*(1), 55–70. doi:10.4018/IJHISI.2018010105

El Morr, C. (2019). Virtual Communities, Machine Learning and IoT: Opportunities and Challenges in Mental Health Research. *International Journal of Extreme Automation and Connectivity in Healthcare, 1*(1), 4–11. doi:10.4018/IJEACH.2019010102

Elahi, B., Kanwal, M., & Elahi, S. (2020). Analysis of Different Image Processing Techniques for Classification and Detection of Cancer Cells. In S. Umair (Ed.), *Mobile Devices and Smart Gadgets in Medical Sciences* (pp. 148–172). Hershey, PA: IGI Global. doi:10.4018/978-1-7998-2521-0.ch008

Etim, A., Etim, D. N., & Scott, J. (2020). Mobile Health and Telemedicine: Awareness, Adoption and Importance of Health Study. *International Journal of Healthcare Information Systems and Informatics, 15*(1), 81–96. doi:10.4018/IJHISI.2020010105

Fishelson, R. I. (2019). Time for a Change: Designing a Mobile Application to Assist People With Intellectual Disabilities. In A. Forkosh Baruch & H. Meishar Tal (Eds.), *Mobile Technologies in Educational Organizations* (pp. 211–232). Hershey, PA: IGI Global. doi:10.4018/978-1-5225-8106-2.ch011

Folami, F. F. (2020). The Influence of Mobile Health Adoption on Medication Adherence on Population Health: Mobile Health Adoption on Medication Adherence. In B. Adeoye & G. Arome (Eds.), *The Roles of Technology and Globalization in Educational Transformation* (pp. 166–175). Hershey, PA: IGI Global. doi:10.4018/978-1-5225-9746-9.ch013

Gasmelseid, T. M. (2016). Improving Pharmaceutical Care through the Use of Intelligent Pharmacoinformatics. In T. Gasmelseid (Ed.), *Advancing Pharmaceutical Processes and Tools for Improved Health Outcomes* (pp. 167–188). Hershey, PA: IGI Global. doi:10.4018/978-1-5225-0248-7.ch007

Giokas, K., Costarides, V., & Koutsouris, D. (2016). Integrated Platform for the Lifestyle Change and Holistic Approach to Personalized Prevention and Self-Management of Patients with High Blood Pressure. In A. Moumtzoglou (Ed.), *M-Health Innovations for Patient-Centered Care* (pp. 72–90). Hershey, PA: IGI Global. doi:10.4018/978-1-4666-9861-1.ch004

Giokas, K., Katrakazas, P., & Koutsouris, D. (2016). A Collaborative m-Health Platform for Evidence-Based Self-Management and Detection of Chronic Multimorbidity Development and Progression. In A. Moumtzoglou (Ed.), *M-Health Innovations for Patient-Centered Care* (pp. 52–71). Hershey, PA: IGI Global. doi:10.4018/978-1-4666-9861-1.ch003

Govinda, K. (2018). Body Fitness Monitoring Using IoT Device. In R. Rajkumar (Ed.), *Contemporary Applications of Mobile Computing in Healthcare Settings* (pp. 154–169). Hershey, PA: IGI Global. doi:10.4018/978-1-5225-5036-5.ch009

Govinda, K. (2018). Clinical Data Analysis Using IoT Devices. In R. Rajkumar (Ed.), *Contemporary Applications of Mobile Computing in Healthcare Settings* (pp. 136–153). Hershey, PA: IGI Global. doi:10.4018/978-1-5225-5036-5.ch008

Govinda, K. (2018). Geo-Location-Based File Security System for Healthcare Data. In R. Rajkumar (Ed.), *Contemporary Applications of Mobile Computing in Healthcare Settings* (pp. 125–135). Hershey, PA: IGI Global. doi:10.4018/978-1-5225-5036-5.ch007

Govinda, K. (2018). IoT in the Field of Healthcare. In R. Rajkumar (Ed.), *Contemporary Applications of Mobile Computing in Healthcare Settings* (pp. 1–20). Hershey, PA: IGI Global. doi:10.4018/978-1-5225-5036-5.ch001

Govinda, K., & Ramasubbareddy, S. (2018). Smart Healthcare Administration Over Cloud. In R. Rajkumar (Ed.), *Contemporary Applications of Mobile Computing in Healthcare Settings* (pp. 34–50). Hershey, PA: IGI Global. doi:10.4018/978-1-5225-5036-5.ch003

Guarda, T., Augusto, M. F., Barrionuevo, O., & Pinto, F. M. (2018). Internet of Things in Pervasive Healthcare Systems. In J. Machado, A. Abelha, M. Santos, & F. Portela (Eds.), *Next-Generation Mobile and Pervasive Healthcare Solutions* (pp. 22–31). Hershey, PA: IGI Global. doi:10.4018/978-1-5225-2851-7.ch002

Gunasundari, E. (2019). Best Practices in the Pharmaceutical Supply Chain Management. In H. Nozari & A. Szmelter (Eds.), *Global Supply Chains in the Pharmaceutical Industry* (pp. 228–247). Hershey, PA: IGI Global. doi:10.4018/978-1-5225-5921-4.ch010

Gupta, S., Goel, L., & Agarwal, A. K. (2020). Technologies in Health Care Domain: A Systematic Review. *International Journal of e-Collaboration*, *16*(1), 33–44. doi:10.4018/IJeC.2020010103

Hoque, M. R., Al Bar, A. M., & Alam, M. J. (2018). Determinant Factors of Physicians' Acceptance of E-Health an Empirical Study: Physicians' Acceptance of E-Health. In J. Tan (Ed.), *Handbook of Research on Emerging Perspectives on Healthcare Information Systems and Informatics* (pp. 467–482). Hershey, PA: IGI Global. doi:10.4018/978-1-5225-5460-8.ch020

Iltchev, P., Śliwczyński, A., Szynkiewicz, P., & Marczak, M. (2016). Mobile Health Applications Assisting Patients with Chronic Diseases: Examples from Asthma Care. In A. Moumtzoglou (Ed.), *M-Health Innovations for Patient-Centered Care* (pp. 170–196). Hershey, PA: IGI Global. doi:10.4018/978-1-4666-9861-1.ch009

Iyawa, G. E., Langan-Martin, J., Sevalie, S., & Masikara, W. (2020). mHealth as Tools for Development in Mental Health. In R. McHaney, I. Reychev, J. Azuri, M. McHaney, & R. Moshonov (Eds.), Impacts of Information Technology on Patient Care and Empowerment (pp. 58-80). Hershey, PA: IGI Global. doi:10.4018/978-1-7998-0047-7.ch004

Iyawa, G. E., Ondiek, C. O., & Osakwe, J. O. (2020). mHealth: A Low-Cost Approach for Effective Disease Diagnosis, Prediction, Monitoring and Management – Effective Disease Diagnosis. In C. Chakraborty (Ed.), Smart Medical Data Sensing and IoT Systems Design in Healthcare (pp. 1-21). Hershey, PA: IGI Global. doi:10.4018/978-1-7998-0261-7.ch001

Kameswara Rao, M., & Santhi, S. G. (2020). Internet of Things-Based Authentication Mechanism for E-Health Applications. In P. Pankajavalli & G. Karthick (Eds.), *Incorporating the Internet of Things in Healthcare Applications and Wearable Devices* (pp. 122–136). Hershey, PA: IGI Global. doi:10.4018/978-1-7998-1090-2.ch007

Kasemsap, K. (2018). Mobile Health Systems and Electronic Health Record: Applications and Implications. In J. Machado, A. Abelha, M. Santos, & F. Portela (Eds.), *Next-Generation Mobile and Pervasive Healthcare Solutions* (pp. 67–85). Hershey, PA: IGI Global. doi:10.4018/978-1-5225-2851-7.ch005

Khan, R., Ullah, M., Shafi, B., Orakzai, U. B., & Shafi, S. (2020). Knocking at Alternate Doors: Survey of Android-Based Smartphone Applications for Alternate Medicines. In S. Umair (Ed.), *Mobile Devices and Smart Gadgets in Medical Sciences* (pp. 22–38). Hershey, PA: IGI Global. doi:10.4018/978-1-7998-2521-0.ch002

Khan, S., Khan, A., Ullah, R., Ali, M., & Ullah, R. (2020). Insulin DNA Sequence Classification Using Levy Flight Bat With Back Propagation Algorithm. In S. Umair (Ed.), *Mobile Devices and Smart Gadgets in Medical Sciences* (pp. 232–252). Hershey, PA: IGI Global. doi:10.4018/978-1-7998-2521-0.ch011

King, H., & Slattery, D. M. (2020). Using Technology to Empower People With Multiple Sclerosis (MS) to Make Shared Decisions About Managing Their Own Healthcare: A UK Case Study. In R. McHaney, I. Reychev, J. Azuri, M. McHaney, & R. Moshonov (Eds.), *Impacts of Information Technology on Patient Care and Empowerment* (pp. 177–198). Hershey, PA: IGI Global. doi:10.4018/978-1-7998-0047-7.ch010

Kirschner, A., Kirschner, S., Seebauer, C., & Bethke, B. (2017). The Potential of Mobile Health in Nursing: The Use of Mobile Communication Technology in Plasma-Supported Outpatient Wound Care in Germany. *International Journal of Reliable and Quality E-Healthcare*, *6*(4), 49–58. doi:10.4018/IJRQEH.2017100106

Koumpouros, Y. (2017). Counterobe: A Mobile and Web Platform for Weight Management Incorporating Unique Behavioral-Strategy Features. *International Journal of Reliable and Quality E-Healthcare*, *6*(4), 59–70. doi:10.4018/IJRQEH.2017100107

Koumpouros, Y., & Georgoulas, A. (2016). mHealth R&D Activities in Europe. In A. Moumtzoglou (Ed.), M-Health Innovations for Patient-Centered Care (pp. 20-51). Hershey, PA: IGI Global. doi:10.4018/978-1-4666-9861-1.ch002

Koumpouros, Y., & Georgoulas, A. (2019). The Rise of mHealth Research in Europe: A Macroscopic Analysis of EC-Funded Projects of the Last Decade. In A. Moumtzoglou (Ed.), *Mobile Health Applications for Quality Healthcare Delivery* (pp. 1–29). Hershey, PA: IGI Global. doi:10.4018/978-1-5225-8021-8.ch001

Kouroubali, A., Koumakis, L., Kondylakis, H., & Katehakis, D. G. (2019). An Integrated Approach Towards Developing Quality Mobile Health Apps for Cancer. In A. Moumtzoglou (Ed.), *Mobile Health Applications for Quality Healthcare Delivery* (pp. 46–71). Hershey, PA: IGI Global. doi:10.4018/978-1-5225-8021-8.ch003

Lobo, J., Ferreira, L., & Ferreira, A. J. (2017). CARMIE: A Conversational Medication Assistant for Heart Failure. *International Journal of E-Health and Medical Communications*, *8*(4), 21–37. doi:10.4018/IJEHMC.2017100102

Malik, J. A. (2020). Effects of Electromagnetic Radiation of Mobile Phones on the Human Brain. In S. Umair (Ed.), *Mobile Devices and Smart Gadgets in Medical Sciences* (pp. 97–120). Hershey, PA: IGI Global. doi:10.4018/978-1-7998-2521-0.ch006

Mande, D. M., & Wigand, R. T. (2016). Information Quality Issues in the Identification and Tracking of Drugs within the Pharmaceutical Industry. In T. Gasmelseid (Ed.), *Advancing Pharmaceutical Processes and Tools for Improved Health Outcomes* (pp. 79–113). Hershey, PA: IGI Global. doi:10.4018/978-1-5225-0248-7.ch004

Mangu, V. P. (2017). Mobile Health Care: A Technology View. In C. Bhatt & S. Peddoju (Eds.), *Cloud Computing Systems and Applications in Healthcare* (pp. 1–18). Hershey, PA: IGI Global. doi:10.4018/978-1-5225-1002-4.ch001

Maniar, N., Donohoe, C., & Troudt, E. L. (2019). The Use of Mobile ECG Monitoring Devices in Embolic Stroke Associated With Atrial Fibrillation. In E. Demiroz & S. Waldman (Eds.), *Optimizing Medical Education With Instructional Technology* (pp. 58–70). Hershey, PA: IGI Global. doi:10.4018/978-1-5225-6289-4.ch004

Manoj, A. S., Hussain, M. A., & Teja, P. S. (2019). Patient Health Monitoring Using IoT. In A. Moumtzoglou (Ed.), *Mobile Health Applications for Quality Healthcare Delivery* (pp. 30–45). Hershey, PA: IGI Global. doi:10.4018/978-1-5225-8021-8.ch002

Mariappan, G., & Kumari, A. (2019). Virtual Screening and Its Applications in Drug Discovery Process. In A. Puratchikody, S. Prabu, & A. Umamaheswari (Eds.), *Computer Applications in Drug Discovery and Development* (pp. 101–126). Hershey, PA: IGI Global. doi:10.4018/978-1-5225-7326-5.ch005

Martins, B., Guimarães, T. A., Santos, M., Frutuoso, S., Portela, F., & Santos, M. F. (2018). Pervasive Computing in Supporting Pediatric and Neonatology Care Unit Decision Process. In J. Machado, A. Abelha, M. Santos, & F. Portela (Eds.), *Next-Generation Mobile and Pervasive Healthcare Solutions* (pp. 86–95). Hershey, PA: IGI Global. doi:10.4018/978-1-5225-2851-7.ch006

Metelmann, B., & Metelmann, C. (2016). M-Health in Prehospital Emergency Medicine: Experiences from the EU funded Project LiveCity. In A. Moumtzoglou (Ed.), *M-Health Innovations for Patient-Centered Care* (pp. 197–212). Hershey, PA: IGI Global. doi:10.4018/978-1-4666-9861-1.ch010

Metelmann, B., & Metelmann, C. (2019). Mobile Health Applications in Prehospital Emergency Medicine. In A. Moumtzoglou (Ed.), *Mobile Health Applications for Quality Healthcare Delivery* (pp. 117–135). Hershey, PA: IGI Global. doi:10.4018/978-1-5225-8021-8.ch006

Metelmann, C., & Metelmann, B. (2017). Can a Mobile Video Communication Improve Patient Safety in Prehospital Emergency Medicine? *International Journal of Reliable and Quality E-Healthcare*, *6*(4), 27–36. doi:10.4018/IJRQEH.2017100104

Moumtzoglou, A. S. (2016). Tailored M-Health Communication in Patient-Centered Care. In A. Moumtzoglou (Ed.), *M-Health Innovations for Patient-Centered Care* (pp. 319–340). Hershey, PA: IGI Global. doi:10.4018/978-1-4666-9861-1.ch016

Moumtzoglou, A. S. (2016). The Nexus of M-Health and Self-Efficacy. In A. Moumtzoglou (Ed.), *M-Health Innovations for Patient-Centered Care* (pp. 341–365). Hershey, PA: IGI Global. doi:10.4018/978-1-4666-9861-1.ch017

Moumtzoglou, A. S. (2019). The Nexus of M-Health and Self-Care. In A. Moumtzoglou (Ed.), *Mobile Health Applications for Quality Healthcare Delivery* (pp. 235–259). Hershey, PA: IGI Global. doi:10.4018/978-1-5225-8021-8.ch011

Moumtzoglou, A. S. (2019). The Science of Individuality and Tailored M-Health Communication. In A. Moumtzoglou (Ed.), *Mobile Health Applications for Quality Healthcare Delivery* (pp. 213–234). Hershey, PA: IGI Global. doi:10.4018/978-1-5225-8021-8.ch010

Muhammad, S., Safaei, H., & Muhammad, T. (2019). Pharmacy Technology to Better Public Health: An Exploration of New Models of Supply and Use of Technology – A Regional United Kingdom Quantitative Study. *International Journal of Applied Research on Public Health Management*, *4*(1), 1–20. doi:10.4018/IJARPHM.2019010101

Narayana Moorthi, M., & Manjula, R. (2018). A Survey of Mobile Computing Devices and Sensors in Healthcare Applications: Real-Time System Design. In R. Rajkumar (Ed.), *Contemporary Applications of Mobile Computing in Healthcare Settings* (pp. 51–57). Hershey, PA: IGI Global. doi:10.4018/978-1-5225-5036-5.ch004

Nizamuddin, I., Basra, R., Vanam, S., & Pirani, N. (2019). Apps and Their Applications: Novel Uses of Technology in the Clinical Setting. In E. Demiroz & S. Waldman (Eds.), *Optimizing Medical Education With Instructional Technology* (pp. 156–176). Hershey, PA: IGI Global. doi:10.4018/978-1-5225-6289-4.ch009

Paglialonga, A., Pinciroli, F., & Tognola, G. (2019). Apps for Hearing Healthcare: Trends, Challenges, and Potential Opportunities. In E. Saunders (Ed.), *Tele-Audiology and the Optimization of Hearing Healthcare Delivery* (pp. 161–195). Hershey, PA: IGI Global. doi:10.4018/978-1-5225-8191-8.ch007

Pistoia, M., Tripp, O., & Lubensky, D. (2017). Combining Static Code Analysis and Machine Learning for Automatic Detection of Security Vulnerabilities in Mobile Apps. In S. Mukherjea (Ed.), *Mobile Application Development, Usability, and Security* (pp. 68–94). Hershey, PA: IGI Global. doi:10.4018/978-1-5225-0945-5.ch004

Ponnusamy, S. K., & Christopher, F. C. (2019). Production Process in the Pharmaceutical Industry. In H. Nozari & A. Szmelter (Eds.), *Global Supply Chains in the Pharmaceutical Industry* (pp. 158–179). Hershey, PA: IGI Global. doi:10.4018/978-1-5225-5921-4.ch007

Ponnusamy, S. K., & Ragini, Y. P. (2019). Product Lifecycle in the Pharmaceutical Industry. In H. Nozari & A. Szmelter (Eds.), *Global Supply Chains in the Pharmaceutical Industry* (pp. 112–132). Hershey, PA: IGI Global. doi:10.4018/978-1-5225-5921-4.ch005

Ponnusamy, S. K., & Saravanan, A. (2019). Characteristics of Pharmaceutical Supply Chains. In H. Nozari & A. Szmelter (Eds.), *Global Supply Chains in the Pharmaceutical Industry* (pp. 181–205). Hershey, PA: IGI Global. doi:10.4018/978-1-5225-5921-4.ch008

Portela, F., Moreira da Veiga, A., & Santos, M. F. (2018). Benefits of Bring Your Own Device in Healthcare. In J. Machado, A. Abelha, M. Santos, & F. Portela (Eds.), *Next-Generation Mobile and Pervasive Healthcare Solutions* (pp. 32–45). Hershey, PA: IGI Global. doi:10.4018/978-1-5225-2851-7.ch003

Pouliakis, A. (2019). Third Age and Mobile Health. *International Journal of Reliable and Quality E-Healthcare*, *8*(4), 67–79. doi:10.4018/IJRQEH.2019100104

Pouliakis, A., Archondakis, S., Margari, N., & Karakitsos, P. (2016). From Telecytology to Mobile Cytopathology: Past, Present, and Future. In A. Moumtzoglou (Ed.), *M-Health Innovations for Patient-Centered Care* (pp. 240–261). Hershey, PA: IGI Global. doi:10.4018/978-1-4666-9861-1.ch012

Pouliakis, A., Karakitsou, E., & Margari, N. (2019). Cytopathology and the Smartphone: An Update. In A. Moumtzoglou (Ed.), *Mobile Health Applications for Quality Healthcare Delivery* (pp. 136–164). Hershey, PA: IGI Global. doi:10.4018/978-1-5225-8021-8.ch007

Ragini, Y. P. (2019). Pharmaceutical Development Process. In H. Nozari & A. Szmelter (Eds.), *Global Supply Chains in the Pharmaceutical Industry* (pp. 133–157). Hershey, PA: IGI Global. doi:10.4018/978-1-5225-5921-4.ch006

Rajasekaran, R., Govinda, K., Masih, J., & Sruthi, M. (2020). Health Monitoring System for Individuals Using Internet of Things. In P. Pankajavalli & G. Karthick (Eds.), *Incorporating the Internet of Things in Healthcare Applications and Wearable Devices* (pp. 150–164). Hershey, PA: IGI Global. doi:10.4018/978-1-7998-1090-2.ch009

Rajkumar, R. (2018). Smart Healthcare. In R. Rajkumar (Ed.), *Contemporary Applications of Mobile Computing in Healthcare Settings* (pp. 21–33). Hershey, PA: IGI Global. doi:10.4018/978-1-5225-5036-5.ch002

Ramakrishna, V., & Dey, K. (2017). Mobile Application and User Analytics. In S. Mukherjea (Ed.), *Mobile Application Development, Usability, and Security* (pp. 231–259). Hershey, PA: IGI Global. doi:10.4018/978-1-5225-0945-5.ch011

Rana, A. (2017). The Immense Potential of M-Care in India: Catering Better to Patients Needs in the Context of a Fragmented Healthcare System. *International Journal of Reliable and Quality E-Healthcare*, *6*(4), 1–3. doi:10.4018/IJRQEH.2017100101

Rastogi, R., Chaturvedi, D. K., Gupta, M., Sirohi, H., Gulati, M., & Pratyusha. (2020). Analytical Observations Between Subjects' Medications Movement and Medication Scores Correlation Based on Their Gender and Age Using GSR Biofeedback: Intelligent Application in Healthcare. In D. Burgos, M. Vejar, & F. Pozo (Eds.), *Pattern Recognition Applications in Engineering* (pp. 229-257). Hershey, PA: IGI Global. doi:10.4018/978-1-7998-1839-7.ch010

Rokni, S. A., Ghasemzadeh, H., & Hezarjaribi, N. (2017). Smart Medication Management, Current Technologies, and Future Directions. In N. Wickramasinghe (Ed.), *Handbook of Research on Healthcare Administration and Management* (pp. 188–204). Hershey, PA: IGI Global. doi:10.4018/978-1-5225-0920-2.ch012

Roman, M., Khan, S., Khan, A., & Ali, M. (2020). Optimizing Learning Weights of Back Propagation Using Flower Pollination Algorithm for Diabetes and Thyroid Data Classification. In S. Umair (Ed.), *Mobile Devices and Smart Gadgets in Medical Sciences* (pp. 270–296). Hershey, PA: IGI Global. doi:10.4018/978-1-7998-2521-0.ch013

Sagahyroon, A. (2016). mHealth: Sleeping Disorders Diagnosis. In A. Moumtzoglou (Ed.), M-Health Innovations for Patient-Centered Care (pp. 115-125). Hershey, PA: IGI Global. doi:10.4018/978-1-4666-9861-1.ch006

Sam, S. (2017). Mobile Phones and Expanding Human Capabilities in Plural Health Systems. In K. Moahi, K. Bwalya, & P. Sebina (Eds.), *Health Information Systems and the Advancement of Medical Practice in Developing Countries* (pp. 93–114). Hershey, PA: IGI Global. doi:10.4018/978-1-5225-2262-1.ch006

Sánchez, Y. K., Demurjian, S. A., Conover, J., Agresta, T. P., Shao, X., & Diamond, M. (2017). Role-Based Access Control for Mobile Computing and Applications. In S. Mukherjea (Ed.), *Mobile Application Development, Usability, and Security* (pp. 117–141). Hershey, PA: IGI Global. doi:10.4018/978-1-5225-0945-5.ch006

Sanzi, E., Demurjian, S. A., Agresta, T. P., & Murphy, A. (2017). Trust Profiling to Enable Adaptive Trust Negotiation in Mobile Devices. In S. Mukherjea (Ed.), *Mobile Application Development, Usability, and Security* (pp. 95–116). Hershey, PA: IGI Global. doi:10.4018/978-1-5225-0945-5.ch005

Seale, D. E., LeRouge, C. M., Ohs, J. E., Tao, D., Lach, H. W., Jupka, K., & Wray, R. (2019). Exploring Early Adopter Baby Boomers' Approach to Managing Their Health and Healthcare. *International Journal of E-Health and Medical Communications, 10*(1), 94–117. doi:10.4018/IJEHMC.2019010106

Shao, X., Demurjian, S. A., & Agresta, T. P. (2017). A Spatio-Situation-Based Access Control Model for Dynamic Permission on Mobile Applications. In S. Mukherjea (Ed.), *Mobile Application Development, Usability, and Security* (pp. 142–165). Hershey, PA: IGI Global. doi:10.4018/978-1-5225-0945-5.ch007

Shipley, N., & Chakraborty, J. (2018). Big Data and mHealth: Increasing the Usability of Healthcare Through the Customization of Pinterest – Literary Perspective. In J. Machado, A. Abelha, M. Santos, & F. Portela (Eds.), *Next-Generation Mobile and Pervasive Healthcare Solutions* (pp. 46–66). Hershey, PA: IGI Global. doi:10.4018/978-1-5225-2851-7.ch004

Simons, L., van den Heuvel, W. A., & Jonker, C. M. (2020). WhatsApp Peer Coaching Lessons for eHealth. In N. Wickramasinghe (Ed.), *Handbook of Research on Optimizing Healthcare Management Techniques* (pp. 16–32). Hershey, PA: IGI Global. doi:10.4018/978-1-7998-1371-2.ch002

Singh, P. (2017). Mobile + Cloud: Opportunities and Challenges. In S. Mukherjea (Ed.), *Mobile Application Development, Usability, and Security* (pp. 260–279). Hershey, PA: IGI Global. doi:10.4018/978-1-5225-0945-5.ch012

Sood, V. R., Gururajan, R., Hafeez-Baig, A., & Wickramasinghe, N. (2017). Adoption of Mobile Devices in the Australian Healthcare: A Conceptual Framework Approach. In N. Wickramasinghe (Ed.), *Handbook of Research on Healthcare Administration and Management* (pp. 662–685). Hershey, PA: IGI Global. doi:10.4018/978-1-5225-0920-2.ch040

Srinivasan, S. (2016). Overview of Clinical Trial and Pharmacovigilance Process and Areas of Application of Computer System. In P. Chakraborty & A. Nagal (Eds.), *Software Innovations in Clinical Drug Development and Safety* (pp. 1–13). Hershey, PA: IGI Global. doi:10.4018/978-1-4666-8726-4.ch001

Sruthi, M., & Rajasekaran, R. (2018). Reading Assistance for Visually Impaired People Using TTL Serial Camera With Voice. In R. Rajkumar (Ed.), *Contemporary Applications of Mobile Computing in Healthcare Settings* (pp. 170–180). Hershey, PA: IGI Global. doi:10.4018/978-1-5225-5036-5.ch010

Stavros, A., Vavoulidis, E., & Nasioutziki, M. (2016). The Use of Mobile Health Applications for Quality Control and Accreditational Purposes in a Cytopathology Laboratory. In A. Moumtzoglou (Ed.), *M-Health Innovations for Patient-Centered Care* (pp. 262–283). Hershey, PA: IGI Global. doi:10.4018/978-1-4666-9861-1.ch013

Suganya, S. (2019). Global Macrotrends in Pharmaceutical Industry. In H. Nozari & A. Szmelter (Eds.), *Global Supply Chains in the Pharmaceutical Industry* (pp. 86–110). Hershey, PA: IGI Global. doi:10.4018/978-1-5225-5921-4.ch004

Sultana, H. P., & Nagendran, N. (2018). Mobile Patient Surveillance. In R. Rajkumar (Ed.), *Contemporary Applications of Mobile Computing in Healthcare Settings* (pp. 58–84). Hershey, PA: IGI Global. doi:10.4018/978-1-5225-5036-5.ch005

Szmelter, A. (2019). Global Pharmaceutical Industry: Characteristics and Trends. In H. Nozari & A. Szmelter (Eds.), *Global Supply Chains in the Pharmaceutical Industry* (pp. 57–85). Hershey, PA: IGI Global. doi:10.4018/978-1-5225-5921-4.ch003

Tamposis, I., Pouliakis, A., Fezoulidis, I., & Karakitsos, P. (2016). Mobile Platforms Supporting Health Professionals: Need, Technical Requirements, and Applications. In A. Moumtzoglou (Ed.), *M-Health Innovations for Patient-Centered Care* (pp. 91–114). Hershey, PA: IGI Global. doi:10.4018/978-1-4666-9861-1.ch005

Trocin, C., & Croda, E. (2020). Empowering Patients Through Digital Technologies: The Case of Mobile Health Applications. In R. McHaney, I. Reychev, J. Azuri, M. McHaney, & R. Moshonov (Eds.), *Impacts of Information Technology on Patient Care and Empowerment* (pp. 34–57). Hershey, PA: IGI Global. doi:10.4018/978-1-7998-0047-7.ch003

Ullah, R., Khan, A., Shah Abid, S. B., Khan, S., Shah, S. K., & Ali, M. (2020). Crow-ENN: An Optimized Elman Neural Network with Crow Search Algorithm for Leukemia DNA Sequence Classification. In S. Umair (Ed.), *Mobile Devices and Smart Gadgets in Medical Sciences* (pp. 173–213). Hershey, PA: IGI Global. doi:10.4018/978-1-7998-2521-0.ch009

Usher, W. (2017). E-Health: Modern Communication Technology Platforms for Accessing Health Information. In A. Moumtzoglou (Ed.), *Design, Development, and Integration of Reliable Electronic Healthcare Platforms* (pp. 49–71). Hershey, PA: IGI Global. doi:10.4018/978-1-5225-1724-5.ch003

Ustun, A. B., Yilmaz, R., & Yilmaz, F. G. (2020). Virtual Reality in Medical Education. In S. Umair (Ed.), *Mobile Devices and Smart Gadgets in Medical Sciences* (pp. 56–73). Hershey, PA: IGI Global. doi:10.4018/978-1-7998-2521-0.ch004

Venugopal, M. (2019). Evolution of Digital Technologies and Use of Virtual Assistants in Drug Development. In N. Bouchemal (Ed.), *Intelligent Systems for Healthcare Management and Delivery* (pp. 1–20). Hershey, PA: IGI Global. doi:10.4018/978-1-5225-7071-4.ch001

Vijay, K., Arti, S., & Suresh, K. (2018). Kernel-Based Machine Learning Techniques: An Innovative Way of Designing Healthcare Systems and Services. In B. Mishra & R. Kumar (Eds.), *Big Data Management and the Internet of Things for Improved Health Systems* (pp. 260–283). Hershey, PA: IGI Global. doi:10.4018/978-1-5225-5222-2.ch015

Vlachopapadopoulou, E., & Fotiadis, D. I. (2016). The Contribution of mHealth in the Care of Obese Pediatric Patients. In A. Moumtzoglou (Ed.), *M-Health Innovations for Patient-Centered Care* (pp. 126–146). Hershey, PA: IGI Global. doi:10.4018/978-1-4666-9861-1.ch007

Vlachopapadopoulou, E., Georga, E. I., & Fotiadis, D. I. (2019). Management of Obese Pediatric Patients in the Digital Era. In A. Moumtzoglou (Ed.), *Mobile Health Applications for Quality Healthcare Delivery* (pp. 72–97). Hershey, PA: IGI Global. doi:10.4018/978-1-5225-8021-8.ch004

Vuković, M., Car, Ž., Pavlisa, J. I., & Mandić, L. (2018). Smartwatch as an Assistive Technology: Tracking System for Detecting Irregular User Movement. *International Journal of E-Health and Medical Communications*, *9*(1), 23–34. doi:10.4018/IJEHMC.2018010102

Waegemann, C. P. (2016). mHealth: History, Analysis, and Implementation. In A. Moumtzoglou (Ed.), M-Health Innovations for Patient-Centered Care (pp. 1-19). Hershey, PA: IGI Global. doi:10.4018/978-1-4666-9861-1.ch001

Wang, Y. K., Gu, J. J., Sun, Y., Jiang, F., Hua, H., Li, J., ... Ding, G. (2020). The Design and Evaluation of an Intelligent Pain Management System (IPMS) in Cancer Patient Care. In R. McHaney, I. Reychev, J. Azuri, M. McHaney, & R. Moshonov (Eds.), *Impacts of Information Technology on Patient Care and Empowerment* (pp. 199–218). Hershey, PA: IGI Global. doi:10.4018/978-1-7998-0047-7.ch011

Weinrib, A., Azam, M. A., Latman, V. V., Janmohamed, T., Clarke, H., & Katz, J. (2018). Manage My Pain: A Patient-Driven Mobile Platform to Prevent and Manage Chronic Postsurgical Pain. In C. El Morr (Ed.), *Novel Applications of Virtual Communities in Healthcare Settings* (pp. 93–126). Hershey, PA: IGI Global. doi:10.4018/978-1-5225-2958-3.ch004

Wickramasinghe, N. (2020). Mobile Health: Precision Post-Operative Wellness Monitoring Solutions. In N. Wickramasinghe (Ed.), *Handbook of Research on Optimizing Healthcare Management Techniques* (pp. 338–349). Hershey, PA: IGI Global. doi:10.4018/978-1-7998-1371-2.ch025

Wilson, M., & Shaw, M. R. (2017). Participant Perspectives on Benefits and Challenges of Engaging in an Online Pain Self-Management Program. *International Journal of Healthcare Information Systems and Informatics, 12*(4), 52–67. doi:10.4018/IJHISI.2017100104

Witzke, K., & Specht, O. (2017). M-Health Telemedicine and Telepresence in Oral and Maxillofacial Surgery: An Innovative Prehospital Healthcare Concept in Structurally Weak Areas. *International Journal of Reliable and Quality E-Healthcare, 6*(4), 37–48. doi:10.4018/IJRQEH.2017100105

Zangão, M. O. (2020). Self-Perceived Health Status. In C. Fonseca, M. Lopes, D. Mendes, F. Mendes, & J. García-Alonso (Eds.), *Handbook of Research on Health Systems and Organizations for an Aging Society* (pp. 1–11). Hershey, PA: IGI Global. doi:10.4018/978-1-5225-9818-3.ch001

Zimeras, S. (2016). Computer Virus Models and Analysis in M-Health IT Systems: Computer Virus Models. In A. Moumtzoglou (Ed.), *M-Health Innovations for Patient-Centered Care* (pp. 284–297). Hershey, PA: IGI Global. doi:10.4018/978-1-4666-9861-1.ch014

Zimeras, S. (2019). Mathematical Models for Computer Virus: Computer Virus Epidemiology. In A. Moumtzoglou (Ed.), *Mobile Health Applications for Quality Healthcare Delivery* (pp. 203–212). Hershey, PA: IGI Global. doi:10.4018/978-1-5225-8021-8.ch009

About the Authors

Kevin Yap is an inter-disciplinary cyber-pharmacist and a digital health researcher at the Department of Public Health, La Trobe University, Australia. He has knowledge in digital media creation, web databases, data mining and analytics. His interests span the whole digital healthcare innovation cycle through the development, utilization, application and/or evaluation of informatics, internet, digital and other health-related technologies in various healthcare settings to enhance medication management in patients, as well as the flow of drug-related information and knowledge to healthcare professionals and patients (e.g. drug databases, mobile apps, telemedicine, social media, virtual platforms, serious games). He is the coordinator of the postgraduate Digital Health Course Suite at his university. He has over 90 publications in peer-reviewed journals, two book chapters, and presented at more than 70 local and international conferences. His work has also been featured in various media channels. He has received many awards, including the Young Investigator Award by the Multinational Association of Supportive Care in Cancer, and the Re-imagine Education International Awards by the Wharton School and QS Rankings organization. He is on several journal editorial boards and also an invited reviewer for over 30 international journals, conferences and grants.

Eskinder Eshetu Ali is a pharmacist by training and has a BA in economics, a MSc in pharmacoepidemiology and social pharmacy, and a PhD in the design and evaluation of mobile technologies for medication management. He is currently an Assistant Professor of Social and Administrative Pharmacy at the Department of Pharmaceutics and Social Pharmacy, Addis Ababa University, Ethiopia. Dr. Ali has practical and research experience in the areas of mHealth, health technology assessment, quality evaluation of medication management mobile apps, healthcare financing and quality assurance of health and pharmaceutical services. He has published numerous articles in international peer reviewed journals. He has also served as consultant on a number of projects of national relevance in Ethiopia and has recently been selected for the Principal Investigator role for the ISPOR Africa Network Research Committee. Dr. Ali is also a member of the editorial support team of the Journal of Pharmaceutical Policy and Practice.

Lita Chew holds concurrent positions as, Head of Pharmacy Department, National Cancer Centre Singapore, and Associate Professor, National University of Singapore. She is a council member of the Singapore Pharmacy Council and sits in numerous committees at the Ministry of Health, Singapore. A/Prof Chew has practiced in the area of oncology for more than 20 years. Her practice and research interests include medication management, medication adherence, pharmacy practice and workforce development. An inspiring pharmacy leader, her work impacts pharmacy practice in Singapore. These include the setting up of a register for specialist pharmacists, establishing training, development and competency frameworks for the pharmacy workforce in Singapore, and leading the National Pharmacy Strategy, a 10-year plan to transform the pharmaceutical landscape in Singapore. A convincing and charismatic leader, A/Prof Chew continues to bridge the profession with her visionary leadership, excellent people skills and passion for her works.

Index

O

P

S

T

U

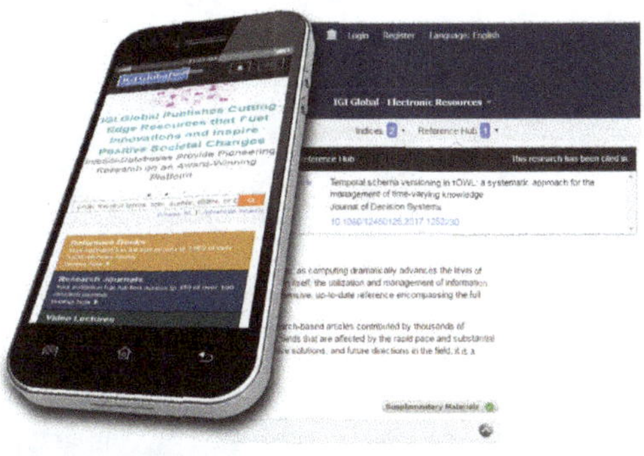

www.ingramcontent.com/pod-product-compliance
Lightning Source LLC
LaVergne TN
LVHW081520300926
849161LV00006B/1237
* 9 7 8 1 7 9 9 8 3 8 3 2 6 *